Coming of Age:
The Evolving Field of
Adventure Therapy

■■■

■■■

Editors:

Scott Bandoroff, Ph.D.
and
Sandra Newes, Ph.D.

Ordering information:
Copies of this and other related books and academic journals are available through AEE's on-line store, which is accessible at www.aee.org. AEE members and quantity purchases are given a discount.

Printed in the United States of America.
Printed on recycled paper using 35% post-consumer waste and soy ink.

ISBN 0-929361-14-8

Publisher
Association for Experiential Education
3775 Iris Avenue, Suite 4
Boulder, CO 80301
Phone: 303-440-8844
Fax: 303-440-9581

The Association for Experiential Education (AEE) is a non-profit, member-based, professional organization dedicated to experiential education.

AEE's vision is to contribute a more just and compassionate world by transforming education.

AEE's mission is to develop and promote experiential education. AEE is committed to supporting professional development, theoretical advancement, and evaluation of experiential education worldwide.

AEE members are students, professionals, and organizations engaged in the diverse application of experiential education in adaptive programming, recreation, leadership development, physical education, adventure programming, corporate training, environmental education, youth service, mental health, corrections and education.

Memberships are available at different levels and benefit structures. See all the details and join online at: www.aee.org.

Contents

Section III: Continuing Evolution

Foreword

It seems fitting that the conference from which this book drew its life occurred on the North American continent. It was there that some of the pioneers of Adventure Therapy had the courage to pursue an exciting new form of adventure-based work that has evolved into what is now known as Adventure Therapy. Strongly influenced by many others before them, people like Rocky Kimball and Steven Bacon somehow began to crystallize Adventure Therapy and, along with many colleagues, contributed to the formation of the Association for Experiential Education (AEE). Now, many years after its formation, AEE has sponsored the publication of this book. The Therapeutic Adventure Professional Group (TAPG) of AEE for many years provided almost the sole international focus for Adventure Therapy (for English speaking people). But by 1990 various forms of Adventure Therapy had evolved in many other countries. The First International Adventure Therapy Conference (IATC) was held in 1997 in Australia, only seven years ago (Itin, 1998). It seems in retrospect that the first IATC emerged at least as much as a response to a growing international demand, as it was something innovative and unexpected. Nonetheless, something was born and the second International Adventure Therapy Conference in 2000 (Augsburg, Germany) found the baby alive and well (Richards, 2003). Subsequently, the third IATC, held in 2003 in Victoria, British Columbia—the conference that spawned this book—seemed a natural progression in the growing maturity of the international field of Adventure Therapy and network of adventure therapists. So the implicit claim in the title of this book, the notion that Adventure Therapy is "coming of age" may at first sight appear fully justified.

But one international conference every two or three years neither signals the existence of, nor keeps alive, a vibrant and maturing international community of practitioners, theorists and researchers. Such impetus to live and grow is, however, just starting to be generated by the recent emergence of regional conferences that have emerged outside the USA (that is, in addition to the pre-existing tradition of AEE conferences in the USA). At the time of writing, two regional conferences had recently been held in Australia, one in New Zealand, one in England, and one is scheduled in the Czech Republic. Additionally, the Nature Therapy movement seems to be starting its own sequence of international conferences. So rather than congratulating ourselves on having successfully come of age, hopefully we will take the title coined by Scott Bandoroff and Sandra Newes as the expression of a wish, toward which we are moving but that we have not yet reached. Perhaps other processes need to emerge before we have come of age. One example of something that seems to still be missing is the existence of an international network of small regional or local networks where practitioners, researchers and theorists can speak together in their own languages and develop work of outstanding quality while at the same time create an influence both locally and internationally.

At an individual level, coming of age signals a transition. Before the transition into adulthood, the child lives a life with few responsibilities. Life is an experiment, a game and a time of continual learning. The child occupies a role where family and society are largely responsible for the welfare of the potential adult whose health and well-being will later help to ensure the survival of that society. The child represents communal hope and at the same time enables the adults to find meaning in their roles of teacher, healer, caretaker, limit-setter and creators of a loving environment. After the transition to adulthood, the neo-adult is no longer able to spend so much time in free play. Now, the young adult is much more responsible for the shaping consequences of his or her own actions. Nor is he/she any longer able to just complain to others about what should be different about the world. This maturing person now has to take action in the world that turns his/her complaints and wishes into remedial actions that help the whole community and not just him/herself.

So, when we view the world of Adventure Therapy, who has come of age? Are adventure therapists taking a place in societies around the world where we are actively shaping therapeutic approaches rather than maintaining our rebellious nature by writing, publishing and talking together about what should be different in the world? Or can coming of age mean many different things? Perhaps focussing on the coming of age of an individual hides a great deal of importance relating to how Adventure Therapy needs to develop. Do we need to come of age as a family perhaps? Do we need to see ourselves as a maturing society where coming of age implies the nurturing of difference and building resilience through diversity? The diversity of points of view expressed in this book suggest that maturity in our field will necessarily involve working constructively with multiple themes, some of which create tension with others.

One such tension is that created by focussing separately on research, theory and practice. With this common subdivision of our work, how can the passionate researchers honour the idea that the practitioners know how to do so much more than can be captured with research—as illustrated by Sean Hoyer and Keith Russell. Are researchers useful forms of life or do they mainly interfere with real life for program operators? The chapter by Elaine Mossman and Colin Goldthorpe provides some practical answers to this question at a literal level. At a meta-level, we could consider this same chapter to have the role of reassuring practitioners that research is a useful activity. The coexistence of theory and practice in the same book can also raise questions like "How do theoreticians remain mindful that their theories can only be rough metaphors for what really happens?" and "How can practitioners accept the existence of the wealth of ideas that come from theory and research but that may even contradict how they work?"

A further glance at the titles of the chapters in this book reveals that other challenges may emerge. Whilst chapter titles are only symbols for something, it may be informative to juxtapose these symbols and to play with some emergent themes. Two of the themes that seem to permeate the substrate of the book are, on one hand the search for certainty, predictability, uniformity and control and on the other hand, the search for curiosity, innovation, exploration, diversity and freedom to explore. Both have their place, but at times it can feel intolerable when our own preferences are challenged. For example, it seems we seek certainty but need to leave a place for "not knowing" and to be "busy doing nothing" as Val Nicholls explores. We need to know enough to enable us to practice and communicate with others but we risk replacing curiosity with knowledge. Is "best practice" as defined by Simon Crisp now prescribed for us all and permanently fixed in place or can we "play with ideas" from different theory bases, as touched upon by Rüdiger Gilsdorf, Blair Gilbert and myself? Can one practice without being the best, or do we owe it to ourselves to follow a blueprint? How prescribed must our work be in order to be ethical?

Perhaps, too, it is not possible to have one "thing" called Adventure Therapy. Perhaps we need to follow Ian Williams' lead and be clearer about what is therapy and what is therapeutic. Putting a firm boundary between what is Adventure Therapy and what is not, challenges our ability to honour the confluence of cultures that Cathryn Carpenter and Anita Pryor explore. The challenge to honour diverse cultural needs is great in the South Pacific but it is even greater worldwide. It seems that we need to believe that Adventure Therapy exists, but as soon as one group of people decides what Adventure Therapy is, others in other cultures may not be able to find their place in our definitions. Even within Western society, Cheryl Willcocks' introduction of ideas from Jungian psychology may create a challenge for some who feel uncomfortable with the role of spirituality in therapeutic endeavours. The introduction of Buddhism from Eastern cultures as described by Norah Trace provides another challenge. I can't help wondering how Western evidence-based empiricism can truly embrace the implicit "not knowing" of Buddhism. Or can we be comforted by the constructivism of Narrative theory, described in a chapter by Jordie Allen-Newman and Reg Fleming, and accept that even as a group of professionals, we need to allow each sub group of this diverse group to find its own meaning? But then is there a place for externally monitored standards, ethics and regulations?

In exploring the themes that seem to me to exist in symbolic nature of chapter titles, I was curious about how the chapter by Guy Lorent, Luk Peeters, and Thomas Debaenst on the topic of working with brain-injured participants on challenge courses fit into the two interwoven themes in the book that I introduced earlier. I am comforted by the idea that this chapter title does not necessarily fit comfortably into a schema that I have chosen to illustrate what are in part my personal concerns in life. What a delight that such an important concept, involving specialist expertise in a specific setting, should not fit my cosy preconception. There needs to be room for innovations and concepts that lie outside our own. And in closing, ever mindful of the adventure element in Adventure Therapy, I hope that we in Adventure Therapy can show congruence between our work and our inter-action with the world. Let us aspire to high-quality practice but not lose sight of Alan Drengson's Wild Way.

Martin Ringer, France, August 2004

Postscript

I want to honour the remarkable effort that Scott Bandoroff and Sandra Newes have put into the production of this book. I have experienced them as profession-al, thorough and understanding in this demanding work. Perhaps they have come of age through the rite of passage involved in such demanding work!

References

Itin, C. (Ed.). (1998). *Exploring the boundaries of adventure therapy: International perspectives. Proceedings of the first International Adventure Therapy Conference,* Perth, Western Australia, AEE/COEAWA.

Richards, K., & Smith, B. (Eds.). (2003). Therapy *Within Adventure: Proceedings of the second International Adventure Therapy Conference;* Ziel Publishing, Augsburg, Germany.

Introduction

This book is the third publication to come out of the International Adventure Therapy Conferences, with the latest occurring in Victoria, British Columbia in April of 2003. This represents an important tradition because both the conferences and the publications serve as vital forums for disseminating information at an international level in a field that has traditionally been dominated by American voices. As Itin (1998) aptly stated in the proceedings of the first IATC, these publications provide "a useful way for our field to move beyond the ethnocentric viewpoints that have dominated the field" (vii).

We have broken with tradition here in choosing not to call this a proceedings manual. There were several factors that led to this decision. First, this collection of papers is only a small sample of the workshops presented at the third IATC, so the book does not provide a fair representation of the conference. Second, not all of the papers submitted for publication were accepted, as they typically are in a proceedings manual. Third, we invited the authors to go beyond what they presented at the conference in addressing the issues that they felt were relevant to the field of Adventure Therapy at this time. Therefore, we do not believe that the label of proceedings accurately reflects the contents of this book. Certainly, the publication was inspired by the conference and the papers were solicited only from presenters at the third IATC. Although this limited the scope of the book, it is our belief that this publication presents a legitimate voice for the field of Adventure Therapy from an international perspective. Clearly, no compendium of papers could purport to speak for an entire field, especially at an international level. However, we feel that this book does indeed offer a snapshot of the field of Adventure Therapy at this point in time in our world.

As the title of this book reflects, it is our belief that the field of Adventure Therapy is "coming of age." This assertion comes with the caveat, also represented in the title, that this is an evolving process. In other words, we would not care to argue that the field has come of age, for clearly, we have not arrived. However, solid and steady progress has been achieved, and it is this development as a field that we wish to illuminate with this publication.

In a keynote presentation in 1997 at the first IATC, Jenny Bunce (1998) identified the developmental stage of the field of Adventure Therapy as adolescence, complete with storm and stress, highs and lows, and search for identity. Many of the issues that she raised to define our adolescent struggle still plague us today such as defining what we do, determining who is qualified to do it, and even what we call that which we do. The real question is this: are we mired in this struggle or are we working toward resolution? Successful resolution of adolescence is not as much a matter of arriving at all of the answers as it is accurately defining the questions. Most importantly, maturity is defined by a willingness to grapple with the issues and a comfort with not having the solutions.

We offer this book as evidence that as a field, we are grappling with the issues and indeed, making progress. There have been clear strides in the development of theory that explains what we do. This is demonstrated by the fact that nearly half of the chapters are devoted to theoretical considerations, the first section of the book. In the introductory chapter by Sandra Newes and Scott Bandoroff, the commonalities and distinctions between Adventure Therapy and more traditional treatment approaches are highlighted in an orientation to the field for newcomers. Blair Gilbert, Martin Ringer and Rudy Gilsdorf engage us in a stimulating discussion of Adventure Therapy from the perspective of three well-established treatment modalities, and encourage us to consider the theoretical approaches that we bring to our work. Sean Hoyer proposes a unifying theory as a framework from which we might develop a comprehensive view of the field and a theory-informed practice of Wilderness Therapy. Cheryl Willcocks draws on the work of Carl Jung to deepen our practice and increase the effectiveness of our programs. Jordie Allen-Newman and Reg Fleming suggest the integration of Narrative Therapy and Adventure Therapy as a means of improving therapeutic effectiveness in adventure therapy contexts. Norah Trace attempts to enhance our understanding of adventure therapy with principles of Buddhist psychotherapy. And finally, Alan Drengson introduces the Wild Way, a comprehensive theory and practice that unites our work with other disciplines, cultural models and whole arts in the development of a unified system by which we can live our lives.

Further evidence of our progress can be found in the second section of the book which is primarily devoted to research developments in our field. Keith Russell summarizes the research on wilderness therapy and describes the latest findings in his efforts to increase scientific rigor in evaluating what we do. Elaine Mossman and Colin Goldthorpe provide another example of sound research in action through a presentation of the findings of their program evaluation, including a much needed focus on process factors. Val Nichols follows suit in her qualitative research study in an effort to advance the field through increased understanding of what exactly it is about Adventure Therapy that works. This section concludes with a look at some innovative programming from Guy Lorent, Luk Peeters, and Thomas Debaenst who share their insights gained from working with traumatic brain-injured patients.

The final section describes the state of the field by looking at where we have been and where we are going. Ian Williams wrestles with some of the issues with which we are still grappling in an attempt to distinguish adventure therapy from therapeutic adventure. Simon Crisp further highlights our struggles and challenges us with a blueprint for the development of our profession. Cathryn Carpenter and Anita Pryor share a working model for dialogue among practitioners across cultures and relate progress from discussions of the difficult issues facing our field. And finally, Denise Mitten critically examines how we fit into the broader field of healthcare and argues that Adventure Therapy should be viewed as Complementary and Alternative Medicine.

So have we come of age? Most certainly, not. However, we are evolving and moving forward. This is an exciting time in the field of Adventure Therapy. We may not be ready to leave home yet, but we are clearly maturing, and this progress deserves our attention and our respect.

See you in New Zealand!
www.adventuretherapy.co.nz

Scott & Sandy

Editor's Note:

We would like to express our regret for the need to require that the chapters in this book be written in English. Although clearly a practical necessity, nonetheless, it falls short of the cultural sensitivity that we would like to model. We did maintain the English of the author, so the reader will note variations in language amongst the chapters based upon the country of origin of the authors. Finally, we would like to direct those readers who are unfamiliar with the initiative activities mentioned in the book to:

http://www.wilderdom.com/games/BooksAboutGames.html
for an extensive listing of resources.

References

Bunce, J. (1998). *A question of identity.* In C. Itin (Ed.), *Exploring the boundaries of adventure therapy: International perspectives. Proceedings of the first International Adventure Therapy Conference:* Perth, Western Australia, AEE/COEAWA.

Itin, C., (Ed.). (1998). *Exploring the boundaries of adventure therapy: International perspectives. Proceedings of the first International Adventure Therapy Conference:* Perth, Western Australia, AEE/COEAWA.

What is Adventure Therapy?

Sandra Newes and Scott Bandoroff

■ ■ ■

The field of Adventure Therapy is experiencing substantial growth and is becoming more well-known. This increased popularity is leading more readers to the literature in search of information. Many of these readers have had little or no prior exposure to the field of Adventure Therapy. This paper is intended to provide an overview for those readers to help them better understand the principles and theories upon which Adventure Therapy is based. This will serve as a foundation for the chapters that follow in this text. At the same time, the authors believe that there is a need to understand Adventure Therapy in the context of broader mental health treatment. Toward that goal, this paper highlights the theoretical constructs that Adventure Therapy shares in common with other treatment approaches, as well as those that are unique to the field.

■ ■ ■

Although the intentional application of adventure education principles to therapeutic populations has been occurring for nearly forty years, many are unfamiliar with the field of Adventure Therapy (AT). It is not uncommon to encounter individuals who experienced great relief upon discovering the field of AT, having thought that they were going to have to create an entirely new discipline. This common experience speaks to both the natural fit between nature and therapy, as well as to the relative obscurity of the field. The numbers of readers of AT literature are growing as more students, traditional mental health practitioners and consumers of AT are attracted to the field. However, while there is an increase in attention focused on AT, it can be difficult for interested individuals to find an overview of the basic essential foundations of this field. In recognition of the fact that many of our readers have had little prior exposure to AT literature, we are providing this overview as a means to introduce the chapters which follow.

Another goal of this chapter is to highlight the commonalities of AT with more traditional mental health treatments. Much of AT may not be particularly unique and it is important to recognize this in developing a thorough understanding of the discipline. Moreover, as AT struggles to gain credibility in the mental health community, establishing commonalities with widely accepted mental health treatments helps to support the growth of AT as a viable mental health approach. It also may allow AT to borrow from the extensive research literature of more widely recognized mental health treatments as a means to provide support for its practices. Naturally, despite commonalities to other approaches, AT has its unique aspects. These will be highlighted as well.

Theoretical Background

Experiential Education

AT is rooted in the tradition of "experiential education" philosophies (Kraft & Sakofs, 1985), defined as "learning by doing, with reflection" (Gass, 1993). Early roots of experiential education can be traced to the educational writings of Dewey (Kraft & Sakofs, 1985). This experiential learning tradition is based on the belief that learning is a result of direct experience, and includes the premise that persons learn best when they have multiple senses actively involved in learning. By increasing the intensity of the mental and physical demands of learning, the participant "engages all sensory systems in a learning and change process" (Crisp, 1998). Psychological research on information processing provides some support of this premise, indicating that multi-sensory processing accounts for a higher level of cognitive activity and increased memory. Applied specifically to the context of AT, the multi-sensory level of the therapeutic experience inherent in adventure activities may account for the high level of change reported by practitioners (Crisp, 1998). This suggests that "integration of experience may be more deeply anchored for the client because of this broad [sensory] base" (Crisp, 1998, p. 67).

Experiential education theory also postulates that active learning is often more valuable for the learner because the participant is directly responsible for and involved in the process. In addition, experiential learning theory is based on the belief that learning is enhanced when individuals are placed outside of their comfort zones and into a state of dissonance. Learning is then assumed to occur through the necessary changes required to achieve personal equilibrium [(i.e., modern dissonance theory), Festinger, 1957]. Kraft and Sakofs (1985) outline several elements inherent to this experiential education process:

1. The learner is a participant rather than a spectator in learning.

2. The learning activities require personal motivation in the form of

energy, involvement, and responsibility.

3. The learning activity is real and meaningful in terms of natural consequences for the learner.

4. Reflection is a critical element in the learning process.

5. Learning must have present as well as future relevance for the learner and the society in which he/she is a member.

In experiential classrooms, individuals are placed in "real life" situations in which it is necessary to employ problem-solving or otherwise creative methods of working with the environment or context at hand. Therefore, effective experiential activities involve the participant in situations in which they must take some form of action to successfully cope with their surroundings. Such activities may take the form of outdoor pursuits such as hiking, rock climbing, or kayaking, but also include team-based initiative activities. Outward Bound is widely recognized as one of the innovators in incorporating the philosophies of experiential learning into adventure activity approaches (Bacon, 1983; Gillis & Ringer, 1999).

The Link to Therapy

In the late 1960's Outward Bound expanded the application of their adventure education model to therapeutic populations (Kelly & Baer, 1968). Gass (1993) has reworked the above experiential education principles and discusses how these principles can be applied to therapy.

1. The *client* becomes a participant rather than a spectator *in therapy*.

2. *Therapeutic* activities require *client* motivation in the form of energy, involvement, and responsibility.

3. *Therapeutic activities* are real and meaningful in terms of natural consequences for the *client*.

4. Reflection is a critical element of the *therapeutic* process.

5. *Functional change* must have present as well as future relevance for *clients* and their society (p. 5).

It is interesting that when examining the ideas stated above by Gass (1993), it is evident to the critical reader that most of these principles are not unique to AT. In actuality, one can see even from these basic statements that the theory of AT builds on the foundations and well-established premises of accepted psychological theory, including cognitive and cognitive-behavioral theory, humanistic theory, and elements of the interpersonal aspects of object relations theory. Therefore, it appears from this definition that what AT may offer is a potentially unique medium for the implementation of therapeutic processes assumed to be present in many therapeutic orientations. Although this may be considered controversial, the remainder of the chapter will offer evidence to support this position.

Definition of Adventure-Based Therapy

Also referred to as "wilderness therapy," "therapeutic adventure," "adventure therapy," "wilderness-adventure therapy," "adventure-based therapy," and "adventure-based counseling," AT is a therapeutic modality combining therapeutic benefits of the adventure experiences and activities with those of more traditional modes of therapy. AT utilizes a therapeutic focus and integrates group level processing and individual psychotherapy sessions as part of an overall therapeutic milieu. While specific types of facilitation occur directly related to the activities, this processing is not associated exclusively with the activities alone. Rather, the activities can also be conceptualized as a catalyst for the processing which occurs before, during, and after activities; a catalyst which provides concrete examples of the immediate consequences associated with individual and group actions that can be referred to by both the client and the therapist. Therefore, therapists may begin with processing exigencies around the activities themselves and branch into other areas related to the issues of the clients. This approach tends to make such discussions more relevant for clients and therefore, arguably, more engaging.

As such, AT lends itself well to multimodal treatment and can be utilized as an intervention independent from other treatments or as an adjunct to other well-established treatments. Importantly, therapists are able to use any type of therapeutic orientation they adhere to in the processing that occurs around the activities. This view contrasts with a commonly held assumption that the postulated change which may occur in AT is singularly related to the activity participation.

Ringer (1994) defines AT as a generic term referring to a class of change-oriented, group-based experiential learning processes that occur in the context of a contractual, empowering, and empathic professional relationship. Notably, elements of this definition are not unique to AT and can be assumed generally in many therapeutic traditions. However, the emphasis on "group-based experiential learning processes" in a typically outdoor and active setting is clearly a combination differentiating AT from other forms of therapy.

Interestingly, Ringer's definition does not mention "adventure." This purposeful omission challenges one common misconception about AT: namely, that in order to accomplish their goals, clients must necessarily subject themselves to adrenaline-fueled feats of daring and technical skill. The fact that "adventure" is not seen as an end unto itself distinguishes AT from other types of outdoor programming devoid of therapeutic focus. In line with this definition, adventure or outdoor experiences alone are not assumed to be sufficient to facilitate deep-level therapeutic growth and change. Instead, it is the processing of the actual experience with the client that promotes the therapeutic process. Therefore, the use of the word "adventure" may in fact be misleading and terms such as "activity-based psychotherapy" may be more appropriate (Gillis, 1992). However, this term has not become one of common usage in the literature and adventure therapy, with all of its connotations, is the name that has become standard.

In examining this discussion, it can be seen that there are problems with delineating distinct and defining parameters of AT. To address this problem, professionals within the field have been involved in an ongoing debate as to how to best articulate a clear definition of what is unique to AT as a treatment modality. Such a definition must necessarily incorporate widely accepted therapeutic principles while also differentiating AT from other therapies and from other types of outdoor adventure programs. In an attempt to focus such definitions, Simon Crisp (personal communication, August 24, 2004) offers the following:

1. Wilderness and/or adventure methods are utilized in the service of therapeutic practice. Therapeutic practice involves:

   a. the identification of a problem the client presents with,

   b. application of a theoretical framework based on a theory of personality, behavioral and psychological problems and process of change that explains the origin and nature of the problem;

   c. selection of strategies of client management and method(s) of intervention which logically and parsimoniously relate to b);

   d. strategies and methods are routinely reviewed and modified according to client need.

2. Professional relationship exists between therapist and client with the following characteristics:

   a. therapist brings to the relationship training and experience necessary and appropriate to meet all foreseeable needs of the client, including a capacity to assess and manage (a) life-threatening and other crises, (b) psychological boundaries, and (c) any potentially competing needs of the therapist,

   b. a contract is formed between therapist and client about the aims, limitations, methods, expected outcomes and risks of therapy,

   c. therapist works towards the best interests of the client and holds this at all times the overriding principle in determining the actions of the therapist, and the therapist acts to protect the client from harm—both physical and psychological.

Once again, the singularly unique aspect of this definition is the emphasis on activities as a means of accomplishing the other common therapeutic goals. This appears to hold true as well for the definition put forth by Alvarez and Stauffer (2001): "Adventure therapy is any intentional, facilitated use of adventure tools and techniques to guide personal change toward desired therapeutic goals" (p. 87). Again, it is also this focus on the use of activities to accomplish said goals which seems to differentiate AT from most other therapeutic orientations. Based on this, perhaps AT can be best be seen as an activity-based approach to treatment that attempts to meet similar goals as do other treatments. Therefore, what must be parceled out as theoretically unique to AT is the mechanism by which AT can accomplish these goals in ways that are more efficacious than other treatments for particular clients. This is a question that remains as yet unanswered. Simply put, it is essential that the field of AT begin holding itself accountable for answering the questions posed to all other treatments: Is this treatment effective? For whom, and under what circumstances?

Thought of in this way, AT can begin to be seen as more similar to other types of treatments than different. The logical assumption should follow then that AT is assumed to operate under the same scientific and clinical umbrella as other mental health treatments, and therefore, practitioners of AT should be held accountable to the same standards as other practicing mental health professionals. However, in reality this is not always the case. AT is often presented by its proponents as though it is a unique and separate entity, an entity somehow not responsible for upholding such standards. This presents a clear contradiction between established standards of mental health practice and AT.

This dilemma is reflected in the ongoing debate within the AT field about the necessary qualifications for an adventure therapist. Let us return to the definitions offered above in an effort to gain some clarity. While Ringer's reference to a "professional relationship" would not suggest that the facilitator necessarily be credentialed, Gillis' inclusion of the word "psychotherapy" clearly indicates the involvement of an academically trained therapist. Crisp attempts to elucidate the issue by defining "professional relationship" but avoids delineating the training, so that uncredentialed professionals might meet the criteria (note that the title of "therapist" is not restricted in many jurisdictions). One can see that clarity is not easily achieved.

The debate surrounding this topic is extensive and heated. It has serious implications since the outcome would prescribe who is qualified to conduct AT programs. Some in the field advocate for a required level of competency as reflected by a specified level of training and accompanying credential, while others advocate "training through experience." This discussion may reflect a presently existing division one finds between those AT practitioners who have followed the more established route of academic and clinical training and those who have learned their clinical skills through direct experience. A related controversy involves the use of the term adventure therapy with some advocating that adventure therapy programs must involve clinically trained therapists, while those programs working with clinical populations without clinically credentialed staff should be referred to as therapeutic adventure. Further discussion of this topic is beyond the scope of this paper. For more information the reader is referred to chapters by Crisp and Williams in this edition.

From the standpoint of mental health practice, the eventual outcome to this debate must involve holding AT to the same standards of care as are other mental health treatments. This would necessarily include a thoughtful examination of ethical practice in AT as well (Newes, 2000). However, in order for this change to occur, there must be further efforts made to establish a foundational knowledge that indicates that AT shares more similarities with other mental health treatments than is commonly believed within the field. It is only with the establishment of such a belief, as well as a clear semantic and theoretical link, that AT will in actuality operate under the aforementioned umbrella of scientific and clinical practice.

Goals of Adventure-Based Therapy

AT proponents have articulated a variety of goals that are recognized as being associated with the modality. While recognizably unsupported by solid empirical data, the following section will broadly summarize these interconnected goals. First, clients are thought to generally increase in self-awareness, leading to an increased recognition of behavioral consequences and available choices; second, clients have a higher level of accountability both to self and others; third, clients are thought to learn healthier coping strategies leading to increased environmental control; fourth, through AT, clients are thought to be provided tangible evidence of success, thereby correcting negative self-conceptions and leading to a more positive self-concept; fifth, clients are thought to learn creative problem-solving, communication, and cooperation skills; and sixth, AT is thought to facilitate realistic appraisal of individual strengths, weaknesses, and self-imposed limitations. Ultimately, this increased awareness is thought to lead to better decision-making abilities.

Overall, AT programs have the overriding goal of an increasing self-awareness in a variety of domains. In line with this, it is thought by AT theorists that connections between behavior and the results of such behavior become more apparent. Therefore, clients can be provided with concrete examples of dysfunctional behavior and shown that alternative behavioral and interpersonal choices can lead to success. Relatedly, Bandoroff (1989) argues that adventure activities, with the feedback and consequences available through such experiences, provide learning that enables participants to begin regulating their own behavior. Amesberger (1998) expands on this goal, noting that AT involves:

...the reflection on internalized norms and values with the aim to support a person to find new and more suitable structures for his or her life. Destructive and dysfunctional behaviors or emotions should be recognized in their effects, as well as helpful and effective ones (p. 29).

Along with this increased insight and capacity for controlling their behaviors comes a higher level of accountability. This goes well beyond the elementary goal delineated in most programs of accepting responsibility for behavior. What we are alluding to here speaks more to integrity. Clients develop an understanding that they have a higher calling than what their prior conduct would reflect. The AT treatment is designed to help them get in touch with that potential and begin to live in alignment with the higher standards dictated by this greater sense of self. Such a life implies an accountability to self that entails, but is more than, accountability to others.

Of note is the fact that the above noted tenets are clearly embedded in the therapeutic process itself, as opposed to embedded within the activities. Taylor (1989) postulates that the exposure to uncertainty or ambiguity accompanied by increases in levels of confidence and skill that can be achieved through the AT process will facilitate a healthier coping response. It is believed that as clients learn and use new modes of coping, they gain greater control of their environment (Nadler & Luckner, 1992). It is hoped that by coping with the treatment environment in new ways, clients can learn to achieve increased personal and environmental control outside of the treatment. This is an experience which may be novel for many clients.

According to Herbert (1996), through AT "persons challenge themselves, and in doing so, (re)learn something about themselves" (p. 5). To accomplish this, mastery tasks, or initial successes, associated with the activities counteract and disprove internally focused negative self-evaluations, learned helplessness, and dependency (Kimball & Bacon, 1993) at a time when such processes may be intensely activated. This heightened activation combined with concrete evidence of success may facilitate further learning. Ultimately, feelings of success and control also associated with the mastery tasks can then serve as additional reinforcers to support changed behaviors. Thus, it is a circular process of interpersonal and intrapersonal activation, success, and reinforcement.

Priest and Baillie (1987) discuss additional possibilities for client change, stating that "The aim of adventure education is to create astute adventurers: people who are correct in their perceptions of individual competence and situational risk" (p. 18). Relatedly, through AT, clients can learn skills related to problem-solving, cooperation, communication, and facing challenge (Herbert, 1996). It is thought that through this process, clients learn to more realistically appraise their own personal strengths and weaknesses, both on a personal and an interpersonal level.

Through this process, clients begin to recognize their own self-imposed limitations and increase in their awareness of available choices, thus becoming better able to accept responsibility for their level of success or failure. As clients increase in this self-knowledge and self-awareness, it is believed that they are ultimately able to make more realistic and healthy decisions. These are important skills many clients lack. Moreover, Taylor (1989) notes that the increased levels of confidence, skill, and self-awareness that participants may gain through AT encourages clients to see uncertainty as a challenge and not a threat, a change with potentially far-reaching positive consequences for clients.

Ultimately, these proposed changes can perhaps be summarized in this inherent underlying assumption embedded within the adventure-based therapy literature: the assumption that by becoming aware of available choices, and by experimenting with different behaviors in a novel environment where one is receiving immediate and realistic feedback, clients can learn to actively influence their probability of success. Furthermore, through AT clients learn to demonstrate personal competencies, build upon skills, accept personal responsibility, more accurately assess themselves, and maintain a higher degree of control over their environment. It is also believed that having an increased capacity to regulate one's own behavior will facilitate further increases in levels of self-awareness, competence and a more internal sense of control of one's own world.

Again, it is important to be aware that these assumptions and goals are common to many other treatment approaches. In fact, statements such as those above with their emphasis on self-awareness and the interpretations of challenge vs. threat carry clear elements of humanistic theory, and the focus on self-knowledge and the increased awareness of available choices directly parallels the humanistic tradition (Csikszentmihaly, 1990; Raskin, & Rogers, 1989; Maslow, 1971). In addition, one can see elements of cognitive, behavioral, and object relations theory embedded in this discussion of the goals of AT.

Characteristics of Adventure Therapy

Having discussed the theoretical background, definition, and the goals of AT, a discussion of the specific characteristics of AT is warranted. Fourteen characteristics, including those delineated by Kimball and Bacon (1993), will be discussed in turn: (1) multiple treatment formats, (2) group focus, (3) processing, (4) applicability to multimodal treatment, (5) sequencing of activities, (6) perceived risk, (7) unfamiliar environment, (8) challenge by choice, (9) provision of concrete consequences, (10) goal-setting, (11) trust-building, (12) enjoyment, (13) peak experience, and (14) therapeutic relationship.

Multiple Treatment Formats

First, adventure programs range in scope from those which incorporate adventure-based techniques with more traditional modes of therapy to those that utilize full-scale extended expeditioning as their therapeutic medium. These types of programs are differentiated based on *where* the therapy is taking place, for what length of time the clients involved, and what types of *programming* are being utilized (Gillis, 1995). As Gass (1993) suggests, three main areas exist within the adventure-based therapy field: (a) activity-based psychotherapy, (b) wilderness therapy, and (c) long-term residential camping.

Given the diversity of programs, it is important to be clear as to what type of program is being referred to under this broad rubric of "adventure therapy" when considering AT from a scientific perspective. Unfortunately, this distinction is not always clearly noted and can be difficult to determine when examining the literature.

Activity-based psychotherapy.

Activity-based psychotherapy (Gillis, 1992) utilizes adventure activities as one type of intervention in the client's overall treatment plan. This type of therapy can occur at the therapeutic facility of the client, at another nearby facility designed for such interventions (e.g., ropes course), or simply in a park or open space using mobile elements. The AT intervention may range from a regularly scheduled one hour group to a full day in duration, which is typical for a ropes course experience.

This type of format is often used in inpatient or residential settings, but can also be used in combination with outpatient psychotherapy. The experiences tend to be contrived (i.e. the facility and initiatives are developed specifically for such an intervention), and focus on teambuilding, trust and problem-solving (Banaka & Young, 1985; Witman, 1987; Witman & Preskanis, 1996). As the group builds upon previous skills and successes to overcome each successive challenge, they increase group cohesion and confidence.

Crisp (1997) more fully defines this type of adventure-based therapy by its "emphasis on the contrived nature of the task, the artificiality of the environment and the structure and parameters of the activity being determined by the therapist" (p. 58). In addition, he notes that the goals of the particular activities are often a specific outcome. These outcomes are typically planned for, and influence the selection of the activities by the therapist.

As previously discussed, it is the activities that make AT unique. However, it is equally important to recognize that the conscious use of therapeutic technique designed to work toward a specific outcome is something that AT has in common with all mental health treatments. In addition, it can be noted that potentially all therapeutic situations can be thought of as contrived, although AT clearly takes this to another level.

Wilderness therapy.

The second format discussed by Gass (1993) is wilderness therapy. This type of program is what most associate with the general term "adventure therapy." Such programs are frequently utilized as an independent treatment and are commonly explored in the efficacy literature for AT. Wilderness therapy interventions have been employed with a wide variety of clients, ranging from military veterans to survivors of domestic violence. However, the vast majority of programs serve adolescents, with diagnoses covering the gamut from developmental disorders to mood disorders.

In wilderness therapy, programs utilize an expedition-oriented format in remote settings and treatment lasts anywhere from 7 to 60 days, although programs may be longer. Some programs employ a basecamp model where clients may spend up to a month in a permanent camp developing skills and participating in clinical assessment before embarking on an expedition. The wilderness therapy intervention is known for its intensive treatment and its capacity to generate dramatic change in a short period of time. These programs typically follow either an Outward Bound or primitive living skills model, and the teaching and practicing of wilderness skills is an important aspect of the intervention. Not only is the learning of these skills necessary for the client's survival and comfort, but it is also believed that this learning provides an opportunity for clients to increase their skill base and thus, their own individual level of perceived competence [(i.e., self-efficacy theory) Bandura, 1977].

The wilderness model allows the development of individual strength within a cooperative framework. Operating as a small, self-sufficient team in a wilderness environment requires mutual decision making which demands trust, cooperation, effective communication and good problem-solving. The members of the group are dependent upon each other for their success as well as their survival. This promotes empathy, sharing, support, and patience and fosters a strong sense of community. This interdependence makes it likely that individual strengths will be maximized and weaknesses minimized. However, the stressful nature of the experience ensures conflict, and the interdependence of the group demands that participants learn conflict resolution (Bandoroff, 1992).

A new term, "outdoor behavioral healthcare," has been coined to describe wilderness treatment programs that are dedicated to upholding standards common to mental health practice (Russell, 2003). This consortium of programs in the U.S. (Outdoor Behavioral Healthcare Industry Council) incorporates a clinical model which includes client assessment, development of an individual treatment plan, the use of established psychotherapeutic practice, and the development of aftercare plans. OBHIC is committed to research as well and launched the most impressive outcome study to date which included 1600 participants from eight programs

(Russell, 2003). These benchmark findings provided support for outdoor behavioral healthcare as an effective treatment intervention for youth. A review of this research along with the results of a two year follow-up study can be found in the chapter by Russell in this edition.

One problem with wilderness therapy programs is that follow-up tends to be limited. Since clients typically come from a wide geographic area, programs generally pass the responsibility for aftercare onto local resources. Thus, aftercare services are provided by professionals who are likely unfamiliar with the client's experience and therefore, less able to build on the treatment gains experienced by the client. From both a research and a clinical standpoint, this lack of follow-up provides significant problems when evaluating long-term treatment gains associated with this type of program (Newes, 2000; Wichman, 1991).

Long-term residential camping.

The third type of therapeutic adventure program is long-term residential camping, also known as therapeutic camping. This format has tended to be used primarily with youth-at-risk and adjudicated adolescents. Program length varies, ranging from several months to as long as two years. Such programs are characterized by Buie (1996) as utilizing considerable acreage, having a permanent base camp, and temporary campsites built by campers (typically tent-covered wood platforms). Clients are responsible for providing for their own survival needs and, according to Gass (1993) "the client change is seen to be associated with the development of a positive peer culture, confronting the problems associated with day-to day living, and dealing with existing natural consequences" (p. 10). The focus on group living as a major component of treatment is similar to other types of treatment programs, as is the reliance on structure. Education in traditional school subjects is also provided during such programs.

These long-term camping programs are less intensive than the short-term wilderness therapy programs described above. They are often more similar to other types of residential programs, such as boarding schools, than wilderness therapy programs. The primary difference between a long-term residential camping program and a therapeutic boarding school is the use of a natural setting and the emphasis on self-sufficiency. Therapeutic camping programs generally utilize wilderness expeditions as well, although they are typically less intense than a wilderness therapy expedition. Moreover, the basecamp phase employed by some wilderness therapy programs resembles the therapeutic camping model. This overlap of programming blurs the distinction between treatment models and makes research comparing these modalities challenging.

Group Focus

The second characteristic of AT is group focus. While some AT programs utilize individual psychotherapy as well, overall AT is considered to be primarily a group process. As in many therapeutic settings, groups typically range from 6 to 14 people (Kimball & Bacon, 1993) and the clients tend to be somewhat heterogeneous in terms of therapeutic issue or diagnostic category. Although the target group could be a family or a multi-family group, this is not the average AT client group. Since the most typical AT client is adolescents, the group focus is especially valuable due to its developmental appropriateness for this population.

As with any group psychotherapy, this group component is a vital part of the overall therapeutic aspect of the intervention. Similar to any therapy group, the group in AT provides support, feedback, and a potent interpersonal context. Uniquely, however, in AT, specific activities are presented to the group as challenges to be overcome, and success depends on each individual member participating in completion (e.g., by standing on a platform, scaling a rock face, or negotiating unmarked terrain to a specified destination). In order to master any of the challenges, the group must cooperate, apply skills, creatively problem-solve, and rely upon each other.

Herbert (1996) discusses more completely the issue of creative problem-solving as it relates to AT. What is expressly different about AT and other problem-solving formats is that in order for the tasks to be completed, all participants must play a role in order for the group to succeed (i.e., utilization of superordinate goals). Therefore, activities require the group to discuss and decide on different strategies, implement such strategies, modify those that are unsuccessful, or implement new strategies: all potentially important skills for clients to practice. Not only does this process involve the successful completion of the task, but group dynamics involved in the decision-making process are closely monitored, and the interpersonal aspects of the activity are then processed by the therapist in a similar fashion as any other type of group therapy.

Drawing from the theory of interpersonal group psychotherapy (Yalom, 1995), it is further thought that group focus leads to the intensive activation of a client's interpersonal patterns, which, in conjunction with appropriate therapeutic processing, facilitates therapeutic change. This assumption also echoes Yalom's "social microcosm" theory of group functioning in which it is assumed that "patients will, over time, automatically and inevitably begin to display their maladaptive behavior in the therapy group" (Yalom, 1995, p. 28). Therefore, this group context provides an environment for the enactment of individual pathology, and the problem-solving associated with the group process may lead to further concrete representations of this, as well as provide an opportunity for the practice of new behaviors.

Also similar to interpersonal group psychotherapy, it is not just what happens during this problem-solving process but how it happens in the group that is of interest. For example, how did the group decide on which strategy to use? Who was the leader? Did some clients participate in the decision-making process more fully than others? Is this a common response for them or a new behavior? What was it like to work through this problem? How did it feel? Each of these components, along with others that can lead into deeper level therapeutic processing, provides a rich opportunity to observe and process a client's relational processes.

It is also thought that the more active and concrete nature of the "task" in AT may lead to greater involvement for all clients than does traditional group psychotherapy. Importantly, such higher levels of involvement have been shown to be a significant predictor of psychotherapy outcome (Gomes-Schwartz, 1978). In a traditional therapy group, certain members can achieve "success" regardless of the level of participation of others. While it can recognizably be argued that a skilled group therapist in any therapy setting can involve the entire group, or in fact involve the entire group around any individuals client's lack of participation, it may be that this type of "non-participation," with its impact on the group, is less likely to occur in an AT setting. Simply put, it is thought to be more difficult for a client to remain unengaged, as the activities themselves necessitate participation by all members in order for the group to achieve success. In addition, one can speculate that clients who process experience in a less verbally oriented manner may participate more fully in this type of intervention. If this were the case, it would perhaps allow for greater growth among those clients for whom traditional psychotherapy feels too threatening or invasive. In fact, it could be argued that traditional "talk therapy" is ill-suited for adolescents in general, and an action-oriented approach is more developmentally appropriate.

Finally, the power of modeling (Bandura, 1986) is an important aspect of the group experience. Naturally, the opportunity to observe and imitate other clients is available in any form of group treatment. In AT the involvement in the activities could provide a tremendous opportunity for modeling of appropriate communication, cooperation, feedback, and help-seeking, again, in what is speculated to be a less threatening format to defensive clients. Thus, such clients may be better able to attend to and utilize such modeling.

Processing

Another descriptor of AT programs is that a great deal of time is spent processing the experience with clients and facilitating the transfer of learning into a client's daily life. It must be noted again that this processing is not necessarily associated exclusively with the activities alone. The activities can be conceptualized as a catalyst for the processing which occurs before, during, and after activities: a catalyst which also provides concrete examples of the consequences associated with individual and group actions. Despite the fact that some of the activities being processed are contrived, the interactions that they create are real and in present time. The opportunity to deal with issues in the here and now provides relevance that is often difficult to obtain in conventional therapy.

To engage in this processing, tools such as individual psychotherapy, group psychotherapy, journal writing, individual time for reflection, modeling, self-disclosure, and metaphoric processing (Gass, 1993) may be utilized throughout the course of an AT program. While the techniques listed above may be familiar to clinicians, the extensive use of metaphoric processing is an aspect of AT which may be fairly unique in its application and thus, warrants further discussion

"The use of metaphors in adventure programming often serves as the key factor in producing lasting functional change to clients" (Gass, 1995, p. 235). Metaphors are vital for linking the learning and growth achieved through the adventure-based experience to situations found in the client's "real life," thereby providing the generalization so necessary for maintaining these gains. It is important to recognize that this perceived lack of relevance to realistic situations that the client may encounter is one of the most commonly voiced criticisms of AT. Clearly, the AT intervention is not about climbing over walls or surviving in the wilderness but about accessing the resources that will allow clients to surmount the walls in their lives and survive the challenges that they face at home.

While the setting and activities utilized by AT programs, whether it be the wilderness or a ropes course, are replete with powerful metaphors, the most effective metaphors are believed to be client-generated. When using metaphor in AT, the therapist takes on the role of conduit, actively helping the client to build such metaphors. Adventure-based practitioners postulate that the use of metaphor helps the client to continue utilizing the learning and growth provided through the adventure experience in ongoing and productive ways. Although the use of nature makes AT a natural fit for metaphoric work, the development of the use of metaphors in adventure programming is associated with the work of Milton Erickson (Bacon, 1983; Itin, 1998). Popularized by Ericksonian psychotherapy, the use of metaphor is common to many therapeutic disciplines.

Applicability to Multimodal Treatment

Another characteristic of AT is its applicability to multimodal treatment. As aforementioned, AT can be used either as an independent intervention or as an adjunct treatment. A wilderness therapy program is the most typical example of AT as an independent treatment, whereas an activity-based group session at an inpatient treatment facility would be considered adjunctive. Importantly, the focus on group level processing in combination with the individual psychotherapy which takes place around the activities provides a therapist with the opportunity to utilize standard and accepted treatment orientations and practices.

Sequencing of Activities

Fourth, in order to allow for the group to develop the skills and the level of cohesion necessary to achieve success in the activities, such activities are incrementally sequenced in difficulty. This sequencing also provides initial successes, or "mastery tasks," fostering feelings of capability while counteracting internal negative self-evaluations, learned helplessness, and dependency (Kimball & Bacon, 1993). This provision of a mastery task (success) concurrent with the activation of negative self-evaluations in the face of challenge is an important component for the therapeutic change thought to be associated with AT. The mastery task provides an opportunity to confront and tangibly disprove such evaluations. It is the therapist's role to facilitate such a transfer as such connections are not presumed to be an automatic reaction to the activities.

Conversely, activities presented with inappropriate sequencing can be counterproductive and reinforce negative self-conceptions for individual participants. The activation of such negative internal processes for a client without the opportunity to counteract such feelings with success can further reinforce existing beliefs in personal ineffectiveness. In addition, such negative conceptions can also permeate the development of a group identity. Therefore, it is vital that the therapist avoid creating a situation in which the group repeatedly experiences failure as it can be recognized that this dynamic can carry the highest potential for emotional harm and would be likely to limit therapeutic potential. By the same token, exclusive success is not desirable either, as failure is useful for the group process and helps to teach frustration tolerance. As with other types of therapy groups, it is recognized that effectiveness is often dependent upon the facilitator remaining aware of where the group is in its development (Yalom, 1995) and taking this into consideration when planning.

Perceived Risk

On the surface, challenges are often structured so as to appear to be impossible or dangerous to the group. In reality, the challenges are in fact low in actual risk but high in perceived risk, with the term "risk" referring to not only physical risk, but also intra- and interpersonal risk as well. A classic example is rappelling, where a participant must descend down the face of a rock wall. As anyone who has ever rappelled can attest, the perceived risk to life and limb is extreme as one steps back off of the cliff edge. However, risk management considerations dictate that all AT activities remain low in actual physical risk. On the other hand, high levels of emotional risk are encouraged. Since emotional risk is more subjective and more difficult to control, it is critical that therapists constantly monitor the emotional risk for each client, as well as for the group, throughout the intervention. This is precisely one of the central arguments for having clinically trained staff involved. The complex interaction between physical and emotional risk is illustrated in the following example. Standing on a platform and falling backwards into the arms of group members (i.e., trust fall) requires more trust than utilizing another person's support to cross a log. However, at earlier points in a group's development, this need to be supported (i.e., depend or rely on someone else) while crossing a log, could be perceived as carrying as high a level of interpersonal risk, along with the associated intrapersonal risk, as any physical activity for some clients.

Conceptually, perceived risk is thought to create tension and disequilibrium within the individual, ultimately leading the client to a position of choice [(i.e., dissonance theory), Festinger, 1957]. With regard to this conviction, Herbert (1996) notes that "In order for a person to achieve equilibrium, persons are challenged to make necessary adaptations" (1996, p. 5). He goes on to state: "Adventure-based work recognizes that it is the effort to overcome obstacles and, in effect, overcoming one's own fears that is critical." (p. 5). Through this combined process of relieving dissonance and overcoming fears, it is commonly believed in AT that clients are shown that old patterns are destructive and new choices can lead to more successful behaviors.

This perception of risk is so central to AT that Amesberger (1998) notes: "The most striking difference between adventure-based therapy and traditional psychotherapy is the client's strong involvement in a reality that is neither harmless nor perfectly safe" (p. 29). Although emotional risk clearly permeates traditional psychotherapy as well, it is the perceived physical risk that is a cornerstone of AT and distinguishes it from other forms of therapy.

Unfamiliar Environment

Another core characteristic of AT is that it is usually conducted in an environment unfamiliar to the client. This use of an unfamiliar and novel environment is thought to unbalance (Minuchin & Fishman, 1981) the client, further activating their underlying inter- and intrapersonal processes. It is hypothesized that the client has no familiar template from which to draw their reactions to the new situation, and thus it is the conviction of AT practitioners that the client must eventually rely on potentially new and ideally, healthier ways of behaving in order to achieve success (Gass, 1993) and equilibrium. In a sense, this can perhaps be conceptualized as providing an opportunity for clients to be free of past determinism. Gass (1990) postulates that this allows clients to explore problems rather than being overwhelmed by them.

The assumption underlying the unfamiliar environment in AT theory is that by taking a person out of their normal context, the client is exposed to new situations where old patterns of coping probably will not work. As social microcosm theory (Yalom, 1995) maintains, it is typical for clients to revert to earlier learned and more dysfunctional ways of behaving in such stressful situations. However, through the AT activities, the client may be provided with more tangible evidence of the consequences of dysfunctional behavior than is typically provided in group psychotherapy. These concrete consequences of dysfunctional behavior in combination with a novel environment, an environment that invites and may even necessitate new ways of behaving, could provide an impetus for change. In addition, the group can also provide reinforcement for new behaviors.

This environmental unfamiliarity in AT is also thought to allow for the client to experience the therapy without drawing from their typical expectations and defenses. Therefore, it is thought that this unfamiliarity may allow for a client to approach the therapeutic experience with less of a defensive posture. The engaging nature of the activities (i.e., fun or challenging), and the surreal environment (i.e., ropes course or wilderness) also help to make AT less threatening. Golins (1978) contrasts AT to traditional therapy methods on this issue of defensive posturing, noting that "traditional individual or group therapy methods may be particularly threatening for persons who have difficulty expressing themselves and/or establishing new relationships" (p. 27). To compare this with traditional psychotherapy research, Orlinsky and Howard (1986) have found "the dimension of the patients openness vs. defensiveness to be related to outcome" (p. 219). If in fact AT does work to lower defenses, this finding suggests that lowered defensiveness may contribute to a more positive outcome for clients.

As with dysfunctional behaviors, it is thought in AT theory that when a client's defenses do inevitably become activated, the therapist and the client may be provided with tangible examples through the activities and the interpersonal interactions during the activities, of the ways in which defenses operate in a client's life. In addition, the unfamiliar and novel AT setting may then provide a situation that is less threatening for some clients to experiment with new and less defensive behavioral and relational patterns. Again, the gamelike or surreal environment may also make it more inviting for clients to "try on" new behaviors (Golins, 1980).

Relationship Between Perceived Risk and Environmental Unfamiliarity

Herbert (1996) discusses how the unfamiliarity of the environment and the high level of perceived risk interact and how this combination is presumed to affect the client. He refers to this interaction as "challenge/stress," and reviews how it is believed by AT proponents that the dissonance created by the unfamiliar environment, in combination with a high level of perceived risk, results in an increased intensity of the activation of interpersonal and intrapersonal processes. Herbert goes on to discuss this interaction and subsequent activation as a potential change mechanism, noting: "Stressful experiences that are likely to occur throughout an adventure-based program serve as impetus for individual change" (p. 5). Gass (1993) also discusses this phenomena in terms of positive stress, or eustress.

It is this belief in client dissonance and the associated intensive activation of intra- and interpersonal processes, the unbalancing based on the lack of familiar "templates," the opportunity for new behavioral choices, the reinforcement provided by the activities, and the associated processing that moves AT most completely away from outdoor adventure programs and into the realm of therapy. While intensity (Minuchin, 1974) is employed in many treatment approaches, it is uniquely inherent in AT.

The AT literature purports that clients who make new behavioral choices in order to complete a novel challenge perceived as high in risk, particularly one they had previously thought themselves incapable of, consequently see themselves in a new light. The ultimate goal of such a transaction is for clients to recognize their own self-imposed limitations. This awareness is believed to increase clients' self-esteem, and such gains have been linked in the psychotherapy literature to decreases in anxiety and depression (Gilbert, 1992). Again, as noted above the AT intervention offers clients the opportunity to confront negative self conceptions and tangibly disprove them. Moreover, Priest (1993) has suggested that participants will be able to influence their probability of success in an adventure experience if they have realistic perceptions of risk involved in the choices they make, as well as a realistic sense of their own competence.

Challenge by Choice

Related to the discussion of perceived risk is the recognition that clients are given the option of "challenge by choice" (Schoel, Prouty, & Radcliffe, 1988). This allows for a client to choose to not participate in an activity for whatever reason. It is important to recognize that the choice to not participate in an activity is not necessarily negative and may have as many therapeutic implications as participation (i.e., choosing to not participate is still a choice). Such an instance may potentially reflect positive steps toward clients asserting their personal boundaries by recognizing and acting on personal discomfort, a potentially important issue for many clients. In such a situation, the therapist makes every effort to include the client in some way, such as "spotting" or observing. According to Royce (1987), "The key to growth in any situation is that the participants should choose to confront their fear rather than being forced to engage in fearful activities. This allows for the individual to take control of one's life instead of being other-directed." (p. 28). It should be noted that while the client ultimately always has the choice to not participate, that option is often not presented as a viable one in wilderness therapy and therapeutic camping programs, where compliance is a primary goal.

Challenge by choice is thought to be based not only on the recognition of risk involved in activities and related boundary issues, but also to an extent on the construct of learned helplessness (Seligman, 1975). Groff and Datillo (1998) discuss learned helplessness theory as it relates to AT, noting that past experiences leading to attributions which result in feelings of helplessness can generalize to other areas of a person's life, potentially resulting in a decreased motivation to engage in activities where one is unsure of the outcome. It is believed that challenge by choice can help lead to the recognition of the power of individual choice that can perhaps begin mitigating learned helplessness (Groff & Dattilo, 1998), thus contributing to the development of a greater sense of control for the client and more realistic cognitive attributions for events. As learned helplessness has also been espoused as a causal element in depression, this may be an important link to explore regarding AT's potential for therapeutic change (Gilbert, 1992).

Schoel et al. (1988) share this example to illustrate the power of challenge by choice:

> A short-term patient [from the Institute of Pennsylvania Hospital], a lawyer, was very depressed, denying his problems, not involved in anything, complaining of a bad back, etc., reluctant to do anything. He eventually tried some of the activities, and on the last day got up on a high element [ropes course] and completed it. According to the therapist, "he felt he never would have attempted the Incline Log at all if we had pushed him. The important thing is that we gave him the decision-making power." (p. 132).

Provision of Concrete Consequences

An additional descriptor of the AT approach is that the activities provide an opportunity for concrete consequences, positive and negative, of a client's behavior to be readily apparent. Beyond those aspects mentioned previously, another important element of this characteristic is that individual actions have consequences for both the group as a whole and the individual in relation to the group. A client who is unable to, or chooses not to, work successfully with the group is impacting the entire group's functioning. Therefore, the client may find his or her place within the group altered, may miss out on the group accomplishment, or even more concretely, may have a wet sleeping bag due to not setting up a tent correctly. Conversely, clients also experience the impact of positive behavior as well within the group. Such consequences at the group level may provide an opportunity for important developmental learning for individual clients. While these consequences are common to all group treatment modalities, the abundance of natural consequences in AT is a hallmark of the intervention. Natural consequences are particularly effective because they do not rely on an authority figure for enforcement, and in AT they tend to be particularly impactful, as the following example illustrates.

As a hypothetical example, at the start of a week-long wilderness expedition, the group leader tells participants to pack rain gear on the top of the pack. The group leader is aware that there is potential for a rainstorm during the course of the day and hopes to help the participants learn to be prepared. Jeff refuses to listen and acts in defiance of the leader, packing all of his rain gear on the bottom of the pack. Later in the pouring rain, Jeff is forced to remove all of the other items from his pack in order to reach his rain gear. The other gear, and Jeff himself, becomes soaked in the process. This gear included some of the dry food that was planned for the group's meal that evening. Justifiably, group members become angry with Jeff and he becomes temporarily ostracized, leading to conflict in the group and consequences for Jeff as a group member. The rainstorm also provided a natural individual consequence to Jeff for not heeding the advice of the group leader. Of course, had the weather not been warm, the leader would have intervened for safety reasons to prevent Jeff from becoming soaking wet.

Goal Setting

Goal setting in AT involves identifying for each client the objectives of program participation, with the ultimate goal being to tie the intervention to specific treatment outcomes for clients. Such goals are not related to the activities, rather, as with any psychotherapeutic treatment, goals are focused on specific problem areas for individual clients. As with any therapeutic intervention, these goals are developed after consultation with the client and/or the referral source and must be held in the therapist's awareness throughout the scope of the intervention. In addition, group goals are also established and often a "full value contract" is agreed upon, specifying the parameters of acceptable behavior within the group. This type of contracting maintains that all participants work together as a group to achieve both individual and group goals, adhere to necessary safety guidelines, and give and receive feedback when appropriate (Schoel et al., 1988). These guidelines are also established to promote physical and psychological safety for all participants.

Trust-Building

As in any therapeutic process, trust-building is a crucial characteristic of AT. Clients must learn not only to trust their therapist, but also to trust and depend on other members of the group, allowing for the closer examination of interpersonal processes related to trust as an ongoing therapeutic issue. This again is not unique to AT but rather mirrors the theory of interpersonally oriented group psychotherapy, and most specifically relates to the stages of therapeutic group development (Yalom, 1995).

The process of building trust is accomplished through the aforementioned sequencing of activities involving an increasing level of cooperation and group interaction. Most adventure-based therapy begins this gradual trust-building process by learning basic level information about each participant, allowing for the trust building process to begin in a way that may feel more natural for clients than does traditional group psychotherapy. As the activities progress, a higher level of self-disclosure is required and participants share deeper level experiences and emotions. As previously mentioned in the discussion of defenses, the activity focus of the group may allow an alternate medium for individuals to gradually share parts of themselves without the fear of being ridiculed or laughed at (Rohnke, 1995). Thereby it is speculated that the activities could provide a vehicle for emotional sharing and closeness for those to whom the more direct approach found in traditional psychotherapy may be overly threatening.

Physical trust is also incorporated and is conceptualized as a gateway to interpersonal trust (Schoel et al., 1988), with the assumption being that as clients increasingly entrust other group members with their physical safety, they will gradually begin to entrust the group with their emotional safety as well. As overall trust increases, the group becomes more autonomous and self-reliant, as well as more willing to openly communicate. As with a traditional therapy group, it is felt that when the group reaches this level of autonomy, that it is the most powerful vehicle for lasting change (Yalom, 1995). Compared to more traditional forms of therapy, AT would be considered unique in its use of physical trust.

Enjoyment

Enjoyment is also a component thought to be inherent in AT, and this is another aspect of AT that may be considered unique. Therapy is not often characterized as fun. Simply put, it is felt by supporters of AT that people are more invested in their treatment when it has positive reinforcement, and allowing for elements of therapy simply to be fun may be one way to provide an opportunity for such reinforcement. An increased level of enjoyment may also help in increasing attention levels and is believed, to take some of the seriousness out of threatening topics. This does not suggest treating such topics lightly, but rather, taking a less direct approach might reduce a client's reluctance to discuss such areas and ultimately lead to more open discussion of frequently avoided issues. This can be seen in some ways as similar to systematic desensitization, where aversive stimuli are paired with relaxation in order to decrease anxiety levels. It seems plausible that in AT this type of enjoyable interaction may function similarly to relaxation in facilitating therapeutic change.

To create such an atmosphere, many activities in the early phases of an adventure-based intervention are designed to increase group cohesion through sharing laughter. These activities "break the ice" and are thought to move the group more quickly and efficiently into the "working phases" of a group's development.

Peak Experience

The final characteristic of adventure-based therapy is peak experience. Herbert (1996) states: "the purpose of the peak experience is to provide an opportunity to practice all of the learning that has occurred and apply it to this one intensive challenge" (p. 6). These experiences can consist of an actual peak ascent or similar climactic wilderness experience, or can take the form of a group activity requiring a high degree of cooperation and trust. In both types of situations, clients perceive the challenge as more intense and complex than prior activities, and these types of experiences are often employed to provide the culmination of the group experience. Of all the characteristics described above, this is the one which may vary the most based upon which type of programming format is utilized.

While the actual therapy setting where the peak experience occurs is certainly unique to AT, this search for a peak experience is clearly something that is shared with other therapies. The emphasis on peak experience as a part of self-actualization is a crucial underlying assumption of humanistic theory (Csikszentmihaly, 1990; Maslow, 1971). Maslow discusses the power for growth embedded in such peak experiences at length, noting that "in a fair number of peak experiences, there ensues what I have called the "cognition of being" (p. 173), noting that this refers to "a technology of happiness" and the avenue to "pure joy" (p. 174).

Therapeutic Relationship

A description of the characteristics that define AT, as well as the change mechanisms that may be operating in AT, would not be complete without a discussion of the therapeutic relationship. Given that the strongest predictor of outcome in psychotherapy research has been shown to be the therapeutic relationship (Orlinsky, Grawe, & Parks, 1994), it is worthwhile to consider the implications of the extended and intensive relationship that is found uniquely in the AT experience. This is particularly true in wilderness therapy programs that last for at least one week and beyond, where the therapists

live together with the clients in the wilderness. Specifically, it is
g to consider the potential effects for the client of continuous
in.   nent with the therapist, as well as the group, that lasts for an extended period of time on an around-the clock basis.

It can be speculated that for some clients this may be immensely threatening. For such clients this may result in their being unable to form positive relationships as their defensive reactions may become intensely activated and further entrenched, essentially making it impossible for them to engage in therapy. However, it may be that just the opposite is true—that such intensive relationships developed on an ongoing basis with no opportunity for withdrawal may in fact facilitate the creation of more positive internal representations based on this all-encompassing level of relationship. Advocates for AT offer much anecdotal evidence to support the latter argument.

Consider the fact that if client and therapist are together for twenty-one days on a twenty-four hour basis, this translates into 504 hours of therapeutic contact, an approximate time equivalent of ten years of weekly psychotherapy. Excluding the hours spent sleeping, that still is roughly 330 hours of contact, an equivalent of approximately six and one-half years of weekly psychotherapy. Obviously a 21-day experience with no follow-up is not the equivalent of 6 or 10 years of weekly psychotherapy. Such a comparison of the numbers is provided merely to illustrate the potential potency of this amount of time between therapist and client spent continuously.

The opportunity for the development of therapeutic relationships in the different, more time intensive, and more multidimensional way provided by the AT experience may facilitate growth in clients based in this relational bond. It also possible that there may be an effect based on this twenty-four hour contact that is simply not available in traditional forms of psychotherapy. Clearly, the access alone is an important factor. Therapists in the field are available to capitalize on teachable moments. The level of support that the therapist can offer with continual presence and during such an intensive experience is another valuable consideration.

From an object relations (psychodynamic) framework, the development of such a potentially unique relationship in AT may provide greater opportunity for corrective emotional experience to occur. That is, the experience helps to heal a prior traumatic event. For example, a caring and supportive relationship experienced with the therapist may help the client to work through abandonment by a parent. If so, such occurrences may become more firmly anchored for the client based on the fact that the relationship becomes a part of their daily existence for a period of time and thus, is grounded in "real experience."

Related to this is the potential power of modeling (Bandura, 1986) that could occur in such a situation. The therapist is living in the same conditions and is required to perform the same tasks as the client.

Opportunities for modeling abound as the therapist faces many of the same daily stressors and must cope with the same hardships as the client. Moreover, the therapist's willingness to expose him or herself voluntarily to these difficult conditions inspires a degree of intimacy, trust, and mutual respect that goes beyond that found in traditional therapeutic settings (Greenwood, Lipson, Abrahamse, Zimring, 1983). Such high regard for the therapist is likely to help the client to be more open to imitating the therapist's behaviors.

It is important to acknowledge that not all wilderness therapy programs maintain a therapist in the field throughout the expedition. In fact, it may be more common for the therapists to visit the field for one or two days per week. Nevertheless, the therapist's willingness to meet the clients in those conditions is very meaningful to many clients and may break down barriers that exist when a client visits a therapist's office. Perhaps more importantly, the AT therapist understands the process that the client is going through and that may be enough to forge a strong relationship when a client is in the midst of such an intensive experience. Of course, with or without the ongoing presence of a therapist, all programs have field staff who are available on a continual basis. For many of the same reasons described above, these staff members are able to develop close relationships with clients and are responsible for much of the therapeutic change that occurs in wilderness therapy programs.

The unconventional therapeutic relationship described above also extends to activity-based psychotherapy and therapeutic camping. Although these formats may not offer the intensity of an expedition-based relationship, therapists are still working outside of an office setting. This alone makes them more accessible for many clients who feel distrusting or defensive in a traditional psychotherapy setting. Moreover, the relationship is activity-based and as mentioned, this is less threatening for many clients.

Illustrative Example

To illustrate, Jane is a hypothetical 32-year-old woman who typically blames others for her problems and often uses threats to get her way. Jane has come to therapy because she "has trouble in relationships" and her ultimate goal in therapy is to both understand and change this problem. Imagine Jane, 30-feet up in the air on a high ropes course element. Her heart is pumping, her fears and anxieties are increasing, and she is beginning to become frustrated because she believes that she cannot proceed. It is likely that if Jane approaches the situation in her "standard way," by yelling at others and blaming them for her inability to complete the task, she will remain where she is and only become more entrenched in her spiraling negativity. This behavior will inevitably alienate members of the group, making it unlikely that they will come to her aid and support her in succeeding.

The level of risk which Jane perceives in the situation has led to an experience of disequilibrium, or feeling unbalanced, leading to Jane's reenactment of previously dysfunctional interpersonal patterns. In this instance, with no further therapeutic intervention, Jane remains stuck on the ropes course and there is tangible evidence of the consequences for her continued maintenance of old ways of behaving. Should she manage to simply get down off the course, she may have learned something, but it is unlikely that the learning will provide lasting characterological change. In fact, an equally likely scenario is that the intervention may be harmful for Jane by reinforcing her negative self-conceptions.

However, if the therapist processes this experience with Jane and the group in a way that helps her to recognize her dysfunctional ways of behaving, as well as assisting her to achieve some level of control and an increased willingness to work with others, she is much more likely to complete the activity successfully. This processing may take place later in individual sessions as well. On the group level, other members also provide Jane feedback as to the consequences of her actions, both while such actions are occurring and afterwards in a group session.

Should Jane succeed, such a success will ideally reinforce for Jane the new and more positive ways of behaving, as well as illustrate for her the negative aspects of behaving in her old patterns. If the therapist were to expand this processing to an exploration of where these dysfunctional patterns originated (using a psychodynamic orientation), Jane could potentially gain insight into these origins and perhaps begin establishing more functional ways of relating to both herself and to others on a level beyond that provided by the activity alone. Should the therapist continue his or her relationship with Jane upon her completion of the AT intervention, such concrete examples provided by the activities could perhaps be referred to as points of reference by both Jane and the therapist. In such an instance, the process of change that began for Jane during the course of her AT treatment component, could potentially be continued and deepened through this ongoing relationship.

What can be seen here is a direct parallel to traditional psychotherapy, with the activity itself simply providing both the catalyst and a concrete external representation of pre-existing issues for Jane. Jane's behavior can be explored, as well as her cognitions, affect, and interpersonal functioning. Repetitions of the activity or participation in new activities can give Jane an opportunity to practice different ways of behaving, thinking, feeling and relating, again, with tangible and easily seen results. Over time, the illustrations provided by the activity can be referenced by both Jane and her therapist. Ideally, a skilled therapist builds upon this learning process, allowing for the activities themselves and the processing associated with them to become an inextricably linked and circular process. This type of model can be used in any of the aforementioned settings when the activities are processed in a therapeutic manner.

Conclusion

As AT becomes more widely recognized as a credible treatment approach, it is important that the literature be able to clearly represent what exactly adventure therapy is. It is also vital that those within the field have a thorough understanding of the theoretical principles that underlie this approach. It has been the experience of the authors that many practitioners, caught up in their enthusiasm for their work, believe that AT is a totally unique treatment approach. This misconception is not helpful in advocating for AT's acceptance in the mental health field. On the contrary, AT shares many commonalities with well-established treatment approaches. In fact, as this paper has attempted to demonstrate, AT is more similar to other types of treatments than different. This is not a liability but rather, an asset that can assist AT in gaining wider recognition among the mental health treatment community and help AT to demonstrate its viability as a treatment approach.

At the same time, there are aspects of AT which are unique and help to make it an effective intervention. Most notably, the activity base which serves as a foundation for AT clearly distinguishes it from other forms of treatment. There is substantial theoretical evidence to suggest that the activities inherent to AT, and more specifically the theoretical process that surrounds the activities, contribute largely to its effectiveness. The research evidence, however, is not as convincing. More process evaluations are needed to substantiate this claim, and future research must address this shortcoming. The field of AT must begin to hold itself accountable for answering the questions posed to all other treatments: Is this treatment effective? For whom, and under what circumstances? To its proponents, AT has long been seen as a powerful treatment intervention; as we "come of age," it is time to garner the evidence to convince the broader mental health establishment.

References

Alvarez, A. G. and Stauffer, G. A. (2001). Musings on adventure therapy. *Journal of Experiential Education, 24*(2), 85-91.

Amesberger, G. (1998). Theoretical considerations of theoretical concepts in adventure therapy. In C. Itin (Ed.), *Exploring the boundaries of adventure therapy: International perspectives. Proceedings of the first international adventure therapy conference.* Perth, Western Australia: AEE/COEAWA.

Bandoroff, S. (1989). *Wilderness adventure-based therapy for delinquent and pre-delinquent youth: A review of the literature.* (ERIC Document Reproduction Service No. ED 377 428).

Bandoroff, S. (1992). Wilderness family therapy: An innovative treatment approach for problem youth. (Doctoral dissertation, University of South Carolina, 1991). *Dissertation Abstracts International.*

Bacon, S. (1983). *Conscious use of metaphor in Outward Bound.* Denver, CO: Colorado Outward Bound School.

Bacon, S. & Kimball, R. (1989). The wilderness challenge model. In R. D. Lyman (Ed.), *Residential and inpatient treatment of children and adolescents.* New York: Plenum Press.

Banaka, W. H. & Young, D. W. (1985). Community coping skills enhanced by an adventure camp for adult chronic psychiatric patients. *Hospital and Community Psychiatry, 36*(7), 746-748.

Bandura, A. (1977). Self-efficacy: Toward a unifying theory of behavioral change. *Psychological Review, 84,* 191-215.

Bandura, A. (1986). *Social foundation of thought and action: A social cognitive theory.* Englewood Cliffs, NJ: Prentice-Hall.

Buie, A. (1996). *National Association for Therapeutic Wilderness Camping: History.* Webpage http://www.natwc.org/history.html

Crisp, S. (1997). *Definition of adventure based therapy.* Unpublished manuscript.

Crisp, S. (1998). International models of best practice in wilderness and adventure therapy. In C. Itin (Ed.), *Exploring the boundaries of adventure therapy: International perspectives. Proceedings of the 1st International Adventure Therapy Conference.* Boulder, CO: Association for Experiential Education.

Csikszentmihaly, M. (1990). *Flow: The Psychology of optimal experience.* NY: Harper Perennial.

Festinger, L. (1957). *A theory of cognitive dissonance.* Evanston, IL: Row, Peterson.

Gass, M. A. (1990). *Adventure therapy for families.* Unpublished manuscript, University of New Hampshire.

Gass, M. A. (1993). *Adventure therapy: Therapeutic applications of adventure programming.* Dubuque, IA: Kendall/Hunt Publishing Co.

Gass, M. A. (1995). *Book of metaphors.* Dubuque, IA: Kendall/Hunt Publishing Co.

Gilbert, P. (1992). *Depression: The evolution of powerlessness.* New York: Guilford Press.

Gillis, H. L. (1992). *Therapeutic uses of adventure-challenge-outdoor-wilderness: Theory and research,* 35-47. Keynote Presentation given at the meeting of the Association for Experiential Education.

Gillis, H. L. (1995). If I conduct outdoor pursuits with clinical populations, am I an adventure therapist? *Journal of Leisurability, 22*(4), 5-15.

Gillis, H. L. & Ringer, M. (1999). Adventure as therapy. In J. Miles & S. Priest (Eds.), *Adventure programming.* State College, PA: Venture Publishing.

Golins, G. (1978). How delinquents succeed through adventure-based education. *Journal of Experiential Education, 1*(1), 26-29.

Golins, G. (1980). *Utilizing adventure education to rehabilitate juvenile delinquents.* New Mexico State University. (ERIC Document Reproduction Service No. ED 187 501).

Gomes-Schwart, B. (1978). Effective ingredients in psychotherapy: Predictions of outcome from process variables. *Journal of Consulting and Clincal Psycholgy, 46,* 1023-1035.

Groff, D. & Datillo, J. (1998). Unpublished manuscript.

Greenwood, P., Lipson, A., Abrahamse, A. & Zimring, F. (1983). *Youth crime and juvenile justice in California* (Report No. R-3016-CSA). Santa Monica, CA: The Rand Corporation.

Herbert, J. T. (1996). Use of adventure based counseling programs for persons with disabilities. *Journal of Rehabilitation, 62*(4), 3-9

Itin, C., (Ed.), (1998). *Exploring the boundaries of adventure therapy: International perspectives.* Proceedings of the first international adventure therapy conference: Perth, Western Australia: AEE/COEAWA.

Kelley, F. J. & Baer, D. J. (1971). Physical challenge as a treatment for delinquency. *Crime and Delinquency, 17,* 437-445.

Kimball, R. & Bacon, S. (1993). The wilderness challenge model. In M. Gass (Ed.), *Adventure Therapy: Therapeutic applications of adventure-based therapy programming.* Dubuque, IA: Kendall/Hunt Publishing Co..

Kraft, R., & Sakofs, M. (1985). *The theory of experiential education.* Boulder, CO: Association of Experiential Education.

Minuchin, S. & Fishman, C. (1981). *Family therapy techniques.* Cambridge, MA: Harvard University Press.

Maslow, A.H. (1971). *The further reaches of human nature.* New York: The Viking Press.

Nadler, R. S., & Luckner, J. L. (1992). *Processing the adventure experience: Theory and practice.* Dubuque, IA : Kendall/Hunt Publishing Co..

Newes, S. L. (2000). *Adventure-based therapy: Theory, characteristics, ethics, and research.* Unpublished manuscript. Pennsylvania State University.

Orlinsky, D.E., Grawe, K. & Parks, B.K. (1994). Process and outcome in psychotherapy. In A.E. Bergin & S.L. Garfield (Eds.). *Handbook of psychotherapy and behavior change* (4th Ed., pp. 270-376). New York: Wiley.

Orlinsky, D. E., & Howard, (1986). Process and outcome in psychotherapy. In S.L. Garfield & A.E. Bergin (Eds.). *Handbook of psychotherapy and behavior change* (3rd ed., pp. 311-384). New York: Wiley.

Priest, S. (1993). A New model for risk-taking in adventure programming. *Journal of Experiential Education, 16*(1), 50-53.

Priest, S. & Baillie, R. (1987). Justifying the risk to others: the real razor's edge. *Journal of Experiential Education, 10*(1), 16-22.

Raskin, N. J. & Rogers, C. R. (1989). Person-centered therapy. In R.J. Corsini & D. Wedding (Eds.). *Current psychotherapies.* (p. 155-196). Itasca, IL: F. E. Peacock.

Ringer, M. (1994). *Adventure therapy: A map of the field: Towards a definition of adventure-based therapy: Workshop Report.* Unpublished manuscript.

Rohnke, K. E. (1995). *Silver bullets.* Hamilton, MA: Project Adventure, Inc.

Royce, D. (1987). Adventure experience and affective learning: Where are we going? *Journal of Adventure Education, 4,* 12-14.

Russell, K. C. (2003a). An assessment of outcomes in outdoor behavioral healthcare treatment. *Child and Youth Care Forum, 32*(6), 355-381.

Schoel, J., Prouty, D., & Radcliffe, P. (1988). *Islands of healing: A guide to adventure-based counseling.* Hamilton, MA: Project Adventure, Inc.

Seligman, M. E. P. (1975). *Helplessness.* San Francisco: W.H. Freeman.

Taylor, F. (1989). The influence of an outdoor adventure recreation class on personality type, locus of control, self-esteem, and selected issues of identity development of college students. *Dissertation Abstracts International, 51*(04), 1122A.

Wichman, T. (1991). Of wilderness and circles: Evaluating a therapeutic model for wilderness programs. *Journal of Experiential Education, 14*(2), 43-48.

Witman, J. P. (1987). The efficacy of adventure programming in the development of cooperation and trust with adolescents in treatment. *Therapeutic Recreation Journal, 21*(3), 22-30.

Witman, J.P. & Presenkis, K. (1996). Adventure programming with an individual who has multiple personality disorder: A case history. *Therapeutic Recreation Journal, 30*(4), 289-296.

Yalom, I.D. (1995). *The Theory and practice of group psychotherapy.* New York: Basic Books.

Authors' Biographies

*Dr. **Sandra Newes** obtained her doctorate in clinical psychology from Penn State University. She is involved in writing about clinical theory and research methodology in adventure therapy, as well as in more conventional settings. She is an active member of AEE and is the past chair of the Therapeutic Adventure Professional Group. She currently maintains a consulting practice in Asheville, North Carolina.*

*Dr. **Scott Bandoroff** is a psychologist with 20 years of experience working with challenging adolescents and their families in wilderness and outpatient settings. He has worked as a clinician, supervisor, internship director, consultant, and trainer. He founded Peak Experience to provide training and consultation in Adventure Therapy and works with mental health agencies, schools, residential treatment centers, and wilderness programs.*

Correspondence

Contact Sandra Newes
(814) 935-2135 or slnewes@yahoo.com

Contact Scott Bandoroff
(541) 951-4329 or scott@peakexperience.org
or on the web at: www.peakexperience.org

Playing with Ideas About Adventure Therapy: Applying Principles of Gestalt, Narrative and Psychodynamic Approaches to Adventure Therapy

Blair Gilbert, Rüdiger Gilsdorf & Martin Ringer

■ ■ ■

Drawing on their backgrounds in Narrative, Gestalt and Psychodynamic Therapy, the authors of this paper propose a number of guidelines and concepts to be considered for the theory and practice of Adventure Therapy. These principles are then discussed to explore different meanings and options for facilitation in the context of a scenario, based on the events in a training workshop. The overall intention is not so much to demonstrate the strength of any therapeutic approach, but to encourage practitioners to reflect on their own backgrounds and philosophies, and to draw on them consciously in the decisions encountered in the practice of Adventure Therapy.

■ ■ ■

Searching for Common Ground

Since 1993, when Michael Gass edited the first book entirely devoted to our young field, Adventure Therapy has come a long way towards developing an identity and place in the therapeutic community. Three different perspectives which have been useful in this respect may be discerned:

1. The search for therapeutic qualities which are inherent in the process of adventure-based learning. From this perspective, the combination of nature, group and adventure activities provides a rich source of healing potential which in a number of ways goes beyond what therapy has to offer in a more conventional setting. Kimball and Bacon's (1993)

"wilderness challenge model" and Foster and Little's (1989) "wilderness quest," both drawing, to a different degree, on the power of rites of passage are examples of such enterprises. In a sense, from this perspective one could regard *Adventure Therapy as an autonomous approach.*

2. The search for appropriate therapeutic contexts within which adventure could play a particularly useful role. From this perspective, adventure activities and the natural setting in which they are experienced have the potential to enrich other therapeutic procedures. The fact that most Adventure Therapy programmes presented at the first two International Adventure Therapy Conferences (Itin, 1998; Richards, 2003) seem to be incorporated into a wider therapeutic context may be seen as an indicator for the predominance of this perspective, which according to Gass (1993) could be labeled *Adventure Therapy as an adjunctive approach.*

3. The search for common ground between concepts developed within and beyond the context of Adventure Therapy. From this perspective, as a member of the 'experiential learning family' Adventure Therapy has quite a few relatives in the world of therapy and may draw on their developments as well as enrich them with its own creations. Along this line of thought, parallels between Hypnotherapy (Itin, 1993), Solution Oriented Therapy (Gass & Gillis, 1995), Gestalt Therapy (Gilsdorf, 1998) or Narrative Therapy (Stolz, 2003) and Adventure Therapy have been explored so far. Simply speaking, from this point of view, one could understand *Adventure Therapy as a synthesis between a number of coherent therapeutic perspectives.*

Clearly, all three approaches offer valuable insights to the field. This article, however, is intended to follow the search for common ground between Adventure Therapy (AT) and other therapeutic approaches. In particular, a number of concepts from Gestalt, Narrative and Psychodynamic Therapy which have affinities to AT and/or are likely to foster a deeper understanding of a therapeutic process involving elements of active exploration, risk and relational learning will be pursued. Obviously, a thorough description and understanding of these approaches cannot be achieved within the confines of this paper. Instead some key concepts from each approach will be studied in relation to a particular segment of practice. In a second part, these concepts will be revisited and their implications discussed via a case study from an experiential program facilitated by one of the authors. Altogether, we'd like to advocate playful moves between different conceptual systems, which often seem to emphasise differences far more than common ground.

Gestalt Therapy

Building on a paper presented at a former IATC conference (Gilsdorf, 1998) and drawing onto an extensive exploration of systemic and process-directive sources for Adventure Therapy (Gilsdorf, 2004), three central areas of Gestalt Therapy will be emphasised: (a) *Presence* as the time, in which our experience is given to us; (b) *Contact-border* as the place, where our experience happens as interplay between organism and environment and (c) *Self-organisation* as the principle, which governs our experience, the way we make sense of it and translate it into further action.

Simply speaking, one could say that Gestalt Therapy has derived three concrete guidelines of practice from these relatively abstract concepts: (a) *Awareness* as a guideline to stay in touch with the presence, the people and the situation in front of us; (b) *Experiment* as a guideline to further explore what happens in a given contact, how we are able to deal with it and how we possibly limit ourselves and (c) *Process-directivity* as a guideline to facilitate a therapeutic process intending to assist such a self-organised exploration.

Awareness.

One of the deepest convictions of Gestalt Therapy is that to develop any real understanding—of a phenomenon, of others, of ourselves —we need to be in touch with the "object" we are trying to understand. Awareness, defined by Rahm (1979) as "a state of attentive awakeness towards the things that happen in the present moment in me, with me and around me" (p. 164), is a way to conceptualize such a "being in touch." As Fuhr and Gremmler-Fuhr (1995) point out, there are at least two contrasting aspects of awareness. On the one hand, awareness can be directed toward whatever we choose to concentrate on. In the language of Gestalt Psychology, it can be *figure-bound*, somewhat sharply focusing on particular details of a given situation. As we are actively attending to something, we may speak in this case of *attentiveness*. On the other hand, there is a rather undirected, almost free-flowing awareness. In Gestalt terms, such awareness is *ground-bound*, sensitive to connections and movements in the whole picture, acknowledging the unsharp and fuzzy character in which it presents itself. As we are somewhat open to receive whatever may appear or happen in the next moment, this kind of awareness may be referred to as *receptiveness*.

However, at best, awareness is not a question of either attentiveness or receptiveness. Rather, it is a kind of oscillation between them, as it appears in Figure 1. Such awareness is active and passive at the same time, "touching out" as well as allowing to be touched. In their emphasis on dualities, Western languages are, as Portele (1992) points out, not well equipped to conceptualize such a *middle-mode*. Furthermore, Western thinking tends to favour active engagement, and as a consequence we may be likely to misinterpret awareness as some kind of mental intervention, overlooking its contemplative quality. In any case, awareness is not something that we can "apply" to a situation. Rather, it involves our body as much as our mind and if anything, we may create a space within ourselves, and between ourselves and others to allow awareness to emerge.

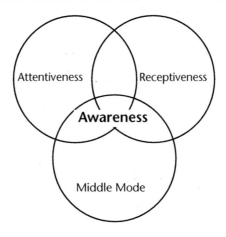

Figure 1. "**Aspects of Awareness.**"

Experiment.

In a sense, experiment is the counterpart to awareness. Awareness refers to the warning insight, that before any change is contemplated, a therapist needs to be fully present and in good contact with the client. In contrast, experiment connotes enthusiasm concerning the realm of possibilities which may lie within reach for discovery and change. According to Zinker (1977), "the creative experiment, if it works well, helps the person leap forward into new expression, or at least pushes the person into the boundaries, the edge where his growth needs to take place" (p. 125). Clearly, Gestalt offers a quite different concept of experiment and experimenting than that which is commonly understood from empirical science. Figure 2 clarifies the essential differences between the two concepts.

Any adventure activity could be understood as an experiment in this sense. In fact, the concept may well serve as a suitable umbrella for different levels of engagement and change found in Experiential and Adventure Therapy. Thus, as Figure 3 illustrates, the client's therapeutic involvement may be understood in terms of deepening levels of experimenting.

First of all, there has to be some kind of agreement about the basic goals, roles and procedures of therapy. This may seem self-evident, but particularly when considering work with adolescents, it becomes clear that the simple question of participation can be a matter of intense negotiation. When requirements and existing choices are pointed out clearly, any client decision can be dealt with as an act of experimenting within a new and strange setting. While some of that may remain abstract in the beginning, experiments become very concrete at the activity level. Confronted with specific tasks, clients repeatedly have to make decisions about their physi-

Empirical Experiment	Gestalt-Experiment
Discovery of universal knowledge	Discovery of personal knowledge and initiation of change
Repeatable	Unique
Standardized	Situated
Test leader striving for control	Not-knowing therapist offering an impulse
Not-knowing test person following instructions	Client making decisions
Result-oriented	Process-oriented
Measurable quantitative results	Tangible qualitative changes

Figure 2. Differences between Empirical Experiment and Gestalt-Experiment.

cal, mental and social engagement. Such engagement has a healthy quality in and of itself in many ways. However, the next step may be seen as most crucial.

Therapeutic adventure activities are meant to help clients get in touch with issues where growth or change needs to take place. Therefore, at the awareness level therapists will encourage clients to make sense of whatever happens to them in an activity, and discover themselves as active agents in that process. Basically, experimenting is understood here as mak-

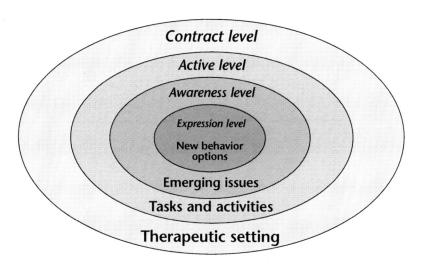

Figure 3. Levels of experimenting in Experiential and Adventure Therapy.

ing connections between outside and inside, physical challenges and emerging personal issues. The ultimate challenge, then, is to move from such understanding to new behaviour. Experimenting can thus be understood as a search for alternative options and as a creative play with new expressions. The therapist will encourage clients to take advantage of the relatively safe space of Adventure Therapy such that they may ideally remember themselves as "new" as the setting and activities to which they have been exposed.

Process-directivity.

Encouraged by self-organisation and constructivist theories, Gestalt holds a strong belief that change may be enhanced, yet never controlled by therapeutic intervention. While it is evident that such a position goes along with certain reservations against a directive style, non-directivity can hardly be a guideline for a process that relies heavily on initiating and facilitating experiments. The answer to this dilemma has been the development of a process-directive therapeutic style (Greenberg, Rice & Elliott, 1993; Peeters, 2003). At first hand, this may appear to be a clear guideline: facilitate a process of exploration, meaning or decision making, and leave decisions regarding its content to the client. However, in the "jungle" of therapeutic interaction, things are usually not as simple as this. At least four dimensions which lend themselves to deeper exploration of process-directivity can be discerned:

1. *The way in which therapeutic power is applied.* When the question of influence and power in therapy comes up, most therapists tend to reflect upon their direct interaction with the client in the therapeutic session. In this sense, influence is exercised basically by the therapist's interventions. However, especially when we think of Adventure Therapy, it becomes clear that a whole range of important decisions concerning the composition of the group, the therapeutic venue, the character and rhythm of the activities and others are made outside of the actual session. Those decisions are powerful in setting a frame for what is possible within the bounds of therapy, and therapists need to acknowledge that many of them are quite directive, leaving clients only marginal influence. In short, one aspect of process-directiveness is that the conscious use of power over the situation allows therapists to apply less power *in* the situation.

2. *The position of the therapist.* In the classic individual therapy setting, the distribution of roles is quite clear; client and therapist are exploring the client's world, and while the former is personally involved in this world, the latter's position is that of an outside expert. One of the main things Humanistic Psychology has emphasised is that any expert influence is likely to remain meaningless in therapy if it is not grounded in a solid relational basis. The therapist needs to be present as a real person. Group therapy and Adventure Therapy, in particular, open up a whole range of possibilities for

real contact to happen. Therapists can, and in fact need to, switch quite often between their position as members of the group—in which they are exposed to similar conditions and events as the clients—and their position as facilitators—in which they take a step back and try to help others clarify what is going on for them at the moment. Process-directivity implies considering the different qualities of interventions from those different points of view, inside and outside, and balancing them in a way that clients end up with the freedom to consider a maximum of new options.

3. *The focus of intervention.* This points to the dimension which is usually characterised by the dichotomy of content and process. Upon closer inspection, Schein (1987) has proposed to differentiate between three levels of intervention: result, procedure and process. As stated above, from a process-directive point of view, interventions will focus on the latter end of this spectrum. An adventure therapist with a Gestalt background is interested in the result of activities only insofar as a client's motivation and self-esteem will be linked to a certain amount of success. The procedures that have been employed to get there are good starting points for exploration, as they can be linked to concrete actions and communications. Process exploration, however, points to the dynamics behind those apparent actions: individual thoughts and feelings, as well as collective rules and norms. An underlying guideline for process-directivity is thus to move from surface to depth. Likewise, the process-directive therapist can be seen as an advocate of ambivalence, questioning any quick explanation of what has been going on, as well as trying to keep him or herself away from such simplified belief systems.

4. *The character and rhythm of intervention.* Process-oriented interventions are meant to touch upon sensible issues. Therefore, therapists need to be careful to intervene in a way that leaves clients the freedom to "pick up" the issue in question, as well as move in another direction if they do not feel ready to deal with it. In this sense, Gestalt encourages interventions that have a rather tentative character. According to the priority of self-directedness and self-discovery, it also encourages therapists not to intervene when in doubt. As a general rule, following the client in a potentially promising direction, rather than taking the lead, should be given priority. However, clients at times turn in circles. In fact, that may well be the reason that they are attending a therapeutic program. From a process-directive perspective, there is an awareness that therapists need to take initiative in critical moments, and there also is an awareness that this needs do be done in a careful way. Once again, the middle-mode, a balance between active and passive, touching out and allowing to be touched, seems to be an appropriate concept to describe what lies at the heart of process-directiveness.

Gestalt Adventure Therapy.

Gestalt Therapy has played a leading role in working toward a recognition of the above principles in the therapeutic community. It is important to note that though its philosophy is deeply embedded in the broader context of Humanistic Psychology, its origins go back to Psychodynamic practice and its latest developments are closely linked to postmodern constructivist and constructionist thinking. If, however, a unique quality of a Gestalt Adventure Therapy had to be emphasised, it would be the "moment-by-moment" character (Greenberg et al., 1993) of therapeutic interventions. Gestalt encourages the adventure therapist to stay connected with his or her experience in the "here-and-now," and to thus consider any diagnosis, method or program as preliminary at best.

Narrative Therapy

In this section three key principles of Narrative Therapy will be presented. While not a complete representation of this theory in its application to the field, they do represent some broad ideas from which to think about Narrative Adventure Therapy. A more thorough account can be found in Stolz (2003), who links postmodern understandings with Adventure Therapy and Monk, Winslade, Crocket & Epston (1997), who offer a full account of Narrative Therapeutic practice. The three principles of Narrative Therapy that will be discussed in this paper are: (a) the problem is the problem; (b) the social construction of reality and (c) the process of deconstruction.

The problem is the problem.

The first principle to be discussed is that "the person is not the problem, the problem is the problem." This simple but powerful first principle opens the door to alternative ways of thinking about human psychology that may not have previously been explored. Traditional counseling has been embedded in modernist models which have often focused on individual pathology. By contrast the first principle shifts the mind set from the person to the problem, thus opening space to explore and understand the issue.

The first principle sits alongside another important Narrative Therapy idea "that people make meaning, meaning is not made for us" (Monk et al., 1997, p. 33). Combined, these two statements encapsulate a major part of narrative therapeutic thinking. When we understand that meaning is made by us, we can become the authors of both the situation and our lives, not victims of the problem itself. This approach highlights the respect shown to the person, or participant, irrespective of the circumstances. With the participant as the author, he or she identifies and names the problem. From this position the therapist can join with the client in exploring and gaining understanding over the problem.

This process is respectful of different cultural perspectives as the person offers his/her own understanding, rather than depending on the therapist's understanding. The therapist comes from his/her own culturally and socially constructed paradigm, one that is often different than the partici-pant's. "People within a culture share a dominant set of discourses, or ways of making sense. But each one of us puts our own individual story togeth-er in our particular way" (Monk et al., 1997, p. 44). The Narrative approach validates the participant's understanding and has no need to either change this or suggest that the person's view is incorrect or inferior to the thera-pist's understanding.

The second characteristic of Narrative Therapy that complements the first guiding principle of "the problem being the problem" is known as externalized conversations. This strategy was developed by Michael White, who is acknowledged as one of the founders of Narrative Therapy (Monk et al., 1997). Externalization gives the participants the opportunity to dis-cuss the problem free from themselves and the often associated blame, judgement and recrimination. When the problem is externalized, the par-ticipants can draw on their resources to work against the problem rather than identify themselves as dysfunctional or unwell. The task of identify-ing the problem rests with the participant rather than the therapist, a major shift from many modernist perspectives where the therapist holds the knowledge about problems and has the power of diagnosis. By contrast, Narrative Therapy recognises that problems are socially constructed and the participant holds the knowledge to identify and address the issue.

The social construction of reality.

The second principle that provides a base to Narrative Therapy emerges from the theories of post-modernism and social constructionism. These theories underpin the view that meaning is created through social interaction. An example of this is encapsulated in the following vignette:

> [Three umpires] are sitting around over a beer, and one says, "There's balls and there's strikes, and I call 'em the way they are." Another says, "There's balls and there's strikes, and I call 'em the way I see 'em." The third says, "There's balls and there's strikes, and they ain't nothing until I call 'em." (Walter Truett Anderson, 1990, p. 76).

This quote clearly demonstrates how words and their associated meanings are constructed within a social context, and to this end can also be deconstructed. So how does post-modernism help with the situations we find in therapy? Some suggest that it provides no answers, but only blurs the parameters of what "is." In contrast, it is this blurring that opens the space for new possibilities, and this can be helpful to the therapeutic process. As a philosophy, post-modernism "challenges generally accepted beliefs about reality, knowledge, truth and transcendence" (Culling, 1996, p. 3). If the truths that people hold about themselves and the problems become contestable, then space can be made available for alternative truths. Only a small proportion of our lived experience is storied and spoken about, but our lives are multi-storied, with most of our lived experience remaining unspoken. These unspoken or non-narrated experiences may provide useful alternatives to the problem story.

One reason that some experiences remain unspoken is due to social norms that are held in place by processes of power. Michel Foucault (1973) believes two types of power operate within a cultural context. These are sovereign power and discipline power. Sovereign power is more easily identified by its open means of operation. The exercise of this power comes from people in "authority" such as chiefs, queens, teachers, governments and police. People tend to know when this power has been enacted upon them. Discipline power is harder to notice. It is pervasive and it acts upon all of us most of the time. Discipline power can be thought of as societal power that seeks conformity of people towards the norm (Stolz, 2003). The practice of externalizing conversations seeks to make this power more transparent. By moving the source of the problem from the individual, Narrative Therapy searches for alternative understandings that take into account both sovereign and discipline power in the construction of the problem.

A process of deconstruction.

The third principle is more tenuous to grasp, but it reflects the need to accept the means by which we make sense of this therapeutic process. Ironically, to state principles of Narrative Therapy invites narrative therapists to take a position within a categorizing structure, thus moving away from post-structuralism and into structuralism. This highlights two concepts within Narrative Therapy—positioning and discourse. Discourse refers to the "taken-for-granted" assumptions that sit just below the surface of a text, or conversation, that enables the text to make sense. Positioning occurs as we place the text and people into a context that fits within the discourses that may be present. For example in an activity-based programme, how do you position an adventure therapist as opposed to an outdoor instructor? The way that you answer this question comes from your discourses and assumptions about the two roles. Narrative Therapy seeks to deconstruct the taken-for-granted assumptions, thereby exposing discourses and positioning. Narrative Therapy tends to ask questions in the process of deconstruction. It is not so much about gaining an answer but rather opening space for new questions and alternative ideas. The third guiding principle, therefore, for Narrative Therapy is the need to accept, search for and acknowledge that which we do not readily see, and to recognise and acknowledge assumptions as contestable assumptions rather than facts.

Narrative Adventure Therapy.

The fundamental difference of Narrative Adventure Therapy from many other approaches is in taking the non-expert position. From this position the therapist explores with the client the meanings the client is making about their experience. Together they notice and track the effect this meaning has on the client's life and on the relationships around them. When a Narrative Adventure Therapist works from the three principles discussed previously (i.e., the problem is the problem, social constructionism, deconstruction), opportunities are created for understanding the problem-saturated story, recognizing the influence of the problem story and noticing lived alternative stories. The power of the adventure approach lies in providing these lived experiences that stand in contrast to the problem-saturated story. The Narrative Adventure Therapist views the group's experience through naive inquiring eyes and joins with the group in their combined exploration of meaning.

Psychodynamic Group-based Therapy

Most of our work in Adventure Therapy occurs with groups, and therefore this section of theory will focus on principles derived from Psychodynamic Therapy that are relevant to group work. It is important to emphasise the group-based approach here because in the Psychodynamic field, there is a clear distinction between group-based approaches and one-to-one approaches (Foulkes & Anthony, 1990). For the sake of clarity, the number of principles described below have been reduced to three from the original eight identified by Ringer (2002). The three principles relating to Psychodynamic group work are: (a) *Mental representations* constitute a conscious and unconscious "truth" about the world that shapes the behaviour of both leaders and participants; (b) *The leader's experience* is a "thermometer" of the group dynamic and (c) *Avoidance of anxiety* is a core (unconscious) motivator of group behaviour.

Overall, Psychodynamic group work is based on the premise that there is a significant part of human functioning that is continually operating outside our awareness (i.e., unconscious). What occurs in this part constantly changes in response to internal and external stimuli. This unconscious functioning has unique elements for each group participant, and elements that exist at the level of the group-as-a-whole (Ashbach & Schermer, 1987).

Mental representations.

Ninety-five percent of the stimulus that affects our behaviour and personality, that is, 95% of our essential emotional, sensory and mental functioning, occurs outside our awareness (Solms & Turnbull, 2002). In other words, our conscious mind only gives us a window on 5% of what is occurring in our internal and external worlds. Hence, for Psychodynamic group practitioners, it is essential to pay attention to the cues that something may be occurring beyond the direct awareness of the group *and also outside of direct awareness of the group facilitator him/herself.*

A significant part of the unconscious material that we constantly have "running in the background" is mental "images" or representations of ourselves, of our world and of the relationship between the world and ourselves (Damasio, 2000). Note that in this context we use the word image to describe an assembly of sensory data and concepts including physical sensations, sounds, smells, feelings, and meanings. The particular mental representations or "internal working models" (Marrone, 1998) that each person has are real to that person but may differ greatly from the mental representations of others around them. (In this way Psychodynamic approaches are very constructivist). However, these mental representations form the basis of reality from which each person operates. For instance, I might believe deeply that I am an honest person with a lot of integrity and that the world is a safe place to be. Another person may perceive me as dishonest and shifty, and this person may see the world as a dangerous place to be. Events *as we experience them* can change our pervasive mental representations (or internal working models) (Bohm, 1996). Therapeutic change almost always involves changing *internal working models.*

Clarity of the leaders' functioning.

Our pre-formed mental representations have a huge influence on what we perceive to be going on at any moment in time. That is, our prior mental models determine how we place meaning on every event. Without any awareness that we do operate automatically from the basis of our existing mental representations, we tend to believe that our perception of events is objective and somehow has a truth to it that should be obvious to everybody else (Bohm, 1996). As soon as we begin to explore our own mental representations, we gain some awareness of our own idiosyncratic ways of seeing the world. Hence, clarity in the leader's own functioning is the key to effective Psychodynamic practice (Maxwell, 1996).

Effective leaders then, are fully aware of the fact that their own functioning is very strongly influenced by unconscious processes—and hence by events of which they will not be aware. To attain effective practice, Psychodynamic leaders will have spent a great deal of time working to build a deep understanding of their own functioning, their own strengths, and their own weaknesses. Conventionally, this is achieved through participating in personal psychotherapy, professional supervision, and in group work for therapy or personal development (Richards & Peel, 2001). Effective leaders develop practice at attuning to subtleties, nuances and not-so-obvious aspects of events in the groups that they run. They use their professional knowledge to guide them, and they are able to revise their opinions quickly when they get evidence that their actions and/or thinking is incorrect or unhelpful. This takes a great deal of courage and a solid belief in oneself that is based on solid experience, many successes, and equally many mistakes.

Anxiety and defenses.

There is a general human tendency and wish to avoid anxiety and this tendency is particularly apparent in groups (Bion, 1961). (It is important to note though, that fear and anxiety are not the same. Fear is related to a specific event and anxiety is more generalized). That is, we consciously and unconsciously seek to minimize the anxiety that each situation provokes. The ways in which we do this are often *defenses*. Defenses are essential strategies for human survival. Healthy defenses enable us to manage our anxiety and get on with life. When defenses do not work, we become overwhelmed, psychotic, depressed, or stop functioning well emotionally and psychologically. When defenses are overdeveloped, we become rigid, wooden, and limited in our possible behaviours (Agazarian, 1997). A part of Psychodynamic practice involves working with clients to explore the way in which they manage the anxiety in their lives—working collaboratively with them to develop strategies for managing anxiety that make room for spontaneity, aliveness, and creativity.

Psychodynamic Adventure Therapy.

The fundamental theme that differentiates Psychodynamic Adventure Therapy from many other approaches to Adventure Therapy is the notion that "all is not what it seems to be on the surface" (Anzieu, 1984; Bateman & Holmes,1995). In other words, much of human functioning occurs beyond rational and conscious awareness. Instead, much of human communication and action can be understood as symbolic and unintentional so that directly approaching everything in its obvious form means that we miss out on a huge therapeutic potential. The main caution is that the therapist needs to always be aware that he/she is working on intuition, hunches and sometimes, guesses. Hence, Psychodynamic adventure therapists need to be able to constantly re-tune their perceptions and re-think their opinions.

A Story

The following event occurred in an Eastern European country. The client is an organisation which provides medical, educational, recreational and psychotherapeutic services within a 28-day, centre-based program for youth with health problems originating from the Tchernobyl catastrophe. Following a recent decision to incorporate experiential and adventure learning into its curriculum, one of the authors was invited to facilitate a 3-day workshop with the staff.

The group consisted of 14 participants, mainly social workers in charge of the recreational/developmental part of the program. The agreement was that participants would be presented a number of experiential activities, such as games and initiative problems, which could be utilized in their work. They would then reflect upon their own experiences, be given some relevant theoretical background and finally, take first steps toward an incorporation of adventure-based learning into their curriculum.

It is important to note that the program was also characterised by the fact that all communication needed to be translated by an interpreter. The program ran quite smoothly on day one and the group had requested a series of activities with increasing challenges. Two of those activities then resulted in very contrasting group processes, which shall be described here in more detail.

Activity one presents the physically demanding challenge to step over a series of ropes which are tied in increasing height between trees. Participants are to stay in physical contact with each other, and verbal communication is only allowed while taking a time-out away from the actual site. In dealing with this challenge, the group develops a high energy level. People are volunteering to take physical risks, with others immediately offering support. The group is thus moving over increasing heights without much hesitation, yet some participants are clearly coming close to their perceived limits. However, the group apparently has established enough cohesion and trust to go all the way through. After the successful crossing of the last rope, a deep feeling of accomplishment is tangible.

After a short break and a reflection that basically allows everyone to express their feelings during the activity, the facilitator asks the group to prepare for another challenge. Every participant is asked to place two stuffed animals somewhere in the surrounding wood, knowing that all of the animals will have to be collected while participants are blindfolded. It is made clear that there will be no time limit, and no specifications are given concerning boundaries. However, the group is told that once blindfolded, within the perimeter defined by their animals, a rope circle will be placed, marking the area where blindfolds may be taken off and where everyone is to gather in the end.

Having finished his presentation and noticing that he has left his backpack with the blindfolds behind at the spot of the last activity, the facilitator leaves the group to itself for a moment. Upon his return, a significant drop in the energy level is already tangible. Participants have split into pairs, most of whom place their animals hesitantly, not far away from the gathering spot. Some discussion about how far they should go is being discouraged by one or two emerging leaders, who urge the group to concentrate their efforts on finding the rope circle. Others, however, are sitting or standing around with a "lost" expression. The group gradually seems to fall apart, unable to draw on some of the energy it has demonstrated only minutes ago, and unable to make a decision. When the facilitator finally checks in as to how everyone feels in terms of their preparation, they somewhat grudgingly agree to start searching. In less than 10 minutes, the task is achieved—all participants finding themselves in the circle with all of their animals. Despite their obvious success, a feeling of discontentment and frustration is prevailing. Further discussion finds the group rather split, as in the activity itself. While some start to discover a connection with profound experiences in their lives, such as the choice between working as an employee as opposed to self-employment, others emphasise that the group has simply been tired after the first activity, and urge to move on without giving too much importance to the experience.

Some Observations and Ideas from Different Perspectives

A Gestalt Perspective

A striking fact in the above story is the temporary absence of the facilitator. He introduces an activity, leaves to amend a technical shortcoming, and finds the mood of the group significantly changed upon his return. It is easy to see that this episode goes along with a complete lack of awareness on the part of the facilitator. There also is virtually no chance for process-oriented intervention when the facilitator is not present. This is not to say that such an intervention would have been the most appropriate choice during the period in question. However, the option to actively facilitate an experience on the edge, as well as the opportunity for the critical observations necessary to make sound judgements regarding a course of action have definitely been lost. Obviously, it is easy to blame the facilitator for this failure. Yet, when we look at all the technical responsibilities that go along with an adventure program, this incident may not be quite as unique as one would wish. It may even highlight an ongoing challenge of the adventure therapist in providing a space where one can be fully present to facilitate the scene one sets for clients.

A second observation relates to the degree to which the concept of experimenting has been understood by the group. Looking at the above levels, there is little doubt as to the group's involvement in the setting, and there also is a clear engagement in both activities. Yet, while it seems somewhat easy for the group to push its limits and thereby develop new forms of contact and support in the first activity, participants are apparently struggling to make sense of the option presented to them in the second case. The critical step, thus, seems to be from the activity to the awareness level, from completing given tasks to dealing with emerging issues. Two options need to be considered. At the outset, the group may have not spent enough time clarifying and discussing what experiential and adventure learning is all about. On the other hand, the second activity may have been too difficult in terms of experimenting with issues participants were not ready to deal with.

The last option relates to a critical aspect of process-directiveness, the power the facilitator exerts via the selection of activities. One of the differences between the two activities is that while both ask the group to make a decision concerning how far they want to go, the second one presents things more open and somewhat ambiguous. This implicitly introduces a conflict between self-organisation, in terms of open limits, and performance, according to exterior criteria in the form of the rope circle placed by the facilitator. This conflict may be particularly difficult to handle for this group, as it touches upon a culturally relevant theme in a country which finds itself struggling with the transition from a communist to a capitalist society. Once again, this raises the question of how appropriate this particular experiment has been for the group in this particular moment. In any case, the facilitator needs to be aware of some possible connections between activity structure and related issues, and he needs to be prepared to deal with strong emotions when deciding to propose tough experiments.

Beyond such analysis, from a process-directive perspective, the facilitator's next move needs to be taken into consideration. However, there are no easy answers. Certainly the connections made by some of the participants between activity and life experiences need to be valued and given space to be explored. In comparison, success or failure in terms of the criteria of the activity is of minor importance. More importantly, the ambivalence which characterises the group and the participants' interpretations of what has been going on must be acknowledged and valued. Thus, the impulse to encourage further and deeper reflection needs to be balanced with patience and with an openness regarding the insights different participants will take with them from those reflections. Finally, the position and presence of the therapist must be taken into account. Considering the fact that the facilitator has left the group alone after initiating such a difficult activity, it would seem appropriate to first have everyone come together for some kind of activity which focuses on re-establishing contact. This would serve to reconnect group members with each other, as well as reconnecting the facilitator and the group. It is a fundamental Gestalt belief that only on such a basis can any further awareness, process-directivity or experiment be developed.

A Narrative Perspective

First we need to establish what, if anything, is the problem? This question needs to be answered by the participants and it will relate to the meaning they have made of the situation. If the therapist answers it, then it comes from the therapist's assumptions and cultural discourse. It would position the therapist as the expert, one who holds expert knowledge over the problem.

For the purpose of this paper it will be assumed that one problem is the difference in the group's energy between the two activities. This problem could be named *lack of energy*. It is tempting to ascribe this problem to the group and the need for a facilitator to have an energized group. This relates to an "adventure-based" discourse on how groups "should" participate in activities. For many, this is an expected norm that is borne out of dominant discourse related to outdoor activity. Rather than ascribing it to anyone, exploring the meaning the facilitator (and group) makes of this change in energy is rich material to work with.

A Narrative Adventure Therapist would be interested in exploring with the group how *lack of energy* arrived in the activity and what effect it had on each group member. It is possible that it may have had a different effect on different members of the group so it could be interesting to know how it came to dominate the whole group rather than just some members. A Narrative Adventure Therapist may also be curious to know the history of *lack of energy* with this group and whether it has existed before, perhaps in their work with their clients or just with them as a group. Perhaps *lack of energy* has links with the nuclear catastrophe. Maybe this is when they first noticed it so powerfully, as one can only imagine the possible sense of hopelessness, when those in authority, including safety operators and the government, could not keep the people safe. Where would you turn?

Somehow this group of social workers has found the energy to work with one of the groups of people most effected by this disaster. It may have seemed overwhelming at times, perhaps even energy-sapping. If this were an accurate interpretation, then it would also be interesting to explore the alternative story of how this group of social workers found, and continue to find the *energy* to work in this area. It may be helpful to learn about the history of this energy that seems to act in contrast to *lack of energy*. Once the history is known, it can be beneficial to explore the future by asking the group to consider what *energy* and *lack of energy* might imply for the group's future. During such an exploration, the group may discover that *lack of energy* gives people a chance to recover and gather up more *energy* for a later time. Maybe *lack of energy* and *energy* actually support each other in their hope for the group to continue its positive work with the young people of the area. Some of the questions at this stage relate to the concept of positioning, with the group noting how they are being positioned by the problem. From here the group could work on positioning the problem themselves, by asking what position the group would like to give *lack of energy* in their workplace, and what resources they have to collectively put *lack of energy* in the position they select.

The narrative concepts involved in the above exploration include naming the problem, externalizing the problem, mapping the history of the problem, establishing the effects of the problem on themselves and their work, and identifying resources that they can mobilize to take control of the problem. This process is often in practice within Narrative Therapy and is only possible by viewing the problem as the problem and understanding that people make meaning, meaning is not a given. Again it is important for the group to name the problem. Then as in the example above, *lack of energy* may not be their problem at all. Regardless, the process of explorative questioning would follow a similar pattern.

Another way to view what is happening in this scenario is to draw on the work of Michel Foucault (1973) related to sovereign and discipline power. The first activity in the scenario was structured in a "traditional" way. The task was about moving from A to B with increasing difficulty, while the facilitator watched the group throughout the activity. It could be suggested that the facilitator and group members played their role as guards in the policing of societal norms (Sarup, 1993). They did what they were expected to do in the expected activity, they succeeded under the dominant cultural understanding of success for that activity. The second activity was different. It was more ambiguous, out of the norm, and then the facilitator left the group for a moment, removing a powerful player in sovereign power from the surveillance of the group. This may have given more space to "society's surveillance," or discipline power, which could have invited the group toward normalized/expected behavior, including a position call such as "adults don't play games with toys." This is often seen when groups are left alone. Discipline power can be recognised when group members say "I hope no one has a camera." The fear of the camera can relate to a fear of judgement from society. Putting on blindfolds and placing stuffed animals around a perimeter could have also offered this dilemma. Once free from the sovereign power of the facilitator, the group may have felt the discipline power more strongly. Society is constructed by our social interaction; with discipline and sovereign power ever-present we begin to understand our world from within the expectations of others. This is summed up by Payne (1997) who states, "people understand things by conforming with socially agreed representations of the world, which they accept as reality" (p. 31).

The narrative approach firstly acknowledges and then attempts to expose these socially constructed realities and opens the door to alternative representations and understandings. This way of seeing the world comes from post-modernism as discussed previously. This is also evident in the way that statements are contestable rather than given as fact. This is supported by using words such as "maybe," "possibly," "could," "explore", and "wondering." These words invite participants to think about and search for their own meaning regarding what is being questioned rather than accept taken-for-granted assumptions posed as fact.

While Narrative Therapy does not subscribe to the psychoanalytical understanding of transference, it does acknowledge that people get positioned in various stories that are known from previous experience. This is how a facilitator can be positioned by the group in terms of power and authority. In the examples above, further questions to explore could relate to how the positioning of the facilitator by the group relates to the group's understanding of people with power and authority. What meaning is made of this authority and how does it position them as social workers when working with young people? It would be especially interesting to link this to issues of power and authority at the time of the Tchernobyl disaster. Finally, to position the above example within the realm of Narrative Therapy is to structure it within a modern discourse; therefore moving away from the post-structuralism and post-modern base that underpins the Narrative Therapy approach. Hence, rather than a definitive statement, the above Narrative-based analysis of the story needs to be read as a tenuous attempt to illustrate a way of thinking that is sometimes called Narrative Therapy.

A Psychodynamic Perspective

The reader must be cautioned that Psychodynamic group work involves the constant forming of hypotheses that emerge from hunches, the critical testing of these hypotheses with constant re-formulation based in second-by-second observation of the group and one's own thinking and feelings. In the story to which we are responding here, there is no opportunity to constantly re-formulate the hypotheses and so if they are inaccurate, there is no chance to change or refine them. With that caveat, we can proceed.

Mental representations and anxiety.

The group participants were themselves leaders of groups and so their experience of the training programme would have been from the point of view of people who would need to take the skills that they had learned and apply them whilst leading their own groups. What seems significant here is that these "trainee" leaders are working with groups of traumatised and damaged participants. For the traumatised youth, the world had proven to be unsafe in completely unpredictable and meaningless ways. Leaders who work with any group (not only with homogeneous backgrounds) become involved in the unconscious mental representations of their group participants. Therefore, the trainee group leaders will have an out-of-awareness perception that the world is unsafe, unpredictable and can deal out death and destruction at any time.

At an out-of-awareness level, these leaders would probably imagine themselves to be the only protection that their traumatised participants had against the world at the present time. This is in itself potentially a traumatizing role and so the trainee leaders would have been in a vulnerable position during this training where their own group leader would be (unconsciously) expected to protect them against the dangers of the world. Overall, there could have been high levels of background anxiety experienced by the trainee leaders, none of which would have made conscious sense in the context of the training group itself.

Successfully completing the first activity involving increasingly high rope obstacles enabled participants to confirm their ability to collectively overcome danger by banding together—even to the extent of being in physical contact. This success is vital given that they need to successfully protect their own group participants from danger. Also, the rope obstacle exercise was held in a physically contained area where the boundaries were defined by the leader. Hence, the physical danger was kept inside a clearly identified area. In contrast, the second activity involving placing and finding stuffed toys not only lacked preset physical boundaries, but also began with the leader absent. The group had to provide all of its own physical boundaries. If the world is unsafe and there is nobody there to protect the group, the natural response is to keep to a small area as a means of managing anxiety. That is just what they did. Furthermore, the first activity involved physical contact but the second involved being alone in the world without any sight. This hypothesis is supported by the fact that participants paired up to place their animals, although they were not instructed to do so. Trauma with the consequent despair create a sense of aloneness in the world and so searching in an uncontained world for a cuddly toy that is lost in the forest, could easily evoke powerful feelings of aloneness and despair. Whilst none of this was voiced, a drop in energy can signal the onset of despair in a group.

The consequent problem was that the participants' way of managing their anxiety was to avoid going a long way into the forest to place their stuffed animals; that meant that the completion of the exercise did not provide feelings of success and subsequent mastery over the environment. This too led to despair, given that one of the roles of these trainee group leaders is to be omnipotent as leaders with their own participants. Often, group participants' strategy to avoid anxiety of one kind leads to them experiencing anxiety originating from another source.

The leader's experience.

The story as we have presented it is basically a description of events and of participants' reaction to those events as experienced by the leader. It does not include much of the leader's experience of himself. While this seems to be common practice for narratives presented in the context of Adventure Therapy, it does not model common Psychodynamic practice. Nonetheless, when Psychodynamic practitioners are leading groups, the task of managing the group may demand so much attention that they may not have access to much of their internal experience in each moment. Therefore, this narrative has been presented in a way that is intended to roughly approximate the immediate information that is accessible to the practitioner—particularly a practitioner who is facilitating a group alone in the midst of the activities.

An integral part of Psychodynamic practice involves the practitioner reflecting on his/her practice in the presence of another practitioner. This retrospective analysis of the practitioner's own functioning enables some of the cues that were missed at the time of running the group to be picked up and subsequently understood. This process resembles what we do here in this paper. In this way, the narrative itself provides some possible clues to the practitioner's functioning. For instance in the narrative, the facilitator notes "...things have run quite smoothly..." Is it possible that the facilitator implicitly values smoothness, "...high energy, cohesion and trust..." and "...deep feeling(s) of accomplishment" in the group? In contrast "...discontent and frustration" in the group may be seen to indicate failure on the part of the facilitator and on the part of the group. On making these observations about himself, a Psychodynamic facilitator would ask himself "what is it about this group that has me placing so much emphasis on smoothness, cohesion, trust, etc. and devaluing discontent and frustration? Could it not be possible that some of the difficult feelings will provide powerful learning?

A first hypothesis would be that the group is acting as if the purpose is to have a comfortable nurturing time so as to help recover from the trauma involved in their work. This may well be a very valuable thing to do, but it would be useful to have it voiced in the group. This might lead to a group decision to keep an overt focus in the group on their need to learn transferable skills for leading experiential activities with their own groups of traumatised youth. This does not allow a full exploration of the psychodynamics of this leader-group system. However, the overall focus of a Psychodynamic group leader in this setting would be to help the group manage their anxiety to a point where they could start to experience some of it more overtly and to talk about how to deal with the stress that is involved in their work with traumatised youth. This could then lead them to be in a more receptive place for learning skills for leading experiential groups of youth. In terms of technique, the main strength required by the Psychodynamic practitioner is the ability to be closely attuned to the group, be appropriately responsive and to maintain a clear strong connection with him/herself.

Closing Remarks

The paper began with a presentation of theoretical thoughts and concepts from the authors' preferred therapeutic backgrounds. While this clearly revealed significant differences in terms of the language we use, it also provided a basis to be used for the exploration of common assumptions and conceptual similarities. To name only a few: Gestalt and Psychodynamic Therapy clearly share a strong interest in the question of consciousness; Psychodynamic and Narrative Therapy both emphasise the necessity for humans to protect themselves against overwhelming feeling; Narrative and Gestalt Therapy invest considerable energy into the exploration of forms of power; and all three approaches highly value and encourage tolerance of ambiguity in the therapeutic process.

Not surprisingly then, our reflections concerning the presented story touch upon a number of common issues such as the crucial role of the presence of the facilitator, the difference between somewhat standard and out of the norm activities and the implications of the cultural and historic background of the participants. In a way, these issues may seem so obvious that one would recognise them from any therapeutic framework. Yet, they frequently go unrecognised. In any case, much of the literature in the field of Adventure Therapy seems to be so preoccupied with the description of standardized programs and the documentation of measurable change in the clients behaviour and/or self-concept that little space is left for an in-depth exploration of the many options from which facilitators have to choose at any moment and of the consequences such choices bring with them.

In this respect, this paper is only a beginning. Clearly, there are also significant differences between the concepts referred to, such as the emphasis on the power of unconscious processes (Psychodynamic Therapy) vs. the strong belief in the possibilities to increase awareness (Gestalt Therapy); the focus on an exploration of defenses (Psychodynamic Therapy) vs. the idea of externalization (Narrative Therapy); and the accent on individual (Gestalt Therapy) vs. social (Narrative Therapy) means to construct reality. All those differences leave plenty of interesting questions open for further exploration.

In sharing our theoretical perspectives and collaborating on this project, we have mused about the reasons that each of us is attracted to the frameworks that we have adapted. Could it be that for each of us, our choice of therapeutic framework is more driven by our values, core sense of identity, and preferred personal styles than it is to do with any so-called "objective" analysis of the merits of the multitude of approaches available to us? Would this be problematic if it were the case? Or, on the contrary, could it be a source to tap on if we intuitively gravitate to therapeutic frameworks that match our pre-existing patterns of perception and well developed interpersonal functioning? Another worthy area that was not addressed in this paper is the notion that therapeutic approaches may need to be matched both to the client group's developmental stage and presenting problems and to the values base of the umbrella or funding organisations within which the programme exists. In sum, it seems useful for practitioners to be able to identify and articulate their therapeutic approaches. However, we must be careful when we take a further step and attempt to claim the superiority of any particular approach without paying close attention to the whole context within which the therapeutic process occurs.

References

Agazarian, Y. M. (1997). *Systems-centered therapy for groups.* New York: Guilford Press.

Anderson, W.T. (1990). *Reality isn't what it used to be.* San Francisco: Harper.

Anzieu, D. (1984). *The group and the unconscious.* London: Routledge & Kegan Paul.

Ashbach, C. & Schermer, V.L. (1987). *Object relations, the self, and the group.* London: Routledge & Kegan Paul.

Bateman, A. & Holmes, J. (1995). *Introduction to psychoanalysis: Contemporary theory and practice.* London: Routledge & Kegan Paul.

Bion, W. R. (1961). *Experiences in groups.* London: Tavistock/Routledge & Kegan Paul.

Bohm, D. (1996). *On dialogue.* London: Routledge & Kegan Paul.

Culling, V. (1996). *Is the postmodernist turn to be applauded or deplored by feminism?* Unpublished paper, Wellington: Victoria University.

Damasio, A. (2000). *The feeling of what happens: Body, emotion and the making of consciousness.* London: Vintage Books.

Foster, S. & Little, M. (1989). *The roaring of the sacred river. The wilderness quest for vision and self-healing.* New York: Simon & Schuster.

Foucault, M. (1973). *The order of things: An archeology of the human condition.* New York: Vintage Books.

Foulkes, S. H. & Anthony, E. J. (1990). *Group psychotherapy: The psychoanalytic approach.* London: Karnak.

Fuhr, R. & Gremmler-Fuhr, M. (1995). *Gestalt-Ansatz. Grundkonzepte und -modelle aus neuer Perspektive* (Gestalt approach. Basic concepts and models from a new perspective). Koeln: Edition Humanistische Psychologie.

Gass, M. (Ed.) (1993). *Adventure therapy. Therapeutic applications of adventure programming.* Dubuque, IA: Kendall/Hunt Publishing Co.

Gass, M. & Gillis, L. (1995). Focusing on the 'solution' rather than the 'problem'. Empowering client change in adventure experiences. *The Journal of Experiential Education, 18*(2), 63-69.

Gilsdorf, R. (1998). Gestalt and adventure therapy. Parallels and perspectives. In C. Itin (Ed.), *Exploring the boundaries of adventure therapy.* Boulder, CO: Association for Experiential Education.

Gilsdorf, R. (2004). *Von der Erlebnispaedagogik zur Erlebnistherapie. Perspektiven erfahrungsorientierten Lernens auf der Basis systemischer und prozessdirektiver Ansaetze* (From adventure education to adventure therapy. Perspectives of experiential learning based on systemic and process-directive approaches). Koeln: Edition Humanistische Psychologie

Greenberg, L., Rice, L. & Elliot, R. (1993). *Facilitating emotional change. The moment-by-moment process.* New York: Guilford Press.

Itin, C. (1993). Linking Ericksonian methods to adventure therapy. In S. Wurdinger & M. Gass (Eds.), *Partnerships: Proceedings of the 21st International Conference for Experiential Education* (pp. 33-45). Boulder, CO: Association for Experiential Education.

Itin, C. (Ed.) (1998). *Exploring the boundaries of adventure therapy: International perspectives. Proceedings of the 1st International Adventure Therapy Conference.* Boulder, CO: Association for Experiential Education.

Kimball, R. & Bacon, S. (1993). *The wilderness challenge model.* In M. Gass (Ed.), Adventure Therapy (pp. 11-41). Dubuque, IA: Kendall/Hunt Publishing Co.

Marrone, M. (1998). *Attachment and interaction.* London, Jessica Kingsley Publishers.

Maxwell, P. (1996). Psychoanalytic psychotherapy: A blank screen? *Psychotherapy in Australia 2*(4) 42-46.

Monk, G., Winslade, J., Crocket, K. & Epston D. (eds.). (1997). *Narrative therapy in practice: The archaeology of hope.* San Francisco: Jossey-Bass.

Payne, M. (1997). *Modern social work theory* (2nd Ed.). London: MacMillan Press Ltd.

Peeters, L. (2003). From adventure to therapy. Some necessary conditions to enhance the therapeutic outcomes of adventure programming. In K. Richards (Ed.), *Therapy within adventure.* Augsburg: ZIEL

Portele, G. H. (1992). *Der Mensch ist kein Waegelchen. Gestaltpsychologie—Gestalttherapie—Seforganisation—Konstruktivismus* (Man is not a cart. Gestalt psychology—Gestalt therapy—Selforganisation—Constructivism). Koeln: Edition Humanistische Psychologie.

Rahm, D. (1979). *Gestaltberatung. Grundlagen und Praxis integrativer Beratungsarbeit* (Gestalt counseling. Basics and practice of integrative Gestalt work). Paderborn: Junfermann

Richards, K (Ed.) (2003). *Therapy within adventure. Proceedings of the 2nd International Adventure Therapy Conference.* Augsburg, ZIEL.

Richards, K., Peel, J.C.F. et al. (2001). *Adventure therapy & eating disorders: A feminist approach.* Ambleside, Brathay Hall.

Ringer, T. M. (2002). *Group action: The dynamics of groups in therapeutic, educational and corporate settings.* London, Jessica Kingsley Publishers.

Sarup, M. (1993). *An introductory guide to post-structuralism and postmodernism.* (2nd Ed.). London: Harvester Wheatsheaf.

Schein, E. (1987). *Process consultation. Lessons for managers and consultants.* Reading: Addison-Wesley.

Solms, M. & Turnbull, O. (2002). *The brain and the inner world: An introduction to the neuroscience of subjective experience.* London, Karnac Books.

Stolz, P. (2003). The unbearable lightness of being. Postmodernism and wilderness-based therapeutic intervention: Confrontation and Change. In K. Richards (Ed.), *Therapy within adventure.* Augsburg: ZIEL.

Zinker, J. (1977). *Creative process in Gestalt therapy.* New York: Vintage Books.

Authors' Biographies

Blair Gilbert is currently the National Programme and Training Manager for Project K New Zealand. He is a Narrative Therapist and was the Programme Leader, Author and Lecturer in the Bachelor of Applied Social Science, (Adventure Therapy) at Waiariki Institute of Technology, Aotearoa/New Zealand.

Contact

Blair Gilbert at:
b-gilbert@clear.net.nz

Rüdiger Gilsdorf, Ph.D., is a psychologist with training in Gestalt Therapy, working for a German institute for teacher training and counseling (IFB). He has published a number of books in the field of adventure and experiential learning, including an extensive research into the theories and concepts of different psychotherapeutic approaches and the promise they hold for a further development of adventure therapy and experiential learning.

Contact

Rüdiger Gilsdorf at:
gutenberg@online.de

T. Martin Ringer is an author, educator and presenter in the fields of experiential learning and adventure-based therapeutic approaches. He currently lives in Aotearoa/New Zealand. Martin's work is widely published and he has an extensive record of international workshops. See www.martinringer.com

Contact

Martin Ringer at:
martinringer@groupinstitute.com

Effective Wilderness Therapy: Theory-Informed Practice

Sean M. Hoyer

■■■

As the field of Wilderness Therapy has developed an identity, we as clinicians consider established theories regarding the individual, the peer group, the role of the clinician, the impact of the environment, and the process of change. The field of Wilderness Therapy must adopt a unifying theory that incorporates a view of the participant, the group, the environment, the clinician, and the interplay among them. This theory will inform our interventions and increase the efficacy of treatment. The Integrated Generalist Model (Parsons, Hernandez, & Jorgensen, 1988) suggests a possible framework from which we might develop a comprehensive view of our field, as well as the individual interventions that we employ. A unifying theory of Wilderness Therapy will describe what is occurring, reveal our operational paradigms of practice, establish a measure of change, and define a standard of intervention.

■■■

What Is the Role of Theory?

This is a discussion about theory. It is also a discussion about practice—specifically, how theory describes and informs practice and how practice exemplifies and modifies theory. Theory and practice are entwined in a reciprocal, symbiotic relationship. Theory provides a common language and framework to describe what we do and say on a regular basis. Theories are explanations for the things that we do or think over and over again that appear to work. At other times, theory clarifies and expands what we should do. A theory creates a matrix within which the clinician organizes the information offered by the participant and the participant system. Theory helps us to make sense of a situation by giving concepts a concrete description and offering a framework for our intervention with the participant.

Understanding and using theory can alter our perception of the work we do and how we intervene. In our discussion, we must recognize that theory serves the needs of the clinician, but benefits the participant. We will examine how our understanding of theory influences what we do with participants in a given situation. We will also gain an awareness of our theoretical paradigm by examining what we do in a given situation.

Developing theory is not an academic, abstract discussion unrelated to the day-to-day interventions that so may of us employ in our work with groups. It allows for a measure of change and a standard of intervention. Bunce (1998) notes, "Therapy is an intentional intervention process designed to address specific individual problems, through the application of mental health principles and practices" (p. 51). Wilderness Therapy is a meta-process of change grounded in real experiences. To reap the full benefit of the experience, we must understand what is occurring so that we can use the tool efficiently.

The Integrated Generalist Model suggests a paradigm of practice consistent with Wilderness Therapy. The wilderness expedition experience provides the context, catalyst, and tools for change. Daily events and activities provide a realistic setting within which individuals and groups can address therapeutic issues. The disequilibrium experienced by the participant due to maladaptive coping patterns creates the internal motivation to examine those attitudes, beliefs, and behaviors (Handley, 1998b). Individuals desire predictability in how the world responds to what they do. When the others do not react as the individual expects, the individual feels an internal desire to adjust or change to achieve a state of emotional comfort. The expectations of the expedition serve as practice sessions for the individual or group to progress towards change meriting positive, reinforcement for incremental pro-social change.

How does theory inform our practice?

Theories often describe participants or problems in behavioral, cognitive, affective, linguistic, relational, or spiritual terms. Other theories describe the impact of the setting upon the individual. Some describe the role of the clinician. And still others describe the process of change. Many theories describe a part or parts of a system. We as clinicians who utilize Wilderness Therapy as a treatment modality, however, are aware of the holistic nature of this style of intervention. Understanding how the individual is affected by the experience, as well as understanding the role of the clinician, the peer group, the activity, and the context in influencing change are paramount to creating effective interventions. If we identify the areas of the individual and system affected by a Wilderness Therapy experience, then we may more effectively tailor our interventions to be most effective in influencing positive change and growth.

Much has been written about the progression and processing of Experiential and Adventure Therapy. However, in the field of Wilderness Therapy, little attention has focused on how the clinician might frontload, debrief, manipulate, or otherwise facilitate the overall experience to achieve the maximum benefit for the participant group. Do we guide treatment by setting the stage for meta-process change through intentional interventions or do we merely respond to participant behaviors that are prompted by their interactions with peers, the environment, and the activity? It would appear from the paucity of writing and discussion on the subject that we as clinicians may be merely reacting to unforeseen circumstances and events and might only assist our participants by co-processing the experience with them. We might also simply manipulate the trip experience for the clinical benefit of the participant.

In contrast, effective clinical interventions within a Wilderness Therapy expedition require that the clinician understand the myriad factors influencing the presenting situation and intervene to change the underlying processes that influence participant behavior. Wilderness Therapy utilizes the tension created by the experience to address the inconsistencies or inadequacies present within the participant system and reinforce assets and competencies. Wilderness Therapy uses this internal tension as the motivator for positive change rather than external influences. Changes made by an individual through their own volition are maintained longer than those caused by outside intervention. Gillis (1998) notes, "We can only direct, guide, and clarify for our participant groups; change occurs when the participant acts." (p. 19). When an individual is ready to change, Wilderness Therapy can be a powerful intervention based on unique opportunities to provide a working context to practice and incorporate change. When the full brunt of the experience is coupled with the deft intervention of the clinician, an individual participant can engage the psychological issues supporting distress. It is in the engendering of skills—not merely coping, but also solving—that empowers participants to effect lasting, holistic, meta-level change. For example, an individual who practices improved interpersonal communication through a cooperative wilderness experience is better equipped to engage positively with her family members. Not only has she learned and practiced communication, she has adopted a belief that effective communication is the key to reducing conflict, not just a means to manage it. A youth who experiences the positive consequences of responsibility will integrate an understanding of interdependence as a key component of beneficial social interactions.

The theories regarding individual functioning, adolescent development, moral development, group development, change theory, the impact of the environment, brain physiology, and learning theory are well developed and accepted as a foundation for understanding how and why indi-

viduals and groups behave. An in-depth examination of the various theo-
ries that describe aspects present within the context of a wilderness activi-
ty or experience is beyond the scope of this paper. Several theories relate to
our discussion: Maslow (Hierarchy of Needs), Kohlberg (Moral Reasoning),
Gilligan (Ethic of Care), Erikson (Adolescent Development), Bandura
(Social Learning Theory), Miller and Rollnick (Motivational Interviewing),
Prochaska and DiClemente (Stages of Change), Yochelson and Samenow
(Delinquency), Yalom (Group Psychotherapy), Gorski (Substance Abuse
Treatment), and Ferrara (Group Counseling with Delinquent Adolescents).
Our discussion will focus on using our knowledge of how these theories
intersect, inform, and describe our practice with adolescents within a
wilderness therapy experience.

The Integrated Generalist Model

A unifying paradigm of Wilderness Therapy incorporates relevant
theories and provides structure to our interventions with clients. The field
has developed its identity consistent with a Systems orientation. Clinical
interventions involve an individual (a system in itself) interacting with
external systems (environment, activity, peers) within a context designed
to address systemic change in a parallel environment (home, school, adolescence). A suitable construct must be congruent with a systems conceptualization of the field. It must be comprehensive enough to explain the
interactions of multiple elements on multiple levels. It must be capable
enough to integrate theories regarding intrapersonal dynamics, interpersonal interactions, and systemic change. It must also be nimble enough to
allow for practical application. This framework outlines a unifying conceptualization of the process of change and details the pathways of change.
Adoption of such a construct allows a practitioner to facilitate intentional
interventions with client populations and also promotes focused development of the field.

Parsons, Hernandez, and Jorgensen (1988) provide a theory that
meets the above criteria. The Integrated Generalist Model of Social Work
views change as holistic, incorporating views of individual change as well
as systemic change. The presence of Systems Theory and a Constructivist
perspective indicate the strong influence of Social Work in this model. The
authors outlined seven components in creating their Integrated Generalist
Model of Social Work.

- The behaviors of the individual are a normal and purposeful
  response to stress given the individual and the stressor.

- Effective interventions must target the problem, not the individual.

- Problems are interactional between the individual and the environment. A "problem" is the dissonance between the individual and

the system. Either can be changed to resolve the problem.

- A clinician may intervene with a system, an individual, or the intersection of system and individual, confident that change will occur in each area.

- The clinician is an educator and mobilizer of resources including skills, motivation, and environmental supports to aid the process of change.

- The clinician's role is to promote competency and empowerment because the individual may not recognize that his or her experience can be different. This view draws upon the work of Friere (1972).

- Differential role taking, teaching problem-solving models, networking, team building, mutual aid, and self-help are the basic tasks of the clinician. It is the aim of the clinician to transfer the knowledge, skill, and motivation to perform these tasks to the participant or system.

The clinician operating within the Integrated Generalist model would recognize that while the participant may be present in the wilderness therapy intervention, he or she might not be the cause of the "problem." The clinician intervenes with the participant to effect change throughout the system. The participant is thus empowered to effect change in the family system and other social systems in which he or she participates. Recognizably, this conceptualization is consistent with current views of adolescent substance abuse treatment, delinquency intervention, and other strength-based, asset development models.

An Integrated Generalist views problems and their solutions as occurring within the individual, within a system, or between the system and individual. This perspective attends to the various aspects of the individual and provides a strength-based, asset development approach to problem solving. The conceptualization of the problem, the focus of intervention, and the context of the intervention may each be different parts of the system. This paradigm differs from models that suggest the "problem" lies with the individual (Cognitive, Behavioral, Psychoanalytic) and therefore focus the intervention on the individual. Other models suggest that the problem lies at the intersection of individuals or groups (Systems Theory). Parsons et al. (1988) offer that a clinician might intervene at any point in the system recognizing that the ensuing change will have an effect upon the problem.

We should capitalize on our understanding of the forces acting within a wilderness experience to create opportunities for our participants to address their treatment goals within these micro-experiences. Gillis and Gass (2000) propose that an "exponentially enlightened professional selects activities based on how they will interact with the participant, knowing the participant's issues. The therapist adapts the experience to meet the needs of the participant. The components are truly interactive, where each element exponentially informs one another" (p. 2). A wilderness therapist who adopts this conceptualization recognizes the options for intervention with participants. Handley (1998b) asserts that "Essential to creating wilderness experiences that provide catalysts for long term change is the ability to incorporate disequilibrium, metaphor, and the processing of the experience into a manageable, effective practice" (p. 207). As seekers of healthy, adaptive change, clinicians may intervene with one part of a system or at one level of consciousness to create change in another part of the system or level of consciousness.

Concurrent Progression

Experiential Therapy has its foundation on the premise that novel situations challenge an individual to draw upon his or her basic coping skills to compensate. The method with which individual participants attempt to get their needs met may be the source of interpersonal as well as intrapersonal conflict during the course of a wilderness therapy expedition. Internal psychological tension arises and peer conflict may ensue as participants struggle with the dissonance between their learned behaviors and the consequences of this new environment. This disequilibrium serves as the internal motivator used by a treatment program to effect long-term behavioral and attitudinal change within an individual. Wilderness Therapy is a powerful catalyst for meta-level change because natural consequences are present for discrepancies in developmental and societal expectations.

Several theorists have proposed models of development that can be used to describe change within the context of Wilderness Therapy. Stages of Group Development (Tuckman & Jenson, 1977), Hierarchy of Needs (Maslow, 1954), and Levels of Moral Development (Kohlberg, 1974) are a few classic models developed to explain change. An astute practitioner may recognize that these models provide parallel and complementary explanations for change within and among individuals on a wilderness therapy trip. As an example, the Forming Stage of group development (Tuckman & Jenson) progresses concurrently with Maslow's first level of Needs and Kohlberg's initial level of Moral Development. An individual is not able to develop a relationship with a peer unless his or her basic need for food and shelter has been met. Likewise, the threat to food, shelter, and safety present within a wilderness context often serves as the catalyst for expression of interpersonal conflict. As an individual develops competence in self-care areas, he or she becomes more aware of and able to address issues related to interpersonal conflict.

An important element of an intentional and theoretically-based wilderness therapy expedition is capitalizing on this concurrent progression. Quite simply, concurrent progression refers to several significant processes that occur during the course of a wilderness therapy expedition (see Figure 1). The individual participant progresses through various levels and stages somewhat parallel to the peer group and the progression of the course. It is in these transition periods that participants' ineffective skills become apparent as they unconsciously replicate the patterns used in their home environment.

To illustrate the concept of concurrent processes on an individual basis, an individual who lacks self-care skills and uses manipulation of her family members to meet her basic needs will encounter resistance from her peers when she uses the same tactics of manipulation to meet basic needs during the wilderness therapy trip. Referring to Figure 1, the reader notes that the individual whose moral development appears arrested at pre-moral, naively egoistic (Kohlberg—Level 1, Stage 2) would attempt to meet her basic needs of food, shelter, and safety (Maslow, 1954) through manipulation of her peers just as she would if she were at home with her parents. The interpersonal conflict that ensues, as her peers do not positively respond in a way consistent with her experience, would be an example of the Norming Stage (Tuckman & Jenson, 1977).

The Integrated Generalist Model further identifies the concurrent processes present between individual and group systems. The participant entering the Preparation Stage of Change (Prochaska & DiClemente, 1983) is at a similar point in development and behaviors to his peer group as they work through the process of Storming (Figure 1). Each experiences discomfort and may soon consider change to achieve equilibrium. This concurrent process becomes more apparent as an examination of individual interactions within a peer process (Tuckman & Jenson, 1977) reveals their stage in individual choice development (Miller & Rollnick, 1991). A peer who is motivated to change his or her own behaviors often influences the peer group's decision to progress. Likewise, the peer group that is at the Transforming Stage (Tuckman & Jenson) often "pulls" an individual along and supports the individual's Action Stage (Prochaska & DiClemente).

With regard to intervention, the clinician responds to the peer group in a way that recognizes each individual's Stage of Change and supports positive progress. Whether one utilizes the Strategies of Intervention (Prochaska & DiClemente, 1983) or follows a particular theoretical model or programming framework, it is appropriate to assist the individual and the peer group through the stages of development and group formation so that each participant may be equipped to explore individual clinical issues and support other peers in their treatment. In application, the effective wilderness therapy practitioner should encourage the peer leadership position of a youth who is demonstrating effective clinical development rather than the individual who is popular but is in the beginning stages of clinical change. The reinforcement of the positive behaviors by staff will engender a positive peer culture (Norming) as other individuals seek acceptance (Maslow—

Category	Theorist / Model	Biological/Physiological (air, food, drink, shelter, warmth, sex, sleep)	Safety (protection, security, order, law, limits, stability)	Belongingness & Love (family, affection, relationships, work group)	Esteem (achievement, status, responsibility, reputation)	Self-actualization (personal growth and fulfillment)
Stages of Psychological Development	Maslow—Hierarchy of Needs					
	Maslow—Hierarchy of Needs – 2nd Revision					Cognitive (knowledge, meaning, self-awareness) · Aesthetic (beauty, balance, form) · Self-actualization (personal growth & fulfillment) · Transcendence (helping others to self-actualize)
	Maslow—Hierarchy of Needs – 3rd Revision					Cognitive (knowledge, meaning, self-awareness) · Aesthetic (beauty, balance, form) · Self-actualization (personal growth & fulfillment)
	Kohlberg—Stages of Moral Development	Level I: Pre-conventional/Pre-moral Responds to external motivation. Obeys rules to (1) avoid punishment, or (2) gain a reward.		Level II: Conventional/Role Conformity Internalizes the standards of authority figures and obeys rules to (3) please others or (4) maintain order.		Level III: Post-conventional/Self-Accepted Moral Principles Internal motivation into making decisions by (5) integrating agreed upon rights or (6) recognizing conflicts and choosing between rights and what is best.
		Stage 1: Obedience and punishment orientation	Stage 2: Naively egoistic orientation	Stage 3: Good-boy/good-girl orientation	Stage 4: Authority and social-order-maintaining orientation	Stage 5: Contractual/legalistic orientation · Stage 6: The morality of individual principles of conscience
	Gilligan—Stages of the Ethic of Care	Individual survival "Do what is best for me".	Transition from selfishness to a sense of responsibility for others.	Self-sacrifice is good to maintain relationships.	Transition from focus on goodness to a realization that he/she is a person too.	Do not hurt others or self.
Stages of Change and Small Group Development	Prochaska & DiClemente	Pre-contemplation	Contemplation	Preparation	Action	Maintenance
	Tuckman & Jenson	Forming	Norming	Storming		Transforming
Strategies of Intervention	McKenna	Denial (External) Blames others and rejects input. Has a reason and explanation for everything.	Compliance (External) Follows rules and expectations but resists real change.	Admission (External) Outwardly admits but inwardly resists. "I won't have to change if I figure out how to beat the system".	Acceptance (Internal) Willing to change rather than resist. Stops trying to figure it out, but still is finding and getting into trouble. Utilizes treatment to make changes.	Integration (Internal) Views self as needing change. Integrates treatment changes into daily life.
	Barrett	Creating a context for change		Challenging patterns and expanding realities		Consolidation
Program Models	Outward Bound	Training		Main		Solo · Final

Figure 1. Concurrent progression.

Level 2). This further reinforces the moral development of the positive individuals and builds a self-sustaining clinical force throughout the peer group during the expedition.

Participants are dependent upon the trip staff to provide direct instruction and behavioral structure to fulfill their basic physiological and social order needs. As the individual and the peer group develop mastery in the area of physical self-care (Maslow, 1954), they begin to establish social structures and group norms. The individual and peer group cannot progress in setting norms for social behavior when they are concerned about food and shelter. Participants begin to test limits consistent with their stage of development as outlined by Kohlberg (1974). Clinicians may recognize that certain stages of conflict and group process occur once the majority of the group members have reached a plateau in their development.

Utilizing awareness of concurrent progression through the stages of individual and group change, the clinician might employ an intervention in one area or domain, recognizing that change can (and does) occur in another. The clinician can readily assess the individual's stage of development by tuning in to the pattern of behaviors representative of a particular developmental stage. For example, an individual who consistently challenges the staff regarding an estimation of mileage left to hike in the day, but refuses to learn how to read a topographic map appears "stuck" at the dependence stage. This behavior is consistent with the clinical issue she presents at home. For this participant to appropriately emancipate from her parents and proceed through normal adolescent development, she must resolve her struggle and invest in learning new skills. Wilderness therapy provides her with the context to learn to cope with uncertainty as well as the catalyst to develop internal motivation and self-efficacy. Therefore, the staff views the teaching of map and compass as supporting psychological and social development rather than merely a transfer of a wilderness skill.

As a participant progresses from a focus on compliance with group expectations (Kohlberg—Level 2) and prepares to examine his or her individual treatment issues (Prochaska & DiClemente, 1983), the clinician recognizes that the participant is shifting from an external motivation perspective to an internal motivation for change (McKenna). Gilligan (1993) and Maslow (1954) share a view of this phase as the individual focuses on the impact of behavior upon self and others. The participant struggles with views of self and the clinician responds by challenging past attitudes and behaviors and supporting examination of healthier alternatives. Referring to the earlier example of the manipulative teen, the clinician would reflect her lack of success in using manipulation to meet her needs and suggest that collaboration may also work at home with her parent.

Contributing Factors

The clinician is constantly assessing the individual as well as the peer group to determine stage of change and phase of development to construct an appropriate intervention. Stauffer (personal communication, October 2002) identifies components of experiential-based clinical services: "assessing the participant, assessing the external environmental norms, engaging with participants and establishing treatment alliances, attending to the environmental norms operating in the setting, and choosing an intervention based on these factors." Aware of the multitude of opportunities for direct and indirect intervention, the clinician is active in using the experience to assist the individual.

This paradigm of intervention is beyond the commonly referred to techniques of metaphoric framing (Gass, 1995) or isomorphic processing (Itin, 1998) of an experience. The clinician's active role and presence within the experience is a critical shift from these previous constructs in which he or she served primarily as an external facilitator. The clinician is not apart from the system impacting the participant, but instead serves multiple roles. Within this dual role as fellow participant and clinical professional, the clinician must be able to conceptualize the concurrent developmental processes occurring within each individual participant along with the group's developmental needs and recognize that an intervention that addresses one domain has an effect in several others.

Importantly, not only does change affect the entirety of the individual, but also a change in the individual affects the system of which he or she is a part. Likewise, a change in any part of the system would have an effect upon the individual. Reflecting the inappropriate behaviors and norms of the group may challenge the individual's moral view and disrupt their perceived safety, leading to regressive behaviors such as food hoarding or increased appetite (Maslow, 1954). Supporting the assertiveness of an individual in fulfilling his or her need for shelter will effect change in another participant's emotion management and still another's sense of entitlement. As each participant progresses, the peer group advances through the stages of development and is further able to support additional individual change. This view of Wilderness Therapy as a holistic approach to change is consistent with the Integrated Generalist Model outlined above.

Furthermore, Wilderness Therapy is unique in that the clinician is not removed from the participant's experience. Rather, the clinician shares and actively participates in the experience, giving direct and indirect feedback to the participant during the participant's interaction with the wilderness and peers. Therefore, an intentional intervention in Wilderness Therapy can happen at any time and can take the form of processing, facilitation (Itin, 1998), or adjusting elements of the system or environmental factors.

Sherman and Freedman (1985) identified critical factors that influenced the efficacy of interventions. Many of these factors are within the power of the clinician to alter or influence the experience of the participant.

- Expand or reduce the number of members in the therapeutic system.
- Vary the time frame for meetings or tasks.
- Change the place in which therapy meetings or tasks occur.
- Alter the activities or introduce a new one.
- Engage different levels of consciousness and thought processes.
- Structure the patterns of communication.
- Alter or reverse the place of members in the system.
- Vary the mode of interacting with the participants.

The following case serves as an applied example of the Integrated Generalist Model by utilizing the concurrent progression of complementary theories. The reader will note the opportunities to explore intrapsychic dynamics, interpersonal conflicts, and identify patterns of behavior and coping skills present on a Wilderness Therapy expedition as well as in a home life.

Case Example

An eight-day backcountry canoe trip will illustrate this concept. Six youth (4 male, 2 female), ages 15 though 17, participated as part of ongoing outpatient therapy at a community mental health agency. They attended the trip with the encouragement of their primary counselor, family member, and/or a probation officer. The three staff (2 male, 1 female) from an agency were cross-trained in Wilderness Therapy, wilderness medicine, and technical skills, and held master's degrees in counseling professions. Treatment issues included mental health (Depression, Attention Deficit Disorder with Hyperactivity, Conduct Disorder) as well as substance abuse (alcohol and/or marijuana). Additional clinical factors included Child of Alcoholic (COA), delinquency, and foster care.

Consistent with the practice of the program, each youth had individualized treatment goals and objectives for the duration of the trip that coincided with their ongoing counseling goals. These included demonstration of assertiveness, appropriate emotion management, identification of cognitive distortions that support delinquent behavior, and identification of ineffective coping skills. Ryan and Melissa (not their real names) were also wards of the State, meaning that they had been removed from their homes due to the substance use of their parent and currently lived in a state supported, temporary group foster home or private, individual foster home. Both were exploring the transition to independent living and the loss associated with not being reunited with their family due to their parent's continued inability to provide appropriate structure in the home. Our case study will focus on these two members of the group.

Ryan was on juvenile probation for retail theft and expressed resentment that he was not allowed to return to live with his alcoholic and abusive mother. Ryan frequently engaged in conflicts with peers and staff at his group home and at his school. He minimized his current alcohol and marijuana use and struggled to consistently relate truthfully with others. Ryan became defensive when the issue of his mother's drug use was raised. He frequently internalized his mother's hostility and inappropriately expressed his emotional needs.

Melissa presented as overly responsible and easily engaged in discussion of her treatment issues. She was active in her school and church, but struggled to maintain healthy connections with her foster parent or comply with household expectations. She struggled in the area of emotional self-management, assertiveness, and interdependence (appropriate reliance on others). These issues typically manifested themselves in periods where Melissa would accept too much responsibility from an adult, become emotionally overwhelmed, unable to ask for assistance, experience failure, and retreat through non-compliance or self-denigration. Melissa also became protective of her mother's drug use and was unable to express her competing feelings of affection and rejection for her mother.

Ryan and Melissa had each participated in counseling for several months before the trip. However, the progress of each had been hampered by difficulty in acknowledging the impact of a parent's substance use upon attitudes, behaviors, and current living situations. Children of substance using parents will often display this internal conflict through patterns of maladaptive behaviors in interpersonal relationships. These roles are often described as Hero, Scapegoat, Lost Child, Enabler, and Mascot in the substance abuse literature. Using the COA role identifiers, Ryan would represent an accurate example of a Scapegoat while Melissa would exemplify a Hero.

Ryan and Melissa had been unresponsive to traditional individual and group "talk" therapies. Their counselors recommended a wilderness therapy experience to catalyze their treatment process by providing opportunities for feedback regarding their errant beliefs. As stated earlier, the process that occurs within a Wilderness Therapy expedition parallels the processes present in a home life situation. Youth receive immediate, tangible feedback for their choices and are provided consistent opportunities to practice new behaviors.

Throughout the first three days of the trip, the peer group progressed through the group development stages of Forming and Norming (Tuckman & Jenson, 1977) as evidenced by challenges of group expectations and interpersonal conflicts. Ryan and Melissa frequently argued with each other and with other peers in a manner that might suggest personality conflicts (Storming). However, the expression of frustration and resentment suggested that each was struggling with internal conflicts. The trip staff hypothesized that their COA roles were being enacted and that the resulting interpersonal conflict was a projection of their intrapersonal conflict regarding their parents.

Application

In this particular example, the clinicians put Ryan and Melissa in a canoe together with one clinician in the center of the canoe. The clinician facilitated a process using the teaching of canoe skills as the context for exploring each individual's need for affirmation, structure, and feedback. The interpersonal conflict arose as each relied on the other for resolution of the immediate discomfort. This realistic situation prompted each to address the internal struggles and beliefs that had kept them stuck in their interpersonal interactions in their home situations. As a staff member was able to interject appropriate skills, Ryan and Melissa adjusted their paradigm to incorporate a concept of healthy interdependence. Each owned their own portion of responsibility for the immediate situation of being stuck in the middle of a lake as well as their role in their family situations.

Operating within the Integrated Generalist model, the Wilderness Therapy clinician might draw the following conclusions displayed in Figure 2 as part of a successful assessment and series of interventions.

Exposition

As can be seen in the above example, Wilderness Therapy provides an invaluable diagnostic feature that helps the ongoing therapist treat the underlying issues, rather than the "dressed-up" problems that the participant often presents within an office context. In the example above, the trip staff acknowledged the meta-level conflicts present and the creation of an isomorphic opportunity (Gass, 1995; Itin, 1998). They sought to create an intervention that would allow the individuals to resolve not only their present interpersonal conflict, but also address their presenting intrapersonal conflict. As Amseberger (1998) notes, "Therapy focuses the reflection on internalized norms and values with the aim to support a person to find new and more suitable structures for his or her life" (p. 29).

Parsons et al. (1988) reflect, "Individual differences and environmental stress are relatively difficult to affect. Situational factors, coping skills, self-esteem, and support systems are more likely to be amenable to change. Change in these factors affects the incidence though not necessarily the cause." (p. 418). Crisp (personal communication, April 21, 2003) suggests, "Improvement in problem-solving skills does not equate with decreased suicidal ideation or increased ability to cope with stressors. Teaching the participant coping skills will moderate the effects of stress and create resiliency."

Integrated Generalist Model concepts	Application examples
The behaviors of the individual are a normal and purposeful response to stress given the individual and the stressor.	The behaviors of Ryan and Melissa are coping skills that have served as ego defenses. The physical stress of canoeing several hours and the emotional stress of interpersonal conflict triggered a need to guard their egos. When their typical responses were met with resistance, their stress increased.
Effective interventions must target the problem, not the individual.	The problem shared by Ryan and Melissa is their maladaptive coping skill of emotional avoidance, verbal aggression, physical acting out, and resignation of personal power.
Problems are interactional between the individual and the environment. A "problem" is the dissonance between the individual and the system. Either can be changed to resolve the problem.	The problem presents as an interpersonal conflict between Ryan and Melissa. For an effective resolution, each must come to an understanding that their issue is not with the other individual, but is with finding an appropriate method of coping with internal stress. The clinician will intervene from a position of alliance with Ryan and Melissa to help them respond to the conflict appropriately and explore the issues that underlie their behaviors.
A clinician may intervene with a system, an individual, or the intersection of system and individual, confident that change will occur in each area.	By identifying several intervention options (individual processing, reallocation of canoe partners, group debrief, silence, etc.) the clinician can chose one that will meet the behavioral and clinical needs of each participant as well as the developmental needs of the group. The clinician adopting the seven Generations of Facilitation (Itin, 1998) will intervene implicitly as well as explicitly to address various levels of consciousness.
The clinician is an educator and mobilizer of resources including skills, motivation, and environmental supports to aid the process of change.	The clinician provides psychoeducation, encouragement, and structure to ensure that Ryan and Melissa can practice an alternative, intrapsychic response to conflict. By practicing the process of change, Ryan and Melissa increase the integration of the new interpersonal skill.
The clinician's role is to promote competency and empowerment because the individual may not recognize that his or her experience can be different. This view draws upon the work of Friere (1972).	Ryan and Melissa had no insight or hope. By supporting a new experience, staff supported the youth through a new paradigm. Staff assisted each in working through a conflict in real time that had implications for their home situations. Ryan and Melissa now consider that their home situations could be different because they have experienced difference, not just discussed a potential difference.
Differential role taking, teaching problem-solving models, networking, team building, mutual aid, and self-help are the basic tasks of the clinician. It is the aim of the clinician to transfer the knowledge, skill, and motivation to perform these tasks to the participant or system.	The clinician shifts to the role of canoe guide by providing the concrete paddling skill that Melissa and Ryan needed to work together, coupled with the interpersonal skill of trust and interdependence. The emotional discomfort of Melissa and Ryan provided the needed internal motivation to risk and adopt a new interpersonal skill.
Through on-going connection, the clinician reinforces the processes used by Ryan and Melissa to address their situational conflict as well as explore their on-going treatment issues.	The impact of Ryan and Melissa working together to paddle their canoe not only reinforced their positive risk-taking, but also affected the tone of the group as their peers saw the results of compromise and cooperation. Each completed the trip with an internalized sense of possibility and hope to resolve other interpersonal conflicts.

Figure 2. **Application of the Integrated Generalist Model.**

Crisp further relates that the effects of stress research indicate, "Learning to appraise the modifiability of a stressor is a critical coping skill." It is not adequate to merely introduce cognitive problem-solving skills. The participant must learn to recognize what can be changed and what must be endured. This strength-based approach is consistent with the work of Friere (1972) in that the "oppressed" often lack the insight into their own situations to identify that alternatives exist. The skilled clinician will intervene directly and indirectly, addressing behavioral change as well as the underlying cause of the stress and aid in developing the participant's appraisal skills. By utilizing the varied opportunities afforded through implementation of a matrix paradigm (see Figure 1), clinicians may intervene overtly or covertly, individually or through the group process, and impact change across the spectrum of individual experience. Participants experience change through the shifts that occur internally as well as those that the group achieves.

Conclusion

As the field of Wilderness Therapy defines itself through the development of theories to explain the process of therapeutic change, it will discover that its strength lies in the complexity of that process. The Integrated Generalist Model provides one perspective of interpreting this complexity. The adoption of an Integrated Generalist perspective emboldens the clinician to intervene with intention upon any point of the system confident of clinical impact. The skilled clinician utilizes his or her awareness of the multiple processes at work to construct and apply intentional interventions. The clinician's awareness of the multiple processes operating within a Wilderness Therapy expedition allows focused interventions, accelerates the change process, and provides participants with tangible results and long-term benefits. By understanding the concurrent processes operating within the individual, group, and expedition, the clinician may intervene at any or many levels to effect that change. The clinician no longer plays a passive role in responding to the clinical needs of the participants. Rather, the clinician is an active participant in the process of therapy, effecting lasting change in real time.

References

Amesberger, G. (1998). Theoretical considerations of therapeutic concepts in adventure therapy. In C. Itin (Ed.), *Exploring the boundaries of adventure therapy: International perspectives*. Boulder, CO: Association for Experiential Education, 201–212.

Berman, D. S. & Davis-Berman, J. L. (1994). *Wilderness Therapy: Foundations, theory, and research*. Dubuque, IA: Kendall/Hunt Publishing Co.

Bunce, J. (1988). A question of identity. In C. Itin (Ed.), *Exploring the boundaries of adventure therapy: International perspectives*. Boulder, CO: Association for Experiential Education, 46–55.

Crain, W. (1980). *Theories of Development: Concepts and Applications*. Englewood Cliffs, NJ: Prentice-Hall.

DiClemente, C. C. (1991). Motivational interviewing and the stages of change. In W.R. Miller & S. Rollnick (Eds.), *Motivational Interviewing: Preparing people to change addictive behavior*. New York: Guilford Press.

Ferrara, M. L. (1992). *Group counseling with juvenile delinquents: The limit and lead approach*. Thousand Oaks, CA: Sage Publications.

Friere, P. (1972). *Pedagogy of the oppressed*. New York: Herder & Herder.

Gass, M. A. (1995) *Book of metaphors: Volume II*, Dubuque, IA: Kendall/Hunt Publishing Co.

Gilligan, C. (1993). *In a different voice: Psychological theory and women's development*. Cambridge, MA: Harvard University Press.

Gillis, H. L. (1998). The journey in oz. In C. Itin (Ed.), *Exploring the boundaries of adventure therapy: International perspectives*. Boulder, CO: Association for Experiential Education.

Gillis, H. L. and Gass, M. A. (November 2000). *Formulas for change with participants in adventure therapy*. Presentation at the 28th Annual Association of Experiential Education International Conference, Tucson, AZ.

Handley, R. (1998a). Provoking thought—evoking meaning. Giving explanation to adventure therapy. In C. Itin (Ed.), *Exploring the boundaries of adventure therapy: International perspectives*. Boulder, CO: Association for Experiential Education, 37–45.

Handley, R. (1998b). The wilderness enhanced model for holistic strategic intervention. In C. Itin (Ed.), *Exploring the boundaries of adventure therapy: International perspectives*. Boulder, CO: Association for Experiential Education, 201–212.

Itin, C. (1998). The seventh generation in adventure therapy. In C. Itin (Ed.), *Exploring the boundaries of adventure therapy: International perspectives*. Boulder, CO: Association for Experiential Education, 201–212.

Kohlberg, L. (1974). *Moral development*. Austin, TX: Holt, Rinehart & Winston.

Luckner, J. & Nadler, R. (1997). *Processing the experience: Strategies to enhance and generalize learning. Second Edition*. Dubuque, IA: Kendall/Hunt Publishing Co.

Maslow, A. (1954). *Motivation and personality*. New York: Harper.

Miller, W. R. & Rollnick, S. (1991). *Motivational interviewing: Preparing people to change addictive behavior*. New York: Guilford Press.

Miller, W. R. (1999). Enhancing motivation for change in substance abuse treatment; Treatment Improvement Protocol—35. *U.S. Dept. of Health and Human Services: National Clearinghouse for Alcohol and Drug Information*.

Parsons, R. J., Hernandez, S. H. & Jorgensen, J. D. (1988). Integrated practice: A framework for problem solving. *Social Work*. Sept.–Oct.

Parsons, R. J., Jorgensen, J. D., & Hernandez, S. H. (1995). Integrated practice: A framework for problem solving. In J. Rothman, J. R. Erlich, & J. Tropman (Eds.), *Strategies in community intervention*, 5th ed.

Piaget, J. (1965). *The moral judgment of the child*. New York: The Free Press.

Power, F. C., Higgins, A. & Kohlberg, L. (1989). *Lawrence Kohlberg's approach to moral education*. New York: Columbia University Press.

Prochaska, J.O., & DiClemente, C.C. (1983). Stages and processes of self-change of smoking: Toward an integrative model of change. *Journal of Consulting and Clinical Psychology,* 51, 390–395.

Prochaska, J.O., DiClemente, C.C., & Norcross, J.C. (1992). In search of how people change: Applications to addictive behaviors. *American Psychologist, 47(9),* 1102–1114.

Rollnick, S., & Miller, W.R. (1995). What is motivational interviewing? *Behavioral and Cognitive Psychotherapy,* 23, 325–334.

Schoel, J., Prouty, D., & Radcliffe, P. (1998). *Islands of Healing: A guide to adventure based counseling.* Hamilton, MA: Project Adventure, Inc.

Sherman, R. & Freedman, N. (1985). *Handbook of structured techniques in marriage and family therapy.* New York: Brunner/Mazel.

Tuckman, B. & Jenson, M. (1977). Stages of small group development revisited. *Group and Organizational Studies,* 2, 419–427.

Yalom, I.D. (1995). *The theory and practice of group psychotherapy, 4th ed.* New York: Basic Books.

Yochelson, S., & Samenow, S. (1976). *The criminal personality (vols. 1-2).* New York: Jason Aronson.

Author's Biography

Sean M. Hoyer*, LCSW, CADC is Coordinator of Experiential and Wilderness Therapy Services at OMNI Youth Services in Buffalo Grove, Illinois. He regularly provides local and regional training on the implementation of experiential therapy. He also presents regionally and nationally on the application and integration of adventure, experiential, and wilderness therapy.*

Contact

Sean Hoyer at:
shoyer@omniyouth.org.

Integrating Jungian Psychology into Experiential Programming

Cheryl Willcocks

■ ■ ■

In experiential learning, participants experience situations that are then linked metaphorically to their living, learning, and working environment. The reflective component of an experiential learning program is enhanced by the use of isomorphic metaphors to connect the insights from the program to the individual's real-life. This paper explores how Jungian psychology can deepen the use of metaphors and increase the effectiveness of experiential learning programs.

Archetypes, the power of mythology, the wisdom of complexes, and the role of symbols in programming are contributions from Jungian psychology. As well, the occurrence of synchronistic events, where two seemingly random events occur in a meaningful way, can be enhanced through the combination of the two disciplines. Jungian psychology provides a perspective that enhances the internal component required for synchronicity; experiential learning provides the programming that enhances the external component required for synchronicity. Combining two disciplines of thought, theory, and method requires vigilance to maintain the integrity of both, to avoid diluting both Jungian psychology and experiential learning and to ensure that a synergistic relationship is created.

■ ■ ■

Overview of Jungian Psychology

Carl Jung was born in 1865 in Switzerland. His relationship and break-up with Freud are legendary: His contributions to the field of analytical psychology are immeasurable. Jung sought to reconcile one's relationship with oneself. Working with both the conscious and the unconscious minds, he established that our conscious experience of ourselves is a small part of a greater experience of the whole—the experience of the unconscious contained by the Self. Our conscious Self, experienced as the ego, is a drop of water in the ocean of the Self.

> If the unconscious can be recognized as a co-determining factor along with consciousness, and if we can live in such a way that conscious and unconscious demands are taken into account as far as possible, then the centre of gravity of the total personality shifts its position. It is then no longer in the ego, which is merely the centre of consciousness, but in the hypothetical point between conscious and unconscious. This new centre might be called the Self (Jung, 1929/1976, p. 45 [CW13, para. 67]).

A lack of acknowledgement by the conscious mind, and a lack of interaction between the conscious mind and the inner world of the unconscious, can result in an individual feeling disconnected and fragmented.

Jung introduced the concept of the collective unconscious as the repository for ancestral legacy. "So far as the collective unconscious contents are concerned we are dealing with archaic or—I would say—primordial types, that is with universal images that have existed since the remotest times" (Jung, 1934/1969, p. 4. [CW9, Part 1, para. 5]). These archetypal images are mythical metaphors that for Jung are the language of the soul. The unconscious communicates in images so that the conscious ego can learn from them when they appear in dreams and active imagination sessions. The shadow, for example, is an archetypal image that lurks in the background of our conscious, showing itself in our projections.

Contributions from Jungian Concepts

This paper will cover some of Jung's concepts in detail; other concepts can be accessed through his own writings and writings about Jungian psychology from other authors. There are many contributions from Jungian psychology that directly impact the process of experiential learning, starting from the initial program design through to the reflective part of the experiential learning process. The metaphorical approach to communication in all aspects of Jungian psychology provides a resource for enhancing the reflective phase of an experiential program. Archetypes bring personal meaning and associations to the experience, which increase a sense of identification with the overall learning process. Active imagination provides a tool to access collective and individual myth-making.

An identification of the shadow at work can also add to the experience of self-responsibility as issues of projection are identified and worked through. The metaphorical signposts created by synchronicity serve to weave a sense of the poetic throughout the debriefing experience. The occurrence of the tension of the opposites and the mediating transcendent function provides an opportunity for creativity and a resolution of the conflict. Watching for symbols can provide the facilitator with rich information about the group dynamic process. Symbols are something that "states or signifies something more and other than itself which eludes our present knowledge" (Jung, 1921, p. 475. [CW6, para. 817]).

These concepts from Jungian psychology provide a sense of possibility that transcends the experience by paying tribute to the imaginal and the validity of the unknown. Jungian psychology works well with experiential learning because inherent in the structure of experiential programming is a space for possibility and meaning.

Metaphors

Use of Metaphors in Outward Bound

Isomorphism: Stephen Bacon (1983) compiled the seminal work in metaphors in his book, *The Conscious Use of Metaphor* in Outward Bound. Bacon discussed metaphors that transcended the allegory or the simile. Allegory and simile approximate the experience; metaphor actually is the experience with all the nuances, affect and richness that represent both the conscious and unconscious components. The metaphor is not an exact representation but a representation that symbolizes rather than literalizes the experience. Bacon wrote: "The key factor in determining whether experiences are metaphoric is the degree of isomorphism between the metaphoric situation and the real-life situation. Isomorphic means having the same structure" (p. 4).

Bacon provides an example of a young woman and a young man belaying. This example contrasts an isomorphic with a non-isomorphic metaphor. The young woman in the example was insecure and having problems engaging with her family. She lacked confidence in her abilities and tentatively approached the responsibility of belaying and catching falls. "When this woman eventually masters belaying and succeeds at catching several falls, it is likely that the experience will profoundly move her" (Bacon, 1983, p. 5). The process of belaying addresses issues of interdependence and confidence that confront the young woman in the example.

The young man in Bacon's example is successful, chooses to spend lots of time alone and is content. Belaying and its inherent metaphors do not reflect his experience of his life and therefore belaying does not provide him with an opportunity for a change in experience.

Catching the falls would give him a mildly pleasant sense of success and interdependency. However, the metaphor "belaying" is so non-isomorphic with his life that it is unlikely it would affect him strongly. The real-life situation must be matched congruently, but a different ending—a new resolution—must also be offered. Otherwise normal behaviour is simply reinforced (Bacon, 1983, p. 5-6).

Transderivational Search

Bacon believed that metaphors allow the client to experience transformation because the client can avoid addressing the issue directly. Instead, the client can address the issue metaphorically. He explained this by a cognitive process called the transderivational search. Bacon (1983) wrote:

> The transderivational search is an outgrowth of the strategy used by human beings to interact with reality. For centuries, philosophers have argued that it is impossible for humans to encounter reality directly....Communication between people requires that the listener decode the set of symbols and behaviours offered him by the speaker in such a way that it makes sense within his own reality map. The process by which another's communication is decoded is the transderivational search (p. 6).

Jungian Approach to Metaphor

The isomorphic metaphor as a key component of the debriefing process is enhanced through the Jungian wisdom surrounding metaphors as a language of the unconscious. Isomorphic metaphors move laterally from the experiential process back to the working, living, and learning situations to which the group members belong. Once that lateral connection has been made, the group can plunge the depths of the metaphor through work with the unconscious. Metaphors are the language of the soul or psyche. It is a means of communication between the conscious and the dreams and active imaginings of the unconscious. "Metaphors are more than ways of speaking: they are ways of perceiving, feeling and existing" (Hillman, 1975, p. 156).

James Hillman (1975), founder of Imaginal Psychology, wrote that his "view of metaphor starts from Vico, who takes the metaphor to be a mini-myth, 'a fable in brief'" (p. 156). The mythic quality Hillman associated with metaphor offers a glimpse of the metaphor's expansive nature, its paradoxes and the richness of expression for both emotions and perceptions. The metaphor's quality of approximating provides texture, depth, and a sense of the numinous to everyday elements and experiences. A metaphor teases, tantalizes, and eludes. Metaphors capture the non-linear by extending beyond the reaches of a linearly entrenched linguistic structure. A metaphorical mindset suggests a curiosity and openness to possibility that allows us to discuss and share our inner experiences. Our ego personifies the metaphors and ultimately catches a glimpse of the unconscious in their nuances.

The textured and cosmological use of metaphor greatly enhances the frontloading and debriefing experiences for an experiential program. Frontloading is a facilitation technique for introducing an experiential activity. It is a strategic technique that may address a wide range of possibilities such as the metaphors that will be introduced, anticipated behaviours, unwanted behaviours and desired results. When setting up an activity, the facilitator begins to weave in the metaphors. The group then experiences the metaphor in a phenomenological way that takes them through to the debriefing. For example, the Spider Web activity, which is explored later in this chapter, can begin with a metaphor about the interconnected strands of the web and how they represent interpersonal connections. As the participants work their way through the web, the strands represent their relationships. How the participants choose to interact with the strands reflects how they choose to interact with their relationships. The care the participants take in moving through the strands can be a metaphor for the care the participants take with their relationships.

While the isomorphic metaphor is used laterally to connect an experience in the moment to an experience in the participant's everyday situation, the imaginal approach to metaphor takes it to a deeper level by engaging the unconscious. Imaginal psychology suggests that the image must speak for itself. Image in this case is not only a visual image but also an experience of the metaphor that can be kinesthetic and auditory. Following the image and allowing it to speak for itself enhances debriefing and therefore, the overall practice of experiential education. An increased emphasis on the primacy of the images and symbols that result from the experience maintains the power of the experience by engaging the unconscious component. In the example of the Spider Web activity, a myth about the spider web from a first nations tradition would bring in a mythic component that amplifies the numinosity of the images through symbolism.

The Power of the Symbol

Jung was very clear regarding his definition of the symbol, which was different from Freud's definition. The symbol, for Jung, was an experience that contains unknown information. Humbert (1988) wrote, "not all images are symbols. Nor are symbols necessarily images. A word, an idea, a gesture can function as a symbol" (p. 38). Symbols have an affective quality that alerts us to their presence. A symbol's numinosity and enigmatic quality defy an individual's ability to fully grasp its meaning.

Whether a thing is a symbol or not depends chiefly on the attitude of the observing consciousness; for instance, on whether it regards a given fact not merely as such but also as an expression for something unknown. Hence it is quite possible for a man to establish a fact which does not appear in the least symbolic to himself, but is profoundly so to another consciousness. The converse is also true (Jung, 1921, p. 475. [CW6, para. 818]).

There is an inclination to reduce these images in order to glean insight and knowledge from them. Hillman (1975) protected these symbolic images as his offspring when he wrote: "We sin against the imagination whenever we ask an image for its meaning, requiring that images be translated into concepts" (p. 39). A warning to facilitators and therapists rests in this admonishment. Interpretations of symbols are in themselves fantastical images. Conscious interpretations cannot avoid being reductionistic due to the very fact that they are created from within the limitations of the conscious mind in relation to the boundlessness of a symbol brought forth from the unconscious.

Reverse Symbolism

Experiential facilitation uses a technique called reverse symbolism. Luckner & Nadler (1997) defined reverse symbolism as "one of the skills of processing where...lived or real experiences are taken as symbols and matched or connected with personal meanings for the individual" (p. 142). In this situation, there is no interpretation or reduction of the symbol. The symbol links to the real life situation of the individual or group. This is similar to the use of isomorphic metaphors; however, instead of viewing the symbol as a metaphor for the real-life situation, the symbol is used as a source of wisdom and a provider of image and language to amplify the experience

Archetypes & Myth

Jung introduced the concept of archetypes in 1912 and then later introduced the word, not as his own concept, but rather attributed it to other writings and concepts including a reference to Plato's Ideal Forms. He continued to revisit the concept and in 1934 wrote:

The ground principles, the archetypoi, of the unconscious are indescribable because of their wealth of reference, although in themselves recognizable. The discriminating intellect naturally keeps on trying to establish their singleness of meaning and thus misses the essential point; for what we can above all establish as the one thing consistent with their nature is their manifold meaning, their almost limitless wealth of reference, which makes any unilateral formulation impossible (Jung, 1934/1969, p. 38. [CW9, Part 1, para. 80]).

For Jung the archetypes of the unconscious had an unknown quality that would ultimately have a unique interpretation as they entered an individual's consciousness. Each image, no matter how primordial, would have its own interpretation, depending on the individual. James Hillman (1975) described archetypes as the "deepest patterns of psychic functioning" (p. xix). For Hillman the archetypes have a collective quality. They transcend culture and time and offer an opportunity for each individual to have a personal connection.

> The root **arche** in Greek meant the "first," and **type** meant,
> "impress," "imprint," or "pattern." Psychological archetypes, then,
> are the pre-existing "first patterns" that form the basic blueprint for
> the major dynamic components of the human personality (Johnson,
> 1986, p. 29).

Archetypes are metaphors. They are the primordial, global images such as Mother, Father, Child, and Hero that can be found in myths, legends and in our dreams. Jung said that:

> ...there is a considerable difference between the archetype and the
> historical formula that has evolved. Especially on higher levels of eso-
> teric teaching the archetypes appear in a form that reveals quite
> unmistakably the critical and evaluating influence of conscious elab-
> oration. Their immediate manifestation, as we encounter it in dreams
> and visions, is much more individual, less understandable, and more
> naive than in myths for example. (Jung, 1934/1969, p. 5. [CW9, Part
> 1, para. 6]).

Polytheism

The polytheistic nature of Greek mythology allows for Gods and Goddesses to take on archetypal roles. Hillman (1975) believed, "Polytheistic psychology refers to the inherent dissociability of the psyche and the location of consciousness in multiple figures and centers" (p. 26). Gods and Goddesses were seen as influencers of human nature. All human experience is included within the multifaceted personalities of Mt. Olympus and their myriad relationships. The Greeks also personified concepts such as Love, Fate and Victory. Hillman wrote that these were "regard-ed as real daemons to be worshipped and propitiated and not mere fig-ments of the imagination" (p. 13). *Daemon* can be another word for *demon*. *Demon* is often associated with evil beings whereas daemon refers to an inner or attendant spirit and was the word used for supernatural beings in Ancient Greece. The word daemon originates from the Greek *daimōn*, which means deity. The use of daemon links the archetypal qualities associated with a deity directly to the individual's internal experience.

Myth as a Comprehensive Metaphor

Myths provide a mirror for psychology with its fantasies, paradoxes, personifications and use of imaginal language. "The comprehensive metaphor, answering our requirements for intellectual puzzlement and explanation through enigma by providing as-if fictions in depth, complexity, and exquisite differentiations, is myth" (Hillman, 1975, p. 153). Mythical metaphors then, are a resource for a personified experience of ourselves through symbols and archetypes.

Archetypes and Archetypal Images

For Jung, the archetypes of the unconscious had an unknown quality that would ultimately attract a unique ontological interpretation as they entered an individual's conscious. He distinguished between archetypes and archetypal images. "The archetypal representations (images and ideas) mediated to us by the unconscious should not be confused with the archetype as such" (Jung, 1946/1969, p. 213. [CW8, para. 417]). The archetypes themselves reside invisible in the unconscious. Their presence is known by the images that the unconscious chooses to put forward. These images are influenced by individual and cultural considerations, whereas the archetypes are timeless structures. Each image, no matter how primordial, would resonate uniquely with each individual. The image takes precedence and each individual must avoid the inclination to allegorically reduce the image that carries with it the wisdom of the archetype.

Archetypes in Outward Bound programs: In 1983, Bacon introduced the idea of archetypes to the field of experiential learning. He saw the presence of archetypes in an Outward Bound program as a key part of success for the clients. In his chapter on archetypes in *The Conscious Use of Metaphor in Outward Bound*, Bacon introduced the archetypes that may be encountered on an Outward Bound adventure. He described their qualities and then discussed how the images were transformative, and in some cases, how the facilitator could enhance the clients' experience of the archetype. He also referred to his understanding that there was an unconscious component involved on the part of the client when choosing an Outward Bound Program.

Hermit Archetype: One of the archetypes that Bacon (1983) described is the archetype of the Hermit. The Hermit represents the isolated journey within. Caroline Myss (2001) presented the lives of Emily Dickinson and Henry David Thoreau as manifestations of the Hermit archetype: "They are among the many others who withdrew from the mainstream of society to make contact with the beauty of life and nature" (p. 257). She expanded on Dickinson as an example, noting that Dickinson's withdrawal from the mainstream of society was not because she believed the world to be hostile but because, as a Hermit, "she chose to live in a way that supported the tranquillity of her soul" (p. 157).

The solo component of an Outward Bound adventure offers an opportunity for the individual to encounter Hermit. Solitude, fasting, and journal writing are all components that create space for Hermit. Bacon (1983) suggested that in order for the solo to be an encounter with Hermit rather than Hero, there must be clear parameters established so that the individual's solo experience is not focussed on overcoming external challenges but rather focussed on overcoming internal obstacles.

Designing an Experiential Program to Include Archetypes

The archetypes provide wisdom in both the construction of an experiential program and in the reflection and debriefing. For example, if a group is looking to increase the effectiveness of their team at work, an activity can be created that addresses the action of completion. The Sisyphus myth (described below) could become an allegorical reference point for the group to work together to move various obstacles and endure the effort. There are many experiential activities that would meet these criteria, including the activity most commonly know as Nuclear Waste. The Marble Tubes (aka Channels) activity would also suffice. For those individuals who are challenged by completion, the movement of the object can metaphorically represent something moving within them. The facilitator can ask the group what the rock or obstacle represents.

Frontloading with Archetypes

Frontloading is prefacing the activity with the metaphor as part of the strategy to create the transference from the experience to everyday situations. The Sisyphus myth can constellate a connection with the archetype in the unconscious and provide space for archetypal images to appear. How Sisyphus arrived at pushing the rock up the hill is a journey of hubris against the Gods. Sisyphus never asked for help and continued to believe that he could move the same rock as Zeus. A transformation that can occur for individuals is the power of asking for assistance. There are opportunities here for the group to work on communicating needs, relying on others in the group and recognizing the different approaches of each group member towards accomplishing the task.

Debriefing with Archetypes

Debriefing a task from an archetypal perspective would take into account an understanding of the story, the lack of resolution in the myth, and what strengths the group displayed that allowed them to shift the energy. The connection back to the workplace includes taking the language of the experience and reconnecting it to everyday life. This connection back to the workplace is the use of isomorphic metaphor. Because this is a group process, not all individuals will experience challenges with this type of activity. Not everyone in the group will have the archetype of Sisyphus wanting to break through from the unconscious to their conscious experience. Therefore, those individuals who do not struggle with Sisyphus challenges can provide the balancing wisdom that helps the group ultimately complete the task. The debrief will allow other aspects of the archetype to be explored as it relates to each participant's unique experience.

Compensation

Jung's theory of compensation describes an intrapsychic process. For Jung, psychic compensation is similar to the homeostatic function of the human physiological systems. Samuels (1986) wrote, "Compensation means balancing, adjusting, supplementing" (p. 32) between the conscious and the unconscious. It is a type of bridge, where the unconscious takes the repressed material from the conscious and returns it to consciousness in the form of a symbol. Within the scope of the activity for a group, compensation could appear as a kinesthetic experience where a stronger person helps leverage the object the group is moving. It could also be an emotional compensation, whereby one individual compensates for the frustrations of another. Working with the idea of compensation, the facilitator can then set up experiential situations that emphasize the compensatory factors as a way to shift any one-sidedness that may exist within a group dynamic situation.

Hermes in the Group

Groups are made up of individuals. Archetypes can provide an understanding of the group dynamic on an unconscious level. For example, the presence of Hermes in the group dynamic provides insight as to how Hermes-energy affects the communication of the group. Hermes is the disruptive, playful trickster who is either shunned for the sporadic nature of his interactions or who is valued for his willingness to question and bring to the surface what is not said but is on everyone's mind—the proverbial elephant in the living room. Hermes is an alchemist, a mercurial figure that can represent a transition between states of being. "Hermes, the luck-bringing messenger of the immortals...a son of many shifts, blandly cunning, a robber, a cattle driver, a burglar of dreams, a watcher by night, a thief at the gates, one who was soon to show forth wonderful deeds among deathless gods" (from the Homeric Hymn to Hermes, www.ancienthistory. about.com/library/bl/bl_text_homerhymn_Hermes.htm). The Hermes in the group may help move the group from one position to the next. It is the facilitator's role to look for the Hermetic images and symbols to incorporate them into the program and facilitation strategy.

Relationships between Archetypes

The archetypes can also point to how different types of people within the group may work together. Two members of the same team may manifest different archetypal energies. Jean Shinoda Bolen (1984) wrote extensively on how the archetypes may occur in different situations. If Artemis and Demeter were colleagues, what would be some characteristics of their working relationship? Artemis brings to the workplace a comfort with conflict, challenge and opposition. An Artemis female will work tirelessly alongside others in the interest of a cause. "The Artemis woman puts effort into work that is of subjective value to her" (Bolen, 1984, p. 58). Demeter, conversely, puts effort into taking care of people in the workplace. A Demeter woman in a position of power in the organization would be likely to nurture it to success through her "maternal energy" (p. 180). Artemis on this team may take advantage of Demeter's nurturing and caring attitude. Demeter would have a difficult time addressing the oppositional energy of Artemis. Demeter may also be challenged by Artemis and try to limit and control her interests as she may think that Artemis' pursuits are not in Artemis' best interests. Beyond the challenges, these two would provide a glimpse into aspects of personality typology to sense how an introvert (Artemis) works as compared to an extrovert (Demeter). The two archetypes would be excellent at managing together if there was an acceptance of their differences and an acknowledgement of the power of the other's strengths. Demeter would be responsible for the nurturing part of the management team and Artemis would be responsible for moving the vision forward and challenging any obstacles.

Observing participants as archetypes in a group is another way of looking at a range of personality types and the ways in which different individuals may approach a group situation or task. Different combinations of archetypes in a working team can allegorically represent different types of councils that may sit on Mt. Olympus. The multiplicity of the human psyche that is represented by the Greek Gods and Goddesses provides a balance that would benefit a group situation. An organization that lacks an individual with Zeus energy may be challenged to move forward in difficult times. The lack of the detailed, focussed Athena (whether in a man or a woman) would suggest challenges with quality and efficiency within an organization. A rich learning opportunity is found in programs that speak to these different Gods and Goddesses to allow participants to experience their qualities within the context of the power provided by the myth.

Shadow

Jung identified three archetypes as having "the most frequent and the most disturbing influence on the ego" (Jung, 1951/1969c, p. 8 [CW9, Part 2, para. 13]). One of these is the Shadow that lurks in the dark recesses of the mind. The Shadow is the part of us that no one wants to know, the part of us that people project onto others until they are ready to fully integrate it into their experience of themselves. When emotions are stirred and an individual responds to a situation with an unnecessarily high degree of affect, then that person may be in the presence of Shadow. Knowing this and acknowledging Shadow's presence can help move conflict within the group's experiential process to a new level.

Any activity that requires planning and collaboration in a situation that has some intensity of time or competition creates fertile ground for the addition of Shadow into an experiential program. An invitation to Shadow into the process allows the opportunity to work with projections. During a team-building program conducted by the author, a participant made the following statement to one of the facilitators, "I realized that when she (another participant) irritates me, it isn't really about her at all, it is something about me that I need to work out." Shadow was named and the individual was able to recognize in herself something that she had previously only been able to see in another.

The facilitator worked with this client on naming the shadow in order to create a conscious image. The creation of a conscious image reduces the chance of the image slipping back into unconscious depths to wait for another opportunity to be projected elsewhere. Projection is defined as one part of the personality transferred onto another individual or external situation. This is a common aspect of relationships and only becomes destructive when the personality becomes impoverished as the individual attempts to control their inner reality by attributing elsewhere their aspects of themselves that they consider unmanageable.

Complexes

Complexes and Free Association

"A complex consists of a cluster of emotionally charged representations" (Humbert, 1988, p. 3). Issues that are traumatic, repressed, or that one is unable to make conscious, eventually form into complexes. These complexes constellate in conscious patterns of behaviour that seem uncontrollable. Jung's work with free association involved providing individual words to which clients would quickly respond with a corresponding word. For example, Jung would say "train" and then the person may respond with 'track.' What he discovered is that when the word relates to a complex, the response time is considerably slower. He measured other physiological changes and determined that the whole body is affected, not just the structures in the brain.

The Role of Archetypes in a Complex

At the core of a complex is an archetypal structure. When this structure is understood, a relationship can begin with the complex and allow it to be made conscious, thereby reducing the degree of affect surrounding the situation. Contained within the complex is the wisdom of the archetypes. This is the main premise upon which archetypal psychology (also called imaginal psychology) was founded. Hillman (1975) wrote: "Archetypal psychology can put its idea of psychopathology into a series of nutshells, one inside the other: within the affliction is a complex, within the complex an archetype, which in turn refers to a God" (p. 104). The complexes bring with them a full experience of the soul. In the grips of the unconscious pathology, as an individual acts out patterns of behaviour that seem beyond our control, one can see the Gods and Goddesses of mankind pointing towards the greater whole.

Complexes in a Group Situation

"Complexes...operate not only as sets of inner tendencies and drives but also as expectations, hopes and fears concerning the outward behaviour of people and objects" (Whitmont, 1969, p. 69). The outward behaviour can impact the group dynamic. Myth-making allows the group to address the archetypes through an imaginal process that invites images and symbols to come forth as representatives of a potential group complex. Understanding the archetypal structure of the myth, which has evolved in a group, begins to make what has been hidden, tolerable to the group. This allows the group complex to begin to shift.

In an experiential program, the phenomenology of a group complex can be observed when repeated patterns of group behaviour arise and continuously affect the outcome of the interaction. The group complex can also be observed through expectations that the participants have of themselves and others. Humbert (1988) wrote: "Upon closer examination, one discovers within the complexes a core element that serves as a vehicle for meaning and that functions independently of conscious will" (p. 3). Complexes typically represent repressed information, trauma or the inability to bring unconscious information into the conscious realm. Groups can have a traumatic experience that carries with it qualities that transcend the sum of the responses of the individual. This experience could be called traumatic synergy. The repression of the group trauma can result in a group complex.

Recognizing the presence of the Gods in a group complex brings back the role of metaphor in accessing the experience of soul. The inclination is to avoid, destroy or befriend the complex. These strategies represent the futile attempt on the part of the ego to remain in control. The wisdom is found in kneeling before the complex to honour the presence of soul: for in the complex of the group may be where the experience of soul is located.

Synchronicity

Jung defined synchronicity as "the simultaneous occurrence of a certain psychic state with one or more external events which appear as meaningful parallels to the momentary subjective state" (Jung, 1952/1969, p. 441 [CW8, para. 850]). He also wrote: "Synchronistic events rest on the simultaneous occurrence of two different psychic states" (Jung, 1952/1969, p. 444-445 [CW8, para. 855]). For Jung, causality is not a factor with the synchronistic events, hence the term *synchronistic* instead of *synchronous*.

Synchronicity is often compared to coincidence. Events that happen in the unconscious are experienced similarly by the conscious. Edinger (1972) wrote: "Such experiences are most likely to occur when the archetypal level of the psyche has been activated and they have a numinous impact on the experiencer" (p. 292). Jung believed that perhaps synchronistic events happen when consciousness is low. This lower level of consciousness may represent a weakening of a barrier constructed by the ego, which then allows an integration of some unconscious images. Synchronistic events are significant as they may provide access to the unconscious that may have been denied until that point. Providing an experiential learning activity that allows for a lower level of consciousness and stimulates the production of images from the unconscious is the aim to induce experiences of synchronicity. The concept of play is present in many experiential activities and contributes to lowering the level of consciousness as the participants, through play, become less defended. The experience of synchronicity is powerful and has a numinosity that is transformational during an individual or group process.

Tension of the Opposites

The Transcendent Function

For Jung, reconciling opposing forces between conscious and unconscious life was the primary function of individuation. Opposites for Jung are paradoxical—it is more than conflict. The opposites represent opposing forces that occur when one accesses the unconscious and then responds to it from the conscious. Reconciliation happens by holding tension between the opposing forces. The transcendent function is an organizing principle developed by Jung to represent the tension of opposing forces. Jung wrote,

> The process of coming to terms with the unconscious is a true labour, a work which involves both action and suffering. It has been named the transcendent function because it represents a function on real and imaginary or rational and irrational data, thus bridging the yawning gulf between conscious and unconscious (Jung, 1917/1966, p. 80 [CW7, para. 121]).

The transcendent function links the conscious and unconscious as part of the ongoing process of individuation where the transcendent function "arises from the union of conscious and unconscious contents" (Jung, 1957/1969, p. 69. [CW8, para. 131]). The conscious is the repository for what is known; the unconscious contains all the rest. The conscious and unconscious contents tend to be experienced as opposites and the transcendent function is the synthesis between these oppositional entities. Jung saw the transcendent function as a symbol. Symbol for Jung was defined separately from image, metaphor and archetype. Humbert (1988) described the symbol as *Darstellung*, which means representation as activity. He further described the symbol as something with an unknown quality that "comes about as a result of a state of conflict or disorientation" (p. 37).

Working with Tension of the Opposites and Symbols in Experiential Programs

The symbol carries with it a psychic impact that identifies it as a symbol. The ramifications on creativity are significant for an experiential program when introducing this concept of the tension of the opposites and the symbolic relationship of the transcendent function. They are significant because the idea of the tension of opposites arises from Heraclitus and his theory of thesis, antithesis and synthesis. His triad is a template for creativity. Groups that participate in an experiential program often identify creativity as one of their primary objectives.

Although Jung's concept of opposing forces does not represent the general notion of conflict, there may be situations for the facilitator where an understanding of larger forces may benefit the group process. There are many experiential activities that are performed with ropes, holding hands, or done in a way that uses tension. A well-facilitated debrief, which may include a symbol, can increase the group's awareness of the tension that is present and can provide an opportunity for a transformational experience.

Observing the group for symbols requires some vigilance and an imaginal perspective on the part of the facilitator. For corporate groups, the corporate logo is an especially powerful symbol. There are often slogans that are part of the company's vision statement that can be incorporated and deconstructed to find their symbolic meaning to the group. The group itself may provide symbols. Symbols are not necessarily images and images are not necessarily symbols. A symbol can be a gesture, a word, or a mode of interaction that carries with it the numinous quality that unmistakably links an unconscious and a conscious experience.

Successful Integration

Jungian psychology and experiential learning, when combined, present an opportunity for facilitators to provide multi-faceted experiences that engage participants on both a conscious and unconscious level. Dual emphasis on the situational and the transpersonal provides an opportunity for transformation on multiple levels. Successful integration of these two methods results from both their shared epistemology and their commitment to metaphor. One of the metaphors that they share is the relationship that both Jungian psychology and experiential learning have with Nature. This relationship also increases the ease of integration of the concepts and warrants further exploration. Avoiding dilution is the primary hurdle for experiential practitioners, whether the programs are integrating Jungian concepts or including interventions from some other school of psychological thought or therapy, (e.g., family systems theory or solution-focussed therapy). Clearly defined program objectives, based on the type of client and their needs, ensure that the newly-introduced concepts can be strategically positioned to maximize effectiveness. An indicator of a strong field of study is its ability to integrate other concepts without being overshadowed. The depth of Jungian Psychology contributes to the strategic integrity of Experiential Learning, and the integration of Jungian concepts highlights the strength of Experiential Learning as an educational and therapeutic discipline.

References

Bacon, S. (1983). *The conscious use of metaphor in Outward Bound.* Denver, CO: Colorado Outward Bound School.

Bolen, J. S. (1984). *Goddesses in every woman: A new psychology of women.* New York: Harper Perennial.

Edinger, E. F. (1972). *Ego and archetype: Individuation and the religious function of the psyche.* Boston: Shambhala.

Hillman, J. (1975*). Revisioning psychology.* New York: Harper Perennial.

Humbert, E. (1988). *C.G. Jung: The fundamentals of theory and practice (4th printing).* Wilmette, IL: Chiron.

Johnson, R. A. (1986). *Inner work: Using dreams & active imagination for personal growth.* San Francisco: Harper.

Jung, C. G. (1921). Definitions. In R. F. C. Hull, (Trans.), *The collected works of C. G. Jung (Vol. 6) [2nd printing].* Princeton, NJ: Princeton University Press.

Jung, C. G. (1966). On the psychology of the unconscious. In R. F. C. Hull, *(Trans.), The collected works of C. G. Jung (Vol. 7) [2nd ed., 4th printing].* Princeton, NJ: Princeton University Press. (Original work published in 1917).

Jung, C. G. (1969). On the nature of the psyche. In R. F. C. Hull, (Trans.), *The collected works of C. G. Jung (Vol. 8) [2nd ed., 3rd printing].* Princeton, NJ: Princeton University Press. (Original work published in 1946).

Jung, C. G. (1969). Synchronicity: An acausal connecting principle. In R. F. C. Hull, (Trans.),*The collected works of C. G. Jung (Vol. 8) [2nd ed., 3rd printing].* Princeton, NJ: Princeton University Press. (Original work published in 1952).

Jung, C. G. (1969). The transcendent function. In R. F. C. Hull, (Trans.), *The collected works of C. G. Jung (Vol. 8) [2nd ed., 3rd printing].* Princeton, NJ: Princeton University Press. (Original work written in 1916, published in 1957).

Jung, C. G. (1969). Archetypes of the collective unconscious. In R. F. C. Hull, (Trans.), *The collected works of C. G. Jung (Vol. 9, Part 1) [2nd ed., 10th printing].* Princeton, NJ: Princeton University Press. (Original work published in 1934).

Jung, C. G. (1969c). The Shadow. In R. F. C. Hull, (Trans.), *The collected works of C. G. Jung (Vol. 9, Part 2) [2nd ed., 5th printing].* Princeton, NJ: Princeton University Press. (Original work published in 1951).

Jung, C. G. (1976). Commentary on the secret of the golden flower. In R. F. C. Hull, (Trans.), *The collected works of C. G. Jung (Vol. 13) [3rd printing].* Princeton, NJ: Princeton University Press. (Original work published in 1929).

Luckner, J. L. & Nadler, R. S. (1997). *Processing the experience: Strategies to enhance and generalize learning (2nd ed.).* Dubuque, IA: Kendall/Hunt Publishing Co.

Myss, C. (2001). *Sacred contracts: Awakening your divine potential.* New York: Harmony Books.

Samuels, A., Shorter, B. & Plaut, F. (1986). *A critical dictionary of Jungian analysis* (reprinted 1993). New York: Rutledge.

Whitmont, E. D. (1969). *The symbolic quest: Basic concepts of analytical psychology.* Princeton, NJ: Princeton University Press.

Author's Biography

Cheryl Willcocks has a master's degree in Jungian Psychology and is one of the directors of Pinnacle Pursuits based in Vancouver, British Columbia, Canada. Pinnacle Pursuits was founded by her husband, Jonathan Willcocks in 1997 and is an experiential learning company that designs and delivers customized, objective-based programs for youth and corporations. Her particular interest is in program design and the development of metaphor as key to the transference of learning for clients. Cheryl is actively involved in the Association for Experiential Education. At the time of publication she had convened the 2003 Annual Conference in Vancouver and was a member of the AEE Conference Advisory Committee.

Correspondence

Cheryl Willcocks
Pinnacle Pursuits Inc.
#200-275 East 8th Avenue
Vancouver, B.C. Canada V5T 1R9
Tel. (604) 876-7535
Fax. (604) 876-0535
Toll-Free in North America. (800) 876-7535
Website. www.PinnaclePursuits.com
E-mail. Cheryl@PinnaclePursuits.com

Making Meaning of Adventures: Narrative Methods in Adventure Therapy

Jordie E. Allen-Newman and Reg R. Fleming

■ ■ ■

Applying narrative methods to the context of adventure therapy can strongly orient clients and therapists to the construction of stories, both in terms of the client's everyday living and within the context of the adventure-based experience. Through the use of the narrative metaphor, clients may be more able to make sense of their experiences, capabilities, and capacities for lasting change. The essential elements of narrative therapy are explored and various applications to adventure therapy are discussed. The integration of narrative and adventure therapy is put forth as an effort to enhance therapeutic effectiveness in adventure therapy contexts.

■ ■ ■

The following analysis explores the application of narrative methods in the context of conducting adventure therapy. A variety of narrative techniques are discussed and seated within areas of potential use for adventure therapists. Adventure therapy is defined and some expressions of adventure therapy are explored: adventure-based challenges, wilderness therapy, and initiative activities. The paper continues with a brief review of the working assumptions of narrative methods. Change is explored in the context of what it might mean to engage in a narrative process in conjunction with adventure therapy. Finally, the central elements of adventure therapy and narrative methods are examined in terms of combining the central ideas and techniques from both healing modalities.

Adventure Therapy

Adventure therapists offer fresh and exciting possibilities for change in the lives of clients: improved self-esteem, change in personal identity, development of maturity, improved communication skills, and progress in personal challenges like substance abuse, disability, and illness (Russell, 2001a; Gass 1993a; Luckner & Nadler, 1997). Extensive debate exists as to the definition of adventure therapy, and agreement on a standard set of therapeutic methods continues to be in development. It is beyond the scope of this paper to explore the nuances of the theory of adventure therapy; however, in order to provide a platform for the integration of narrative therapy techniques, a specific definition of adventure therapy is offered. Also a description of some of the expressions or tools of adventure therapy is provided.

Alvarez and Stauffer (2001) state that: "...adventure therapy is any intentional, facilitated use of adventure tools and techniques to guide personal change toward desired therapeutic goals" (p.87). This definition is based on the following theoretical assumptions: (a) the therapy is intentional and experiential, (b) it involves the facilitated use of adventure therapy tools, (c) the facilitation process guides personal change for clients, and (d) the change is in line with desired therapeutic goals (Alvarez & Stauffer). Adventure therapy programming has expanded to serve people with techniques that are grounded in adventure-based challenges, wilderness exploration, and initiative activities or games (Gass, 1993b).

Adventure therapy is based on the philosophy of experiential learning. Experiential learning processes are defined as learning through doing with a therapeutic intent (Luckner & Nadler, 1997; Gass, 1993b; Bunce, 1998). Experiential learning involves the idea that when people are in a situation that is somewhat outside of their comfort zone, they experience states of dissonance and make efforts to adapt in order to reach equilibrium (Gass, 1993b). The main goals of the techniques of experiential processing are: to support the learner to become a participant in the learning process; to utilize meaningful activities that generate natural consequences; to create opportunities for reflection; to create situations for choice and challenge; and to define current and future relevant change for a person (Gass, 1993b). The techniques of experiential processing may be used in a variety of settings beyond adventure-based and wilderness contexts, including traditional psychotherapy settings, classrooms, and worksites.

What follows is a discussion of some forms of adventure therapy prevalent in the literature. It must be noted that these forms often over-lap — for instance, adventure-based challenges are often used on wilderness trips or may have initiative exercises incorporated. Processing techniques common across adventure therapy will also be discussed.

Adventure-based Challenges

One form of adventure therapy is the use of adventure-based challenges. Adventure-based challenges use adapted natural or contrived physical structures as a basis for a therapeutic intervention (Gass, 1993b). Adventure-based activities can occur in both urban or wilderness contexts, but the key is the focus on a specific physical, psychological and social challenge using some type of adventure challenge (e.g., a high or low ropes course, indoor or outdoor climbing, skiing or snowboarding, canoeing, etc.). What sets adventure-based challenges apart from wilderness trips or initiative activities is the focus on short-term, intensive physical and psychologically demanding activities that create opportunities for interpersonal and intrapersonal growth (Luckner & Nadler, 1997).

Wilderness Therapy

A second expression of adventure therapy occurs in the wilderness. Wilderness therapy typically occurs in a natural setting that is isolated or distant from modern services and settlements. The significance of isolation is that it can create varying degrees of physical, psychological, and spiritual intensity, as well as connection with nature. The difference from other expressions of adventure therapy is that the intensity of the wilderness experience is used to explore personal or social challenges and transformation as opposed to an emphasis on a leader-constructed initiative activity (e.g., the human knot), or an adventure-based activity (e.g., indoor climbing).

Wilderness therapy utilizes adventure pursuits in nature to enhance personal and interpersonal development (Kimball & Bacon, 1993). According to Todesco (2003) a nurturing experience is created in the relationships that surface between practitioners, nature, and clients. Wilderness exploration attempts to provide psychological healing to participants—based on individual and group processes—through the use of story telling, initiative activities, adventure-based strategies, and reflective learning (Gass, 1993b; Todesco, 2003; Russell, 2001b). The reader is referred to Russell (in this publication) for a more in depth discussion regarding the elements of wilderness therapy.

Initiative Activities

A third form of adventure therapy occurs in the use of initiative activities or games that focus on the promotion of fun and interaction with a therapeutic intent. Problem solving, communication and trust are common goals of initiative-based interventions. The use of initiatives does not rely on a contrived structure like a rock climbing gym or high ropes course, nor a natural setting like that found in the wilderness. Instead, initiative activities emphasize the facilitation skills of the adventure therapy leader, a contrived, process-based activity, and group interaction or reflection. Initiative activities are most effective when they are linked with a clients' everyday experiences (e.g., an obstacle course based on symbolic objects should reflect back to the client's experience of a problem like substance misuse), and promote a resolution of their everyday problems (e.g., a shift toward cooperation and healthy risk taking through the use of trust falls).

Processing Activities

A variety of innovative processing techniques have emerged that are common across the various expressions of adventure therapy outlined above including: reflective learning, front-loading, debriefing, exploring isomorphic connections, and group process witnessing or observing. For a complete discussion of these techniques, the reader is referred to Gass (1993d) and Gass, Gillis and Priest (2000). Briefly, reflective learning is a broad process of looking back at an experience to extract lessons with a focus on applying these to the client's future experience (Gass, 2000). This builds upon theories of experiential learning (Warren, Sakofs, & Hunt, 1997). Frontloading involves the use of activity or language that flows into a challenge or experience; it is thought of as a staging process that prepares clients for an activity and can result in enhanced learning by providing learning markers and frames of reference. Debriefing is a common facilitation technique that involves exploring client experience directly after an activity (Gass et al., 2000). The creation of isomorphic connections is a process of making parallels between areas of resiliency, problems or possible change in the clients' everyday lives and their experience in an adventure activity. This is often accomplished with the use of metaphor and reflection of meaning. Finally, witnessing involves drawing on the group as an audience for acknowledging and heightening change. The technique uses the group as a support to solidify an area of change (e.g., the group being a witness to a client's success in leading them to a solution in a low ropes course).

In summary, adventure therapy as an intentional, facilitated use of adventure tools and techniques promotes the following practices: trusting the learner to make sense of his or her experience, intentionally facilitating a process that aims to create change and supporting the client in exploring his or her perceptions of their experience. The discovery and transfer of preferred ways of being into the client's everyday life is a central task of all expressions of adventure therapy (i.e., adventure-based challenges, wilderness therapy, or initiative activities). Overall, adventure therapy leans towards a practice of healing that favors the client's meaningful construction of experience. This leads to a discussion of narrative therapy.

The Essential Elements of Narrative Therapy

Overall, narrative therapy is based on the theory of social constructivism, which states that what is real evolves out of social interactions and agreements about what is fact, as opposed to an objective, unchanging and fixed reality (Cottone, 2001). It is beyond the scope of the paper to fully explain the practice and theoretical foundation of narrative therapy. In general, social constructivism is embraced by narrative therapists who understand that the way people make sense of their experience is through the contextually-shifting influence of culture, meaning-making attributed to events through language, and social interaction that fosters paradigm development. The construction of stories that place people in positions of empowerment and continued growth in desired directions is the preferred outcome of narrative methods.

A number of elements or assumptions have emerged over the past 25 years in the field of narrative therapy including: (a) the idea that narrative therapy is a social process that is best accomplished as a collaborative effort between therapist and client, (b) that clients are viewed as experts in their own right regarding their lives, (c) that the focus of helping ought to be on the construction of meaningful stories that serve the client in their process of change, and (d) the client experiences the desired change once a story of personal agency or empowerment is discovered and supported.

A narrative perspective assumes that the client and the professional helper can be thought of as co-writers, crafting a meaningful change in the client's life story. Practitioners of narrative therapy highlight the importance of the client-therapist relationship, and assumptions held regarding change come from a post-modern perspective. Similar to the process of co-writing a story, the development of a therapeutic relationship within a narrative framework involves the attention to the creation and maintenance of a collaborative partnership. Important aspects of creating a co-working relationship are the assumptions, attitudes, and positioning of the therapist in the relationship with the client. In addition, several writers in the field of narrative psychotherapy have emphasized the importance of developing a therapeutic attitude that reflects a position of being curious, as opposed to problem focused (Duncan & Miller, 2000; Rowan & O'Hanlon, 1999; Monk, Winslade, Crocket, & Epston, 1997).

Gerald Monk has aptly discussed the positioning of the therapist as a positive and reflective collaborator in relation to a client. He states the following:

> Narrative therapy requires an optimistic orientation. The main character in this plot is frequently positioned in the therapeutic conversation as the courageous victor rather than the pathologized victim, as a colorful individual who has vivid stories to recount rather than a hopeless individual leading a pathetic life. The stories will not only change the teller in the telling but will also change the counselor as a privileged audience of the tale (Monk et al., 1997, p.4).

Underlying the need to be curious is the positioning of the therapist as a person who is fundamentally intrigued and genuinely interested in exploring the client's perspective about their experience, their sense of a problem, or what they have done to improve their lives. The conversation that occurs with the client—because it is based on the client's content—becomes a reworking of his or her dominant beliefs that impede change. Re-storying within the collaborative atmosphere is assumed to be more probable when the client feels empowered, acknowledged, and supported. For example, a therapist might work with a client struggling with depression to highlight what ways they have stood up to depression. The client's answer may provide the unique outcomes or exceptions to the dominating effects of the depression. Furthermore, the conversational story is influenced in the direction of the client being in a more powerful position in relation to depression, which is treated as a problem that can be influenced by the actions taken by the client.

A second element identified in narrative methods applies to the assumptions regarding power, knowledge, and therapeutic change. Specifically, the client is seen and respected as an expert about his or her past, current and future storied experiences. A core element of this idea is that people have the resources and capacities within them and through their relationships to alter their life circumstances and to solve problems (Monk et al., 1997). Furthermore, it has been argued that change is more likely to happen when it is the client's ideas that are worked with, as opposed to those ideas held by the therapist (Duncan & Miller, 2000). This is not to say that therapists using narrative methods cannot assist in the process of change by offering their insights or ideas, but change is more likely to occur when we get behind the client's own perception of his or her experience and assist with a narrative process of writing, rewriting, or editing stories.

In the context of doing therapy within a narrative framework, the ideas of the therapist are less about the diagnosis or assessment and more about facilitating the rewriting of debilitating life-defining stories. In other words, therapists contribute to change by paying attention to the process of meaning-making by the client, assisting the client to question "taken-for-granted" notions or practices of disempowerment, and providing acknowledgement for positive gains within their stories of change. Many narrative therapists argue that when offering an insight, it is better to take a tentative posture—offering insights within a descriptive context rather than prescriptive ideas from an authoritative position (Freedman & Combs, 1996; Monk et al., 1997; White & Epston, 1990). From a narrative perspective, the therapist's position is transparent, and therefore is thought less likely to be understood by the client as mysteriously authoritative. A therapist being transparent may, for example, explain his or her prior experience with a similar struggle, and wonder aloud whether the client has had a similar experience. By providing more information about the therapist's comments or tasks, the client is put into a position of greater understanding and freedom to accept or reject the therapist's input.

A third important element of narrative therapy is the need to identify and emphasize the specific stories that are more likely to assist the client in the process of therapeutic change. A key task is one of shifting the client's view from "problem-land" into "solution-land" (O'Hanlon & Weiner-Davis, 1989). O'Hanlon has emphasized that it is much easier to do something than to not do something. Working with a client to develop an alternative or preferred story to the problem is key, in terms of change. For example, a client's desire to quit drinking is much more likely to be accomplished when they have developed alternative activities that compete with the drinking such as meditation or kayaking. Stories that are about client strengths, valued qualities, and preferences tend to move forward in direction over time. In contrast, stories about limitations, problems, and deficits can have stagnating and perhaps debilitating effects on clients.

A final assumption refers to the position of the client as an empowered protagonist in his or her own story development. White and Epston (1990) have written in detail about this concept of "agency." These authors explain that our cultural practices, including therapies that assume a more scientific and positivistic stance, put clients in a passive position reacting to forces internal or external to them (e.g., depressive illness or alcoholism). The narrative mode puts the client in a protagonist or participant position—to be an agent of change. Specifically, the client engages in meaningful and productive change when he or she begins to put into thought and action stories about his or her influence on problems. Reclaimed or newly discovered abilities that influence lifestyles reflective of their preferred directions are highlighted in the therapeutic process, which utilizes experiences found in or outside of the therapy. Additionally, sources of support beyond the therapeutic relationship are found or clarified, and life courses are plotted in the direction of desired change. Once the client comes to an awareness of specific thoughts and feelings—that are attached to a narrative process and are then confirmed by accounts of lived experience—the emerging story can continue to take hold, shaping their life in preferred directions with felt experiences of positive change.

According to the assumptions of narrative therapy, change is more likely to occur when the details of people's problem stories are articulated and understood in a collaborative, respectful and transparent context. In addition, change may begin when the effect of problems shrink with the exploration of stories that run counter to the plots that describe the problem, and with the encouragement of dialogue/action that supports preferred directions and ways of being in everyday life.

Creating Client Change: Linking Narrative Concepts in Adventure Therapy

The application of narrative approaches in adventure-based work can provide a theoretical basis for therapists to guide their work with clients. Narrative methods provide a structure or "road map" for the therapist, enhancing client change in adventure therapy by clarifying problems as a changeable story, engaging in a re-storying process, and highlighting alternative-storied knowledge or experience. As will be discussed, narrative therapy techniques can draw on the unstoried experiences that are prevalent in adventure-based challenges, wilderness therapy, or initiative activities and assist the client's formulation into storied experience that can be generalized beyond the adventure therapy intervention.

People's views of themselves and their world reflect a lifetime of stories that have been told about them, stories that they have told about themselves, and stories that are part of an interactive effect with dominant societal stories or grand narratives, and the experiences that support these notions. As noted above problems happen, in part, when the truths people understand about themselves are limiting, pathologizing, victimizing, or destructive.

An important first therapeutic task of an adventure-based experience informed by narrative methods is the clarification of the dominant problem. Dominant, problem-saturated stories can become so pervasive and developed that they can represent a felt-sense or identity story within a person (White & Epston, 1990). A client could, for example, have developed a dominant story about himself or herself as a "troublemaker." Such a client may have also adopted the story of being a troublemaker as described by others. In this case, it would not be surprising to observe the troublemaker posture surfacing through a client's participation in adventure therapy. This might be expressed through a disruption in the preparation or experiencing of an activity, through self-descriptions that highlight a troublemaker identity during debriefing processes, or in descriptions other participants have for the client.

The identity of the troublemaker can surface in the context of doing adventure therapy in diverse ways. For example, the person may find "trouble" inviting them to be critical of an activity or the leader, placing them in a position of being consequenced for their behavior. This reaction could then reinforce a shared story of the client as a "troublemaker." Using narrative methods to externalize the problem from the person can create an opportunity for the client to collaborate with the leader in the discovery of ways to "distance themselves from trouble" and discover ways they are successful in reducing the effects of "trouble" in the activity. More generally, the way some stories are constructed or perpetuated can blind a person and others to the possibility for change, but they can also open up possibilities for change and growth when reconstructed into a new story.

The second therapeutic task of a narrative informed adventure thera-pist is to engage in a re-storying process with the client's input. The reflec-tion of past experience in narrative therapy is very similar to the process of debriefing commonly used in adventure therapy (e.g., creating metaphori-cal links between solutions or struggles in an activity and the person's every-day life and exploring what each person noticed about the group in an activity). Eron and Lund (1996) have described the therapeutic re-storying as a process that involves the client moving from his or her current struggle to development of a narrative reflecting being at their "best." Furthermore, Eron and Lund suggest that exploration of the "gap" between the current story of where the client is at and the preferred story can create a strong motivation for change. It can also be a motivator to do more of the same in terms of the person's everyday life. In adventure therapy, for example, a client may be assisted to change his or her ideas about fear when a therapist asks questions that help a client understand the effects that fear is having on him or her in an activity, or would ask the client to reflect on elements of the experience that surfaced when the client was at "their best."

Finding evidence of change is a common theme in adventure thera-py. People are challenged to push beyond the limits imposed by their day-to-day lived experiences and to make metaphorical links with possible alternative ways of being. White comments that constructing a narrative requires recourse to a selective process in which people prune from their experience those events that do not fit with the dominant evolving stories that are held by other people in the person's life or by the client themselves (Bruner, 1986, cited in White & Epston, 1990). These prunings can become the essential ingredients of new stories developed in narrative-informed, adventure therapy experiences. For example, such re-storying can occur in moments of immediacy during initiative activities (e.g., a trust fall), adven-ture-based challenges (e.g., succeeding in creating a solution to a high ropes problem), and at various points of responsibility during wilderness trips (e.g., setting up a camp, cooking a meal for a group, or occupying a leader-ship role on a backcountry hike). In such instances, a person potentially engages in a new set of previously unexplored behaviors. When processed, this is then used as evidence of change and provides a concrete example that can be generalized to the person's daily life outside of the adventure therapy experience.

A third therapeutic task when conducting adventure therapy from the narrative perspective involves assisting people to reclaim their lives, to stand up to problems and to build communities of support for preferred stories about themselves. As mentioned previously White refers to agency —the personal expression of power and autonomy in a society—as a story line encoded with discursive elements of direction and power (Epston &

White, 1992). Narrative methods provide an opportunity for the client to articulate and make sense of adventure-based experiences using stories that reflect self-efficacy. For example, "I was able to fight my fear by trusting my partner on the ropes course," and have that preferred story witnessed by the group. These stories of ability or strength run as counter-plots to the client's prior accounts of themselves, made more powerful by the audience who supports these accounts. In an adventure-based context, the group and the leaders act as the supportive culture for the client's new direction reflecting personal power and autonomy. It is this story line that provides a significant platform for ongoing change, and opens an invitation to the entire group or community to support the desired story.

A structured celebration or graduation at the end of an adventure-based experience is an example of using narrative methods within a group context to promote change for the client's future. Celebrations of achievement can highlight the specific qualities or characteristics of the client that support a preferred description of his or herself, recognize achievements that fit with a story of struggle against the dominant problem, and invite the client and the group to speculate on how this story may unfold in the future. Change can be punctuated or reinforced by verbal announcements and written certificates of client achievements, tailored to their unique preferred story. Social recognition of these events further supports the change, with the audience supporting the emerging preferred accounts of the client.

Developing empowering stories can run as counterplots to stories that dominate or oppress; these preferred stories usually have elements of an emerging set of ideas that can be heard as stories of authentic power, growth, and personal capabilities. For example, a client may receive a certificate recognizing her or his efforts to "take her or his life back from fear," "demonstrating leadership and cooperation with problem solving," and "showing the courage to directly state her or his needs." It is not uncommon for clients to value these documents, hang them on a wall, and refer to them as symbolic reminders of their capabilities when faced with challenging situations.

In summary, the narrative methods discussed above provide a therapeutic frame of reference for adventure therapists to assist clients in a change process. Utilizing a position of collaboration, being tentative and transparent with questions and observations, and assisting the client to identify preferred stories about themselves begins the process of change. Recognizing positive exceptions to problems or preferred stories creates the possibilities for actions that support changes identified as important to the client. These new directions can be supported and solidified by journaling, letter writing or celebratory rituals led by counselors that recognize gains or strengths, and the development of communities of concern (i.e. the people who care about the person). Audiences that acknowledge reclaimed or preferred directions are critical to a social process that supports the client's future growth (Monk et al., 1997).

Complementary Paths: Exploring Common Ground

Narrative methods and adventure therapy are complementary in a number of ways. First, both dwell on optimism and openness by emphasizing client strengths, resources, and capacities for growth. Second, both involve a collaborative process between client and practitioner. Third, both have the potential to remove the stigma garnered by constructing people as problems. Fourth, narrative and adventure therapies share a potential use of narratives and metaphors as therapeutic tools in the exploration of experience. Fifth, the subjectivity of both approaches is another area of commonality. Finally, both narrative and adventure therapy approaches can be combined into a process that uncovers storied experiential knowledge and transfers wisdom to everyday life.

First, narrative methods and adventure therapy share a sense of optimism and openness—and are grounded on the fundamental belief that people are capable of change. Individuals are not perceived as problems, but as creative collaborators with an ability to construct life-defining stories. Adventure therapy provides the setting to explore and identify new capacities, talents, and solutions to interpersonal problems. Adventure-based challenges, wilderness therapy, and initiative activities also provide various opportunities to break through previously held limitations. Leaders and participants can join together to support the development of transformational stories through adventure processes. These stories can become new paradigms based on competence and potential for growth.

Second, collaborative approaches are common to both narrative and adventure therapy. Adventure therapy provides opportunities for lived experiences regarding the social elements of collaboration, cooperation, and interdependence. The client, group and leaders form a temporary cultural climate that can challenge problematic positions held by the client's previously held notions and lived experiences by using strength-based, cooperative approaches to situations found within the adventure. An adventure therapy approach that values the client's beliefs about his or her problems, the nature of change, and preferred direction in life is complemented by narrative-based adventure leaders who can assist in the deconstruction of limiting and debilitating stories. Effective leaders in adventure therapy are more likely to be those who demonstrate the qualities of respect for the client, providing tentative and transparent feedback, and encouragement of even the smallest gains.

A third area of intersection between narrative and adventure-based work lies in a belief that problems are separate from the people who experience them. The externalization of problems allows the client an opportunity to not only understand the dominating effects and influence of the problem, but more significantly, the client's ability to influence the problem or to create preferred outcomes. Clients often begin the adventure-based activity with problem-saturated stories about themselves, believing that the location of the problem is within, and therefore difficult to change. Adventure therapy and narrative practices are informed by an attitude that emphasizes the relative influence that people can have on their problems, rather than seeing people as being powerless or passively helped by solutions external to them. In other words, working with problems as external and separate from the client's identity allows for story development with the client in a more active, influential and positive position. The adventure that highlights the client as a "cooperative problem solver," for example, is a lived experience that can be remembered and retold and could influence their future dealings with interpersonal problems.

The idea and use of metaphor is a fourth area of commonality between narrative approaches and adventure therapy. The use of metaphor in adventure therapy lends itself to re-storying a client's view of him or herself, stories about others, and perhaps the client's understanding of life's larger issues that generalize beyond the immediate experience. A metaphor —which can be constructed collaboratively between client and therapist— may be found in a group cooperative task like rappelling down a rock face. The metaphor of rappelling down a rock face could be likened to other experiences in the clients life, for example, stories about interpersonal trust, feelings of being cared about, and meeting one's needs for protection. Importantly, what can be found in the metaphors and narratives of such a powerful experience is the potential to deconstruct, write or rewrite a client's story about trust.

A fifth commonality found between narrative and adventure therapy lies in the nature of human experience and ways of knowing. Narrative methods begin with the posture that all understanding is subjective, whereas, adventure-based therapy is grounded in the idea that experience is the central locus of knowledge. Narrative therapy is a discursive process of making sense of everyday life. Adventure therapy is based on the fundamental assumption that therapy takes place in an experiential context and learning comes from experience (Allen-Newman, 2003; Hunt, 1997; Crosby, 1997). While seemingly different, the intersection of these approaches is that narrative begins with the discursive terrain and then moves out into lived experience, while adventure therapy begins with the experiential ways of knowing and then moves to the exploration of meaning. Both therapies share the same terrain of understanding, but acquire this knowledge from different directions. The strength of integrating narrative methods into adventure therapy is the exploration of meaning captured by the client's stories — ones that are constructed, told and witnessed.

Likewise, adventure therapy offers a unique context to literally bring the client's storied knowledge to life through activity and interaction. The client can use the resulting stories as sources of wisdom applicable to life's adventures beyond the therapy.

Over time, and with some experimentation, it is possible for the adventure practitioner to identify various narrative techniques that can help guide interventions with clients in an effort to integrate narrative and adventure therapy. Figure 1 provides a brief description of six dominant narrative concepts, which have been discussed. As can be seen, the type of question provides the possible direction for conversation, debriefing, and experiencing client narratives. The third column offers some contexts for the potential uses of the concepts in adventure-based work.

Conclusion

In summary, the complementary use of narrative methods with adventure therapy can enhance the construction of preferred future stories. Both therapies are grounded on the lived reality of experience and the social construction of meaning. Possibilities for change are more likely when the details of problem stories are explored in a collaborative, respectful and transparent relationship between client and therapist. Adventure therapy offers a rich context for clients to explore their stories. Narrative methods can enhance this process by helping people understand stories that partially maintain a problem, engaging people in the production of new stories, and by highlighting an alternative story that does not fit with the problem storied account.

The client's experience of a preferred story comes alive within an adventure-based, wilderness, or initiative activity context. Each person is given the opportunity to question previously fixed ideas about themselves, as well as to develop new meanings about their lives, their relationship to others, and even dominant cultural and societal practices. The use of narrative methods can assist in the meaning-making process of clients' experiences by providing their stories with a structure that encourages empowerment, acknowledgement of new and more effective ways to be an active participant in their lives, and direction for their present and future growth. Finally, the adventure therapist and the other participants become an active support system in the lives of clients. The emergence of a support system involves each person offering their assistance as important witnesses to the telling and retelling of powerful stories of change and by providing a supportive community that can nurture the gains experienced by clients.

Through the use of these methods in adventure therapy, clients will be better able to make sense of their lives and to develop their capabilities and capacities for lasting change. Narrative methods provide a map for a therapeutic process characterized by optimism, collaboration, and the iden-

Narrative Method	Examples of Relevant Narrative Questions	Potential Uses in Adventure Therapy
Introducing the person from a posture of curiosity	What is one quality about yourself that might be a surprise for others to learn about you? When you were doing [the desired way of being or doing a particular change], what small things would you have noticed about yourself that were different? When you were at 'your best' today, what were you doing?	Forming a group Experiential Games Therapeutic conversations Visualizing preferred outcomes as a group
Listening to the dominant problem description and externalizing the problem.	What is the problem that seems to get the better of you? When did this problem first appear? Who does it affect, how? In what ways have you stood up to the problem?	Frontloading an activity Assessment Group activities Debriefing activities.
Identifying cultural supports involved in maintaining a problem.	How might ideas about the problem be supported in your school, on TV, etc.?	Group talking circles about societal stories e.g., body image, relationships, culture, and so on.
Identifying Unique Outcomes	How do you resist an invitation from the problem [to do a certain behavior or practice]? What characteristic do you have that doesn't fit with the problem?	Frontloading an activity e.g., what the client hopes to use as qualities on this trip.
Exploring the relative influence of problems.	What ways does this problem get the better of you? When do you stand up to the problem?	Assessment Interviewing Debriefing a perceived high-risk activity.
Understanding oppression	If [the problem] was alive, what would you say [this problem] tries to convince you to do or be?	Integrate into a group activity e.g., cooperative games.

Figure 1. **Six ways to generate stories in Adventure Therapy.**

tification of problems as separate from the person, along with strategies that encode preferred stories for current and future directions. The adventure therapist, who is informed by narrative methods, is engaged in a process of questioning, listening for important details, and directing clients to develop new, dominant narratives or ways of being in their worlds. The construction of new meaning found through adventure-based events can become a key source of developing alternative stories to the problems that brought them to therapy in the first place. New meanings can be shaped and reshaped into preferred and liberating stories, stories that help inform clients about actions that are consistent with the changes that they desire.

References

Alvarez, A.G. and Stauffer, G.A. (2001). Musings on adventure therapy. *Journal of Experiential Education,* 24(2), 85-91.

Allen-Newman, J. (2003). *A critical analysis of the theory of adventure therapy: From a helping modality based on experience towards an emerging theory of change.* Unpublished manuscript, Department of Education, University of Victoria, Canada.

Bruner, J. (1986). *Actual minds: Possible worlds.* Cambridge, MA: Harvard Press.

Bunce, J. (1998). A question of identity. In C. M. Itin, (Ed.), *Exploring the boundaries of adventure therapy: International perspectives.* Boulder, Colorado: Association for Experiential Education.

Cottone, R. R. (2001). A social constructivism model of ethical decision making in counselling. *Journal of Counselling and Development,* (79), 39-45.

Crosby, A. (1997). A critical look: The philosophical foundations of experiential education. In K. Warren, M. Sakofs and J. S. Hunt (Eds.), *The Theory of Experiential Education.* Boulder, Colorado: Association for Experiential Education.

Duncan, B. & Miller, S. (2000). *The heroic client: Doing client-directed outcomeinformed therapy.* San Francisco: Jossey-Bass.

Epston, D. & White, M. (1992). *Experience, contradiction, narrative & imagination: Selected papers of David Epston & Michael White 1989-1991.* Adelaide, Australia: Dulwich Centre Publications.

Eron, J. & Lund, T. (1996). *Narrative solutions in brief therapy.* New York: Guilford Press.

Freedman, J. & Combs, G. (1996). *Narrative therapy: The social construction of preferred realities.* New York: W.W. Norton & Company.

Gass, M. A. (1993a). *Therapeutic applications of adventure programming.* Dubuque, IA: Kendall/Hunt Publishing Co.

Gass, M. A. (1993b). Foundations of adventure therapy. In M. Gass (Ed.), *Adventure therapy: Therapeutic applications of adventure programming.* (pp. 3-10). Dubuque, IA: Kendall/Hunt Publishing Co.

Gass, M. A. (1993c). The theoretical foundations for adventure family therapy. In M. Gass (Ed.), *Adventure therapy: Therapeutic applications of adventure programming* (pp. 123-139). Dubuque, IA: Kendall/Hunt Publishing Co.

Gass, M. A. (1993d). *Adventure therapy: Therapeutic applications of adventure programming.* Dubuque, IA: Kendall/Hunt Publishing Co.

Gass, M. A. & Gillis, H. L. (1995). Focusing on the solution rather than the problem: Empowering client change in adventure experiences. *Journal of Experiential Education, (18)*2, 63-69.

Gass, M. A., Gillis, H. L. & Priest, S. (2000). *The Essential Elements of Facilitation.* Dubuque, IA: Kendall/Hunt Publishing Co.

Gass, M. A. & Priest, S. (1997). *Effective Leadership.* New Hampshire: Human Kinetics.

Hunt, J. S. (1997). Dewey's philosophical method and its influence on his philosophy of education. In K. Warren, M. Sakofs, and J.S. Hunt (Eds.), *The theory of experiential education* (pp. 23-33). Dubuque, IA: Kendall/Hunt Publishing Co.

Kimball, R. O. & Bacon, S. B. (1993). The widerness challenge model. In M. Gass (Ed.), *Adventure therapy: Therapeutic applications of adventure programming* (pp. 11-42). Dubuque, IA: Kendall/Hunt Publishing Co.

Luckner, J. L. & Nadler, R. S. (1997). *Processing the experience: strategies to enhance and generalize learning.* Dubuque, IA: Kendall/Hunt Publishing Co.

Monk, G., Winslade, J, Crocket, K., & Epston, D. (Eds.) (1997). *Narrative therapy in practice: The archeology of hope.* San Francisco: Jossey-Bass.

O'Hanlon, W. & Weiner-Davis (1989). *In search of solutions: A new direction inpsychotherapy.* New York: W.W. Norton & Company.

Rowan, T., & O'Hanlon, B. (1999). *Solution oriented therapy for chronic and severemental illness.* New York: John Wiley & Sons.

Russell, K.C. (2001a). Ideas about ideas: Exploring the genesis and movement of conceptual boundaries. In C.M. Itin, (Ed.), *Exploring the boundaries of adventure therapy: International perspectives.* Boulder, Colorado: Association for Experiential Education.

Russell, K.C. (2001b). What is wilderness therapy? *Journal of Experiential Education. 24*(2), 70-79.

Todesco, T. (2003). Healing through wilderness. *The BC Counsellor: Journal of the British Columbia School Counsellors' Association. 25*(1), 53-63.

White, M. & Epston, D. (1990). *Narrative means to therapeutic ends.* New York: W.W. Norton & Company.

Authors' Biographies

Jordie Allen-Newman is an adventure therapist with Power to Be Adventure Therapy Society (Victoria, British Columbia) and an adolescent and family clinician with the Vancouver Island Health Authority. Jordie uses climbing, backcountry hiking, snowboarding and sea kayaking as part of the helping process with people with brain injuries, life threatening illnesses, and mental health and substance use issues. He recently circumnavigated Vancouver Island by sea kayak as part of his own healing narrative relating to his relationship with his father.

Reg Fleming has been a childcare worker in residential treatment settings, a child protection worker, and a family therapist. He holds a bachelor's degree in Psychology, and a master's degree in Clinical Psychology. He has been working with young people and their families who are affected by drug misuse for the last 11 years. Reg is interested in many outdoor pursuits, martial arts, and photography. The intersection of these interests and therapeutic work with young people has lead to many rich experiences.

Correspondence

Contact Jordie Allen-Newman
(250) 721-2669 or
jordie.allen-newman@caphealth.org

Contact Reg Fleming
(250) 721-2669 or
reg.fleming@caphealth.org

Adventure Therapy as Opportunity for Self-Reorganization: A Journey with Buddhist Psychology

Norah Trace

∎∎∎

Novel contexts available through adventure therapy offer opportunities to recreate sense of self. Adventure therapy is defined as a practical combination of ecopsychology and psychotherapy. Understanding of adventure therapy can be enhanced with some principles of Buddhist psychotherapy. Buddhist psychology adds to the understanding of fluid sense of self with concepts of "no-self" and "mindfulness." Mindfulness is discussed through four distinct foci: embodiment; emotional regulation; effect of thoughts; and experiences of "Inter-Being" and impermanence. Adventure therapy can allow us to slow down the entire nervous system, access calm emotions, and form new neural networks and patterns which in turn, influence our perceptions, emotions, and cognitions. This makes experiences of embodiment more likely to occur than those of dissociation. Emotions are easier to self-regulate, and the mind slows down and looks more deeply into what is present in self and the world, and is more able to consider how to create well-being. This requires and allows a reorganization in sense of self. Adventure therapists can help integrate the subsequent sense of self through narrative dialogues onsite and afterwards, to ensure ongoing growth and integration. Two types of meditation are looked at that are readily practiced in Adventure Therapy contexts: slowing down and looking deeply at who we are, and mindfulness of how we Inter-Be.

∎∎∎

Adventure Therapy offers a good opportunity for facilitating a changing sense of self. Buddhist psychology can be used in describing the processes of changing sense of self that often occurs through Adventure Therapy where the environment itself becomes the context for changes in the individual's self-reorganization.

Mindfulness practices are integral to bringing the ideas of Buddhist psychology to life. In mindfulness practice sense of self can be witnessed through: experience of being in a body (Varela, 2000); emotional regulation (Siegal, 1999; Varela, 1993); conceptual maps and strategies for organizing and reexamining them; means and degrees of integration among body, heart and mind (Dalai Lama, 1995; Hanh, 1998); expression of feelings and conceptualizations of expanding sense of self in terms of interconnectedness (Macy, 1991).

A simple definition of Buddhist psychology is the attempt to break through the solid static separate sense of self by revealing the bigger deeper ground that lies beneath out feet (Varela, 2000). Focus is often on beliefs of self and how, as we mature, the idea of individual selves dissolves. Inter-Being is a term introduced by Thich Nhat Hanh, to describe our sense of interrelatedness with all else. Self is "made only of non-self elements...the air, the water, the forest, the river, the mountains, the animals" (Hanh, 1998, p. 126). Over the last 40 years the concept has been adopted and adapted for psychology by Buddhist thinkers and social activists from all around the globe (Capra, 1996; Macy, 1991). The term Inter-Being signifies how all things are connected in a flow of time and space.

Wilderness as a Context For Slowing Down and Looking Deeply

Adventure therapists can provide a safe interpersonal environment that encourages noticing embodiment of spirit, heart, and mind in the context of an optimally challenging physical journey. Outdoor adventure offers us opportunities to experience our selves in a unique context, disembedded from our daily lives. This can support us in slowing down and looking deeply at who we are and developing insight into our Inter-Being within our ecological context.

We live in a culture where most people are challenged to be steadily evolving within the complex and high speed worlds in which we live. Technology increases our sense of possibility; self is constantly thrown into question by exposure to multiple realities at both the sensory and social levels. Sometimes there is the feeling of being overwhelmed by the view of new possibilities. Saturation (Gergen, 1991) occurs as there is only so much experience our bodies, minds, and hearts can integrate in any space of time. Slowing down and looking deeply becomes an attractive experience when self is saturated and caught in patterns that keep being repeated. In any given context, a person may experience a sense of limitations, and a dissolution of various possible selves that do not get to manifest in the context. Consequent feelings of overwhelm, groundlessness, and loss are common in our culture, even in highly functioning people.

When we step out of the everyday world and slow down, we slow down everything—our nervous systems, our minds, our emotional rhythms, and our sensory intake. When our bodies are not so overwhelmed, we can move more toward embodiment and away from dissociation. A feeling of being more alive is common to many people who participate in wilderness adventure therapy. For many people it is this very sense of being alive that gets lost in a high-paced, urban life (Ogden, 2003). If we put ourselves in a gentle wilderness situation, we can slow down our entire being. From here we can attune our own bodies with the natural world, and walk through the saturated self and arrive at the sense of self that feels and understands Inter-Being.

Changing Sense of Self in a Novel Context

By accessing a novel wilderness context, we can hope to arrange for the emergence of new aspects to be integrated into the global sense of self (Trace, 2003). When we move away from the familiar physical and social environments, and attend to who we are in the novel context, an awareness of effects of specific social and physical environments can occur. Also, there is chance to notice the inner emotional field (e.g., feelings of love, fear, joy, angst, etc.). Another place to focus attention is the ongoing streams of thoughts. On an Adventure Therapy experience, we can do mapping exercises every day on the journey. This requires half an hour with a blank piece of paper and a pen to make a "map" of the current experience of self. The map could offer names for dominant or novel thought patterns; emotional states and patterns of containment and expression; physical experiences; and interactions with the physical world, nonhuman life forms, and interpersonal worlds. Mapping on a regular basis helps people see that over time, we all have experiences of many possible selves, each reflecting specific inner and outer contexts in which we live (Harter, 1999; Siegal, 1999). Context may vary as a result of psychological history, emotional state, and environmental conditions. Each possible self has a chance of being lived at any given moment.

A biographical history shapes particular patterns of feelings, attitudes, and meanings that are most likely to be enacted in the future, especially if people are in a basically familiar context, with similar tasks and social scenarios. Through repetition, these patterns for experience and expression of sense of self become engrained both neurologically and psychologically (Cozolino, 2002; Grigsby & Stevens, 2000; Siegal, 1999). Distinct selves acquire stability because they are highly practiced; other possibilities can be practiced with changed internal and external environments (Grigsby &

Stevens, 2000). This is a key concept when we consider one of the opportunities offered through adventure therapy is moving oneself into a novel inner and outer context, so that a new sense of self can be experienced.

Bringing our attention to focus on following changes in self as they naturally occur, and intentionally making changes in who and how we are in the world is what we do in psychotherapy. The outdoor context itself necessitates being and doing in different ways. If the adventure therapist invites expression of new versions of the self, in dialogue or through journal exercises, the participant can more intentionally integrate and maintain a new sense of self. We can mindfully invite participants to notice how a novel context allows a unique sense of self to be present, to be practiced over a length of time, and to be named in dialogue within self and with other participants.

Buddhist Psychotherapy and Ecopsychology: Inter-Being and Interconnecting

The main principles of ecopsychology are about making conscious our experience of our lives as lived within the greater flow of life unfolding. Ecopsychology proposes the idea of interconnecting as a reciprocal relationship between people and the environment in which they live (Roszak, 1998). This is similar to what is referred to in Buddhist psychology as Inter-Being. Mindfulness of Inter-Being is about feeling more fully the deep connections among self, world and spirit.

In considering Inter-Being and Adventure Therapy, we see that feelings of interconnectedness often naturally emerge by being in the wilderness. If a facilitator invites participants to slow down and look deeply, and to bring the insights forward for reflection with the self or other participants, often the theme of feeling connected is named. A practitioner who believes that this is an integral part of adventure therapy can give participants opportunity to attend to images, emotions, sensations, and thoughts. One practice could be for participants to have conversations wherein they tell the stories of who they are when living in this deeply connected sense of self. This allows for more integration of experiences of Inter-being into sense of self, and to slow it down and notice that the feeling of being connected is with them, even while they are talking about the feeling of Inter-Being.

The healthy development of the embodied human spirit was long ago defined as one of the main concerns of psychotherapy by William James (Varela, 2000). In discussing the practice of psychotherapy, we talk about the relational context that influences the therapeutic outcome. In Adventure Therapy we are referring not only to the interpersonal context but also to the relational context at the Inter-Being level. The integration of ecotherapy (Clinebell, 1996; Macy, 1991; Roszak, 1998) and Buddhist psychotherapy into Adventure Therapy introduces mindful embodiment as part of the journey. We count on the environment to stimulate a self-organizing process that the adventure therapist helps the client to notice and embody through mindful reflection and expression.

When we are in new territory, inside and outside, we can progress toward an expanding of sense of self. Buddhist psychology offers a framework to use as we look at new forms of perceptions, feelings, sensations, mental formations and consciousness that will emerge during Adventure Therapy. The challenge at a physical level, be it gentle or extreme, is a big part of opening to new possibilities and realizing them, unwinding and strengthening values and beliefs and personal strengths, re-embodying at a deeper level, bonding mind, heart and body together. We can return with novel experiences and the potential for a shifted sense of self that we may not have been able to specifically predict. If we attend to these aspects of self mindfully, slow down and look deeply, then new forms of self become more known and can intentionally be brought to life. When we intentionally attune and align ourselves inside and outside with a wilderness ecology, we also attune and align ourselves with that which is much bigger and older than ourselves. In Adventure Therapy contexts we can step into the opportunity to name these as part of an ongoing self-narrative, and engage with these stories as descriptions of our sense of self as it is changing over time.

The Power of Telling Our Stories

As noted above, we can intentionally access variations in sense of self by placing ourselves in novel physical environments and activities. Whether or not one consciously experiences Inter-Being, at the very least there are numerous opportunities to add to or change the self-narrative. Hence the adventure therapist invites expressions of the new, more complex version of the self.

In psychotherapy we are asked to find words or images for our experience of sense of self and being in this world (Freedman & Combs, 1996; Mahoney, 2002; Peavy, 1996). As we speak, we become conscious of links and mutual influences, or co-creation of our inner and outer worlds. We form categories and frames through which to view this experience. We can practice reflecting upon and describing our experience and the frames and maps through which we view our experience.

In Adventure Therapy we access the emergent self-narratives to promote mindful conversation about change in sense of self by making the most of both spontaneous conversations and group circle times, where we tell impromptu stories about the immediate recent moments. After climbing the face of a mountain, we have many vignettes, each describing our current sense of self. We can redefine ourselves in increasingly healthy forms. If we bring mindfulness to what we focus on and how we tell the story, we are intentionally shaping our sense of self. What we, as therapists, promote and encourage in the chats or more formal check-ins influences how sense of self will define itself (Mahoney, 2002; Siegal, 1999).

Mindfulness: Adventure Therapy as a Context for Discussing "No-Self"

To Study Buddhism is to study the self.

To study the self is to forget the self.

To forget the self is to be one with others.

(Zen Master Dogan)

In the practice of mindfulness, moment to moment awareness of changing perceptions can be practiced. This way, we experience self as transient. We can also gather information about the flow of our lives within the whole of life. Here are four basic forms of mindfulness practice: (a) awareness of body senses; (b) awareness of heart and feelings; (c) awareness of mind and thoughts; (d) awareness of the principles that govern life—Inter-Being and impermanence among them (Varela, 2000). The goal is to harmonize all and bring each of the forms of mindfulness into greater presence long enough to gain a fuller and more integrated insight into the nature of self.

Awareness of Body Senses

We can use mindfulness to build awareness of our experience of being in a body. Varela (2000) described mindfulness as when the mind is present in embodied everyday experience. Just as "the mind is not in the head" neither is sense of self experienced only in the mind (p. 72). "Cognition is actively embodied" as sense of self is experienced through being in a body and through perceiving and sensing (p. 73). Sense of self arises through an immediate experience of being in a body that is active, moving, and coping with the world (Goleman, 2003; Harries-Jones, 1995; Hayak, 1952; Lakoff & Johnson, 1999; McNaughton, 1998; Schore, 1996; Siegal, 1999; Varela, 1993, 2000). We are constantly reorganizing as part of the process of making meaning of the information relayed by and through the body (Cozolino, 2003; Kelso, 1999). Just as perception influences cognition, so cognition influences perception by noticing it and naming it and constructing maps for noticing it in the future. If we put ourselves in unusual situations, our body develops new neural networks and musculature in adapting to the new scenario. If we are paddling, we develop paddling muscles; if rock climbing, then rock climbing muscles. The human brain itself has become an organ that maintains sense of self in a fluid form. "Like a river whose eddies, vortices, and turbulent structures do not exist independently of the flow itself, so it is with the brain" (Kelso, 1999, p. 1).

If we focus on our experience of being in a body, then a sense of ourselves as part of a physical world begins to be evident. We can then redefine ourselves in terms of interconnectedness within various dimensions of a whole ecosystem. Sometimes, if we can intentionally attune ourselves with the rhythm of the landscape, we are able to trust the connection we feel with the trail.

Being in the wilderness with a pack, living in a tent, hauling and filtering water and dealing with equipment is all about attending to our bodies. Our bodily awareness and the situation we are in comes first or we dissociate. Because of neurological plasticity (Cozolino, 2002), we are able to take on greater demands: learn and self-organize in more complex ways, and find simpler ways to be comfortable. We quickly form new patterns and routines. In this way we embody new images and stories about ourselves.

Awareness of Heart and Feelings

The second focus of mindfulness practice is awareness of heart and regulation of emotions. Emotion and its regulation are a fundamental part of what influences sense of self at any specific moment in time (Ogden, 2003; Siegal, 1999). Strengthening embodiment gives increased consciousness of possibilities for increasing intentional emotional regulation, and increased emotional regulation increases our ability to be in our bodies. As part of the interaction between a person and the environment, emotional responses to the world influence and reflect the way the sense of self is shaped (Schore, 1996; Siegal, 1999; Varela, 2000).

Strong emotion and novel experience are the necessary preconditions to memory, and memory influences self-narratives (Schore, 1996; Siegal, 1999; Varela, 2000). Self-narratives are created within the processes that organize the experience of the whole person in interaction with the world. Emotion is a key aspect in integrating these processes (Combs, 2002; Goleman, 2003; Grigsby & Stevens, 2000; Harter, 1999; McNaughton, 1998; Siegal, 1999; Varela, 2000). Balanced expression of emotion reflects psychological health (Goleman, 2003). Optimal emotional regulation allows the mind to be present, conscious, and flexible in interaction with the environment.

Strength of emotion bonds us with our physical and interpersonal environments and hence, a particular sense of self. Strongly positive emotional experiences strengthen the bond with a wilderness environment, just as they do with people or other places. The strength of the emotion also influences the sense of self that we experience, remember, and name in our conversations with others (Siegal, 1999). In the Adventure Therapy context, the inner emotional landscape reflects our interactions with the physical landscape. When we remember a trip, we remember the felt-sense of the trip, as well as the physical part of the journey itself. We remember stories about ourselves on that trip. The stories contain and evoke emotional themes. Just as trauma can "leave an individual with a profoundly reorganized sense of self" (Grigsby & Stevens, 2000, p. 336), so too, strong positive emotional experiences alter sense of self.

In Buddhist psychology, the concept of equanimity refers to a balanced, yet expansive emotional field of which we are aware. When practicing equanimity, we witness emotions moving through, but the emotions do not control or direct our entire experience (Dalai Lama, 2000; Hanh, 1998). Emotional responses to the external environment give us important information about that environment and of ourselves in it. It is the emotional experience of Inter-Being that inspires us to integrate it into our ongoing sense of self.

Awareness of Mind and Thoughts

The third focus of mindfulness practice that is useful on a wilderness trek is awareness of mind and thoughts. In novel situations that require mindful embodiment and emotional regulation, new forms of thinking about the self are possible. By watching thoughts we can mindfully witness the change and redefinition of who we are. Keeping the mind focused on the present moment keeps us attuned to that current sense of self. As we become aware of the coming and going of discontinuous feelings, sensations, and perceptions, we can focus on attending to the experience of what the mind is doing. The thoughts we have about our being in the world are representations of the information we receive through sensations and perceptions, through body, and emotional response to the world. In the cognitive world we name, describe, and make meaning of information brought to us through our bodies. Our cognitive worlds are heard in the stories we tell. Our cognitive worlds are representations of how we organize and integrate what we experience at the basic perception, sensation, and emotional levels of ongoing experience. Their primary function is to hold a steady sense of self which can respond to the world.

Climbing the side of a mountain requires total focus. We know that even brief periods of such focus leave a sense of invigoration and liberation, which reflect neurophysiological responses that go with reorganization (Grigsby & Stevens, 2000; Goleman, 2003; Hanh, 1998). When a plateau is reached and people stop to drink water and snack, there is most often a sudden increase in narrative conversations about the physical, emotional, and cognitive experiences of the past minutes. Everyone drinks and shares a bite, tightens boots, changes layers in clothing, and in general takes care of the immediate sense of self. This is all part of practicing mindfulness of self through witnessing of the embodied, emotional, thoughtful beings that we are.

Awareness of the Principles That Govern Life—Inter-Being and Impermanence

Do not be attached to the sign;

The mountains and rivers around are our teachers

(The Diamond Sutra)

The final focus of mindfulness practice is remembering impermanence and Inter-Being. Sense of self is a function of embodiment, emotional regulation, intentional thought, and Inter-Being with the ecological scenario. Alignment within the body, equanimity of the emotions, quieting of
the mind, and attunement with the environment are discernable goals in
this form of Adventure Therapy. Mindfulness reveals the continuous, yet
transitory nature of our experience of self. In this way we get a sense of our
own impermanence in terms of physical, emotional, and cognitive experience. When we have an experience of Inter-being, we know "no-self."
"From the point of view of time we say 'impermanence,' and from the point
of view of space we say 'no-self'" (Hanh, 1998, p. 132). If self is experienced
as impermanent and "not," then there is a greater possibility that we will
reach for a bigger ground through our interconnectedness with all that is.
From this sense of Inter-being, rather than sense of self, we will value and
protect everything, not just our separate selves (Dalai Lama, 1995).

When we have an experience of interconnectedness we see and feel
how self and world arise together, co-create each other, and support each
other as facets of a whole that endures through time. We see that "the self
that I am" is transitory both immediately and in the long term, yet is
always connected with something bigger than itself. With this moment of
awareness, the fact of our own impermanence is far less a threat to our
identity. The sense of spaciousness becomes a felt experience, directly influencing and influenced by the state of our mind and the regulation of our
emotions. We can approach the mountaintop with various forms of meditation, as well as the intention of basic mindfulness. When we return to our
usual worlds, there remains some strengthened inner part of us that instills
standing on top of a mountain with much space, varied terrain, and multiple life forms all around. We carry this perspective with us throughout our
lives. In this way the adventure has taken us to new territory, and we take
that new territory back with us to our daily lives.

Mindfulness allows us to have some degree of control over the effect
of thoughts and emotions on our sense of self, and to become more embodied. This inner alignment (Ogden, 2003) allows us to attune with life. To
develop and integrate insights, we first slow down our thinking, habits, and
strong emotions so that we can see them more clearly. Slowing down
accesses a calmness and openness to seeing what is here and what is new
in our immediate experience. Then we can practice looking deeply to

understand self, and to generate choices regarding how best to be, and what to do and what not to do to create well-being (Dalai Lama, 2000).

Conclusion

When we intentionally put ourselves in a novel situation such as an "adventure," we are often seeking a means of recreating a sense of self by calling up a strong affective experience, a strong embodiment experience, and a different social and physical context that will allow us to feel, interact, and think differently about self and relationship to life. This makes an adventure therapeutic. We take the saturated self on a journey into new terrain in an inner and outer wilderness. This encourages self-reorganization: physiological, emotional, psychological, sociocultural, and psychospiritual. The journey necessitates adaptability and flexibility because we do not have the familiar sensory world, nor do we have routines and structures that hold us in our familiar selves. The flexibility that begins in the wilderness context where we perceive unusual things and processes, and respond in unusual ways, then globalizes to the rest of our sense of self. We see everything with fresh eyes because everything is fresh; we become refreshed.

The self is an emergent process created within the body-mind in its self-organizing capacities. As body and mind integrate in a novel context, self reorganizes itself. Self is a process and not an entity (Grigsby & Stevens, 2000; Siegal, 1999). Even though we only experience one form of sense of self at a time, the psychological experience of self-continuity is re-created from moment to moment. We can use both intentionality and mindfulness to create slight shifts in sense of self. In daily life, as a function of the familiar environmental context, we can lose some of our larger scale adaptability, flexibility, and fluidity in sense of self. We can, however, count on the emergence of a unique sense of self when in a unique environment, and intentionally promote a sense of integration of this new, partly chosen, partly random outcome. The goal is to help an individual achieve an increasingly balanced and functional form of self-organization. Then we work to mindfully integrate it.

In Adventure Therapy we have an opportunity to redefine ourselves in terms of interconnectedness within a bigger dimension of existence. We have situated ourselves within a non-familiar group and a non-familiar context, and we have an abundance of choice points through which to redefine ourselves. A youth becomes someone good at building a well-contained, yet effective fire; another loves to get the water, finding she likes watching the water at the stream and noticing and protecting dragonfly larvae. In each case a new self concept with increased differentiation and integration is developed.

As adventure therapists, our job is to ensure opportunities for mindfulness of new behaviors and experiences of self: to access affirming and evolving qualities and to mindfully integrate them through narrative dialogues. Our job is to encourage mindful attunement with the environment, aligning the body, heart, and mind, and trusting the new possibilities that emerge as the individual reorganizes in the novel context. We do not necessarily have to try controlling the "outcome"; we may choose to simply guide and then trust that the new form will take the shape needed. "The process of shifting self-representations takes place consciously for the most part, occurring automatically and habitually, and in accord with fundamental dynamic patterns" (Grigsby & Stevens, 2000, p. 335). We can, however, bring as much mindfulness as possible to this journey.

Bibliography

Andersen, T. (1991). The lived experience of transformation. Unpublished Doctoral Dissertation. University of Alberta. *Dissertation Abstracts International*.

Butz, M. (1997). *Chaos and complexity: Implication for psychological theory and practice*. Ann Arbor, MI: Taylor & Francis.

Capra, F. (1996). *The web of life: A new scientific understanding of living systems*. New York: Anchor Books.

Chamberlain, L, & Butz, M. (Eds.). (1998). *Clinical chaos: A therapist's guide to nonlinear dynamics and therapeutic change*. Ann Arbor, MI: Taylor & Francis.

Clinebell, H. (1996). *Ecotherapy: Healing our selves, healing the earth*. New York: Haworth Press.

Combs, A. (2002). *The radiance of being: Understanding the grand integral vision; Living the integral life*. St. Paul, MN: Paragon House.

Cozolino, L. (2002). *The neuroscience of psychotherapy*. New York: W.W. Norton & Company.

Dalai Lama, (1995). *The heart of the Buddha's path*. London: Thorsons.

Dalai Lama, (2000). *Transforming the mind: Teaching in generating compassion*. London: Thorsons.

Drengson, A. (1995). *Shifting paradigms: From technocrat to planetary person*. Berkeley, CA: North Atlantic Books.

Eve, R., Horsfall, S. & Lee, M. (Eds.). *Chaos, complexity and sociology: Myths, models and theories*. Thousand Oaks: Sage.

Francis, S. (1998). Chaos, complexity & psychophysiology. In L. Chamberlain and M. Butz (Eds.), *Clinical Chaos* (pp. 147-163). Ann Arbor, MI: Taylor & Francis.

Freedman, J. & Combs, G. (1996). *Narrative therapy: The social construction of preferred realities*. New York: W.W. Norton & Company.

Gergen, K. (1991). *The Saturated Self: Dilemas of identity in contemproary life*. New York: Basic Books.

Goleman, D. (2003). *Destructive emotions: A scientific dialogue with the Dalai Lama*. USA: Bantam Books.

Grigsby, J. & Stevens, D. (2000). *Neurodynamics of personality*. New York: Guilford Press.

Hanh, T. N. (1993). *Inter-being*. Berkeley, CA: Parallax Press.

Hanh, T. N. (1998). *The heart of the Buddha's teaching: Transforming suffering into peace, joy and liberation*. New York: Broadway Books.

Harries-Jones, P. (1995). *A recursive vision: Ecological understanding and Gregory Bateson.* Toronto: University of Toronto Press.

Harter, S. (1999). *The construction of the self: A developmental perspective.* New York: Guilford Press.

Hayak, F .A., (1952). *The sensory order: An inquiry into the foundation of theoretical psychology.* Chicago: University of Chicago Press.

Heath, R. A. (2000). *Nonlinear dynamics: Techniques and applications in psychology.* London: LEA.

Kauffman, S. (1995). *At home in the universe: The search for the laws of self-organization and complexity.* Oxford: Oxford University Press.

Kelso, J. (1999). *Dynamic patterns: The self-organization of brain and behaviour.* Cambridge, MA: MIT Press.

Lakoff, G. & Johnson, M. (1999). *Philosophy in the flesh: The embodied mind and its challenge to western thought.* New York: Basic Books.

Macy, J. (1991). *World as lover; World as self.* Berkeley: Parallax Press.

Mahoney, M. (2002). *Connecting: Self, other, and spirit.* Public Lecture at University of Victoria, July 2002.

Masterpasqua, F. & Perna, P. (Eds.). (1997). *The psychological meaning of chaos: Translating theory into practice.* Washington, DC: American Psychological Association.

McNaughton, I. (1998). The narrative of the body-mind—Minding the body. In I. McNaughton, (Ed.), *Embodying the mind & minding the body.* Vancouver: Integral Press.

Peavy, V. (1996). *Sociodynamic counselling: A constructivist perspective.* Victoria, B.C.: Trafford

Roszak, T., Gomes, M. & Kanner, A. (Eds.). (1995). *Ecopsychology: Restoring the earth, healing the mind.* San Francisco: Sierra Club Books.

Roszak, T. (1998). *Ecopsychology: Eight principles.* Retrieved from http://ecopsychology. athabascau.ca

Schore, A. (1996). *Affect regulation and the origins of the self.*

Siegal, D. (1999). *The developing mind: Toward a neurobiology of interpersonal experience.* New York: Guilford Press.

Trace, Norah. (2003). Adventure therapy as intentional self-recreation in a novel context. *B.C. Counsellor.*

Varela, F., Thompson, E. & Rosch, (Ed.) (1993). *The embodied mind: Cognitive science and human experience.* Cambridge, MA: MIT Press.

Varela, F. (2000). Steps to a science of inter-being: Unfolding the dharma implicit in modern cognitive science. In *The psychology of awakening: Buddhism, science and our day-to-day lives.* Maine: Samuel Weiser.

Wilber, K. (2000). *A theory of everything: An integral vision for business, politics, science, and spirituality.* Boston: Shambala.

Author's Biography

Norah Trace *is a lover of wilderness journeys and has been a practicing Buddhist for 25 years. She lives in the last greenbelt outside of Victoria, British Columbia. She graduated with a Ph.D. from University of Alberta in 1991. For the last 14 years she has worked as a Graduate Program Coordinator and Visiting Professor in Counselling Psychology at University of Victoria, and as a registered psychologist in private practice. She has frequently led small groups out into wilderness settings, and never misses a season for an adventure herself.*

Correspondence

Contact Norah Trace at:
trace@uvic.ca

The Wild Way

Alan R. Drengson

■■■

The Wild Way is a learning and practice system. It is a synthesis of several unifying disciplines and whole arts. The design draws on many cultural models (e.g., the martial arts of China and Japan, yoga forms of India, and shamanic practices of aboriginal cultures). Experiential journeying set in wild nature has evolved into the art of the Wild Way. This article surveys the development of the Wild Way, and systematizes its features, techniques, and practices using journey, adventure, and healing narratives. The Wild Way has many levels of meaning grounded through adventure in wild areas. Its metaphoric and mythic narratives unite our journeys communally and personally, from physical to spiritual, and theoretic to practical. Practicing the Wild Way gives us deep meaning as we reconnect with wild energies in wilderness and our home places.

■■■

This paper explores the conceptual and practical features of wild journeying as a unifying discipline and whole art. It describes how four approaches to Nature found in contemporary wild journeying are blended through the formal and practical articulation of a whole art called the Wild Way. These four ways are: (1) the unstructured ways of spontaneous spirituality, such as wilderness wandering and life in the free open air; (2) the ordered practices of primal spirituality found in shamanic journeying, trance dancing, and Nature ceremonies; (3) the formal disciplines of concentrated flowing movement exemplified by Tai Chi and Aikido; and (4) the ways of organized wilderness journeying developed in North America under these and other influences. Some core values of these approaches are respect and nonviolence toward wild Nature in all its forms. The features of wild journeying are described here along with its practice as a spiritual discipline called the Wild Way.

Whole arts as spiritual disciplines use grounding and centering practices such as body movement, focus on breath, and mindful sensitivity to attune us to the feelings and energies of particular mediums, beings, and places. When practiced by a group, they create community spirit, centered connection with the earth, and harmony with place and other beings. Their practice makes us more receptive and spontaneously open to new experience. The Wild Way integrates and unifies our fourfold self-nature of sense, emotion, intellect, and spirit as embodied in a place. Its practices help us to create and nurture positive relationships with others based on mutual respect and consideration. It helps us to deeply know ourselves and others.

The Wild Way whole art system is distilled from the evolution and development of wild journeying as practiced in North America. It is drawn from personal perspectives and shared narrative experiences. There are important cross-cultural elements in this art, and it has a role in furthering ecological paradigms in industrial society. For purposes of exposition, this paper focuses mostly on wild journeying in Canada and the United States. The development of the Wild Way is contextualized through personal, communal, and local knowledge gained from wild journeys. This article explores how tradition and practice embellish and elaborate on basic spiritual themes that emerge from our spontaneous experience in wilderness places. It describes ways to integrate and unify ourselves through practicing harmony with wild beings and energies. It explores how through wilderness wandering as a simple natural practice, we spontaneously experience the unity of life to become more sensitive to diverse wild energies and beings.

Overall, the Wild Way is explored in depth by comparing it with other arts. The Wild Way can be practiced in many kinds of work, leadership, farming, forestry, relating to animals and so on. One goal of this paper is to help others to find their personal Wild Way practice that is appropriate to their local place and community.

Whole Arts

"Art" here refers to the practical skills and knowledge forming a coherent unifying discipline. Fine arts can be considered whole arts when they are ways of life used to make daily value choices that cultivate the spiritual integration and growth of the artist. So are martial arts when they are practices for the unification of the whole person. Art in this sense transcends science, since science depends on the art of imagination to proceed. The dedicated practice of a whole art completes a person as a self-conscious being. Many whole arts can be done without tools or materials (e.g., dancing, singing and acting).

Whole arts, as spiritual disciplines, are ways to embrace the whole. Whole arts can be distilled into a kata or koan, and embodied in a person or tribe. Their practice creates a high quality of life, even with few material possessions, as we learn from wild journeying in wilderness using minimal gear. The metaphoric complexity of wild journeying reveals the holographic nature of whole art systems of practice. These arts perfect and improve the practitioners, and also have other products and benefits. Wilderness journeying as a whole art is an ordered system of physical and mental skills for living and traveling through the unsettled wild areas of our planet.

Creative imagination is a source of our dominant cultural myths and patterns of meaning. Science provides skills for finding out about aspects of the world not evident to our unaided senses. Science uses conventional modes of awareness, whereas arts are open to all modes of awareness. When we talk of the art of life, or art as a way of life, we refer to the fact that we can have a unified aesthetic approach that is a complete or whole way of life. In this sense, farming can be a whole art (Imhoff, 2003). Life and farming are filled with creative possibilities, and wise farmers welcome these. In the Wild Way system we are positive and creative in response to the world as it is. We discover many ways to journey in daily life and also in the wilderness.

Wild journeys in progress embody the art in our actions and narratives. As a whole art the Wild Way is self-realizing and expansive. It orders our lives and gives them beauty and meaning. It is a recursive art. By doing it, we become better, and by doing it better we improve ourselves as whole persons, which enables us to practice ever more beautifully, and so on. In summary, whole arts are self-organizing and self transcending ways of continuous learning and growth.

In Quest of Wholeness

Many years ago, it was my good fortune to teach basic mountaineering and wild journeying. At that time, I knew the value of wild journeying, but didn't fully appreciate its rich cultural and international connections. I loved the mountains, had mountaineering and wilderness skills, and a deep appreciation for the joys of wild mountain living. I wanted to share these treasures with others who had not experienced them. I acquired wilderness skills and knowledge with a neighborhood tribe of teens led by a neighbor elder mentor. Our spirited group shared fun, adventure, and knowledge. When younger children joined the group, the more experienced helped them learn new skills and acquire knowledge. We shared our enthusiasm for the joys of wilderness hiking, which for us was a way to improve character and well-being. When I taught basic mountaineering, I appreciated the unifying effects of what we were doing. At that time, only a few people fully appreciated the deep integrated values learned through wild journeying and similar outdoor engagements.

While teaching this course, I also began to understand the role that serious play and outdoor activities can have on furthering personal competence and wholeness. Young people often came to the first classes with a lot of fear, lack of confidence, and little signs of leadership. As they participated in the course they often experienced a change in themselves through increased personal confidence and initiative.

As part of this, I relied on more experienced students, with practice in roped climbing, to share their skills with others. I taught new leaders to replace those who were leaving the college to work or study elsewhere. This participatory leadership process led to deep changes in those who stayed with the program for more than one season. They developed greater self-esteem, not just in climbing, but also in other areas. Their increased integration and wholeness were obvious to others.

Through teaching the mountaineering course, I came to see that wild journeying is a learning practice for life, and can be a way of life, that is, a unifying Way or Tao. A Tao is a route, path, or way of holistic practice that is in harmony with Nature (Lao Tzu, 1971). Following or practicing a way expands our horizons and helps us to become well-integrated, whole persons. In other words, whole arts make us whole persons. Learning whole arts develops our intuitive and emotional intelligence, creative spontaneity, cognitive clarity and cultivates deep feelings and balance. Their practice integrates body and mind, reason and emotion, and generates spiritual strength, resilience, and kindness. Their practices give us values, skills, and spiritual communion through mindful actions together. When we are fully aware and at one with our activities, we transcend our small self-willfulness in an authentic way. We communicate nonverbally through shared experiences. This is a realization in everyday life of compassionate awareness in our relationships (Dalai Lama, 2001).

Elements of the Wild Way in Practice, Mastery, and Metaphor

People use wild journeying both literally and metaphorically. We can take a journey in the wilderness or we can journey within ourselves. For example, this symbolic use is implied when one says "be a wild journeyer in daily life," knowing one works in the city. In both daily life and in wild journeying, we climb and descend many mountains and follow and cross many valleys, ridges, trails, and routes. In journeying we know a mountain through seeing and sensing it with all our capacities, from many perspectives and under a variety of conditions; so in daily life we come to understand the dynamics of love and hate, work and rest, roles and role models. Just as in wild journeying the routes can vary, some are difficult, some easy, some have no paths. So too with the routes open to us in daily life. Just as in wild journeying we learn the value of balance, pace, and attention to details, so in daily life we learn the value of balance between home and work, sustainable work pace, and care for details with a love for our places.

Wild journeying used descriptively refers to the outdoor activity of cross-country travel and trail hiking, while living in wilderness or semi-wilderness practiced for days at a time. Its practice over time can lead us to integrated unity as wild spontaneous persons, to abiding together in harmonious ways, sharing beautiful actions and stories.

Wild journeying as a form of mountain touring requires the skills of basic mountaineering. The first elements include the development of basic skills such as use of the ice-ax for self-arrest, belaying, and step chopping; the selection and skilled use of appropriate alpine boots and personal equipment and the selection, and use of climbing equipment, such as crampons, ropes, slings, carabiners, and assorted anchors. Alpine journeyers must have a wide range of skills for outdoor living and travel. These include knowing how to find or set up shelter, select and use proper clothing, prepare sustaining provisions, plan trip itineraries, cook meals, and arrange transport. Other desirable skills are first aid, orienteering, stellar navigation, map reading, wilderness survival, route finding, glacier climbing, ridge climbing and descending, snow and glacier travel, basic rock climbing, and negotiating steep vegetated terrain. The wild journeyer must be able to handle a variety of situations such as storms, injuries, and personal conflicts within the group.

The next elements are that journeyers need knowledge of wild animals and weather conditions. In winter and early spring they need to assess avalanche hazards. They need to know what to do if caught on a peak during a sudden lightning storm. They need to recognize the danger and symptoms of hypothermia, and know how to prevent and treat frostbite. They should know something about the area's trees and plants. Skills in photography, sketching and describing mountain terrain are valuable to help further personal development and knowledge of whole landscapes and places. This list of skills gives us some idea of the wide range of knowledge in wild journeying.

People who achieve competence in these skills, along with their appropriate attitudes and values, can live outdoors in a self-sufficient capable way. Most people can master these skills. Masters of the whole art have an elegant simplicity in their actions and equipment. For them to journey is to dwell in authentic states of value. They journey safely, with playfulness, and are kind to wilderness, companions and self. Their mastery is a continuous learning process, not a fixed state. It is ongoing self-development. They know that sincere practice is more important than reaching an arbitrary level of flashy skill in techniques.

All whole arts are activities loved for their own sake. Learning continues, even at the highest levels of mastery and old age. Learning with increasing awareness is life with the highest quality. Through mastery of the art, we better understand ourselves, each other, our place, and how we are in the natural world. We appreciate the world as a dynamic, changing and creative process. We can ever expand and deepen our respect, insight and love. Appreciation has no limits. Whole arts realizing this complete unification are called spiritual disciplines. Through their practice we actualize our indwelling spirit as we continue to learn more about ourselves and others. Mastery of wild journeying is like the mastery of a language and its dialects. With holistic unity, mastery of skills has coherence, depth, meaning, and insight. It is not like fragmented specialization.

The Wild Way's comprehensive themes and framework deal with subtle energies, attitudes and ultimate values. Its spiritual narratives are about ultimate purposes and meanings, and are means for perfecting ourselves and communities. The practices transform the negative elements in our awareness and life into positive feelings. The completion or fulfillment of the art is in the journeying process as an ongoing integrative practice, and hence as a transformative art. Finding footholds, skillfully moving in balance across a steep slope, or using a compass effectively are part of a total activity that has a larger meaning in mastery of the whole art or way. At a high level of mastery, skills are just part of a natural unity in the flow of a meaningful whole life journey. They are like notes and voices in a whole choral symphony, or steps, poses, and movements in spirit dance or ballet. Each can be very informal and intuitive, or highly organized in stylized patterns with basic forms and explicit values. The essence of a whole art can be distilled into a single system and its significant gestalts symbolized through, for example, the mountain climbing or adventure story, or an outdoor adventure therapy program. A whole story can encapsulate a whole art.

Flexibility is a key feature of the Wild Way art. Mastery transcends the guide and instruction books, which are often written for beginners. Master wild journeyers understand the art as a whole. They internalize it as an organic reality. It is part of who they are. They identify with it and it shapes their identity. Detailed descriptions of methods call attention to aspects of the art for the purpose of learning, but eventually they are part of a fluid activity of creative improvisation, like jazz. At this level of mastery, we appreciate the significance of each act and its variations within a place and its larger context. Mastery opens unlimited possibilities for creativity; no two trips will be exactly the same. Most importantly, what we learn through this mastery is directly applicable to daily life in the city.

Deep Lessons in Feeling and Knowing

Let us explore some lessons gained through mature wild journeying experience. All of life is approached as an art like wild journeying. We develop a unifying story embodied in its practices. We see how its skills, values and practices are used in other contexts, such as sailing a boat or teaching school. Actions in daily life are part of the whole art as a way of life.

Wild journeying engenders unity in a wide range of personal and communal relations. It develops emotional, intellectual and practical skills. Each of us is unique and lives in a specific place and ecosystem. The practice of the Wild Way helps us to become integrated, confident, whole persons who appreciate a wide range of values. We strive to live in harmony with others and Nature. Through wild journeying we create community with human and nonhuman beings in our home places.

Active Participation

Wilderness education is a participatory process. The educator helps others to develop their capacities to engage in creative action, inquiry, and practical actions in cooperation with others. The educator guides others to discover their own native intelligence and creative freedom. They learn to examine their experiences for distorting theories, preconceptions, dysfunctional beliefs, conflicted emotions, and crippling fears. The skills, techniques, and methods used to aid this process are not themselves the end or aim of education. Through their active fruition we gain a sense for human life as a whole, for our relations to all beings. We become attuned to the wild natural way, the way of no force, a way with heart. The Wild Way is deep in ecocentric values and involves learning as a way of life.

Wilderness learning makes a profound contribution to our first-hand experience of knowing the natural world and our deep ecological self through time. The wild journeying art can be used as a model for education, since it furthers self-knowledge and deep understanding of our relationships in our whole context. It helps us to understand that we are part of the natural context and can decide how we shall contribute to it. It engages us from the physical to the spiritual. Wild journeying involves complete immersion in wild land, life-and-death situations. These places demand practical action rather than emotional withdrawal, disengaged speculation, or abstract theorizing. Thus, journeying carries risk, as does all genuine personal growth. The art of the Wild Way, like the very nature of life, is dynamic, creative, and open-ended. It requires responding appropriately with all of our physical, emotional, intellectual, and spiritual energies as these are unified through practicing this art. Its values are woven together with action and meaningful themes oriented to Nature by means of a multi-purpose Wild Way narrative.

Wilderness experience deepens our spirited appreciation for all forms of life and for the sentient energies that pervade the natural world. Wilderness brings us into direct contact with this more than human conscious reality. It helps us to transcend doubt, fragmentation, alienation, and nihilism in our subjective lives. These conditions reflect our urban lifestyles, which cut us off from natural communities and our deeper ecological sensibilities and wild energies. In industrial society we tend to become personae filling stereotyped roles and specialized functions. In wilderness, we discover our larger personal resources and deeper spiritual connections. Modern industrial culture stresses competition which undermines community spirit, whereas journeying together inspires cooperation and nurtures a cohesive community spirit.

Spiritual Depths in Daily Life

Wild Way journeying as a spiritual practice leads to unity of self through deep appreciation for the wild aesthetic qualities of the natural world and natural selves. This compares to Rasa Yoga, the way of beauty and aesthetics championed by Tagore (1971). As we journey through the deep silence of wilderness, with its rich ecological diversity, we awaken to the creative source of life. The radiant starry night sky enhances the whispered sounds of a stream; on a dark night a bugling Elk serenades our camp in a high alpine basin. These, and so many other experiences, intensify our wonder at the mystery of all things. The sounds of falling water and rushing streams, the cycles of rain and snow, and the wind high in the trees are all part of the natural world's wild spontaneity. Abiding with them helps us to stop intellectualizing, worrying about the future, and painfully reliving the past. We know how to be fully in the present.

After many days of mountain journeying, we take on the rhythms of Nature's wild ways. When hungry, we eat; when sleepy, we sleep; when tired, we rest. When under way, we are intensely alive, totally involved in what we are doing. We are not divided as we so often are in the city. When at home, eating is often accompanied by tension, worry, argument, watching TV, talking on the phone, or reading, but in the mountains we just sit together and eat. This total involvement makes each experience intensely satisfying. It takes us out of the haste and tyranny of clock time and into the unlimited presence of wild time that is open and alive. Wild Way mountain journeying has mythic stature and universal symbolism. It joins the personal and the communal with affective adventure stories.

Affinity with Other Practices and Simplicity

The Wild Way has affinities with the Laung Gompa walking of Tibet (LaChapelle, 1978) and the marathon walking of the Japanese Buddhist monks of Mt. Hiei (Stevens, 1988). It gathers elements from Shamanic Journeying (Harner, 1986) to connect with the spirits of Nature. Its ceremonial journeying visits the lower and upper worlds of Nature spirits, ancestors and gods. It resonates with the aboriginal Australian walkabout, and North American vision quests (Sun Bear, Wabun, & Weinstock, 1987). Many have contributed to the visionary, practical and spiritual development of wild journeying as a whole art called the Wild Way.

The breathtaking beauty of the natural world, with all its unhurried cycles, has been a source of inspiration for all people, including sages and religious leaders. God spoke to Moses from a burning bush on a mountain. Jehovah appeared to Job in the form of a whirlwind. Jesus prayed and fasted in the wilderness for forty days and nights. Buddha meditated under the Bo-tree for several days and nights attaining enlightenment under the glowing morning star.

Wild journeying teaches us voluntary simplicity. For wilderness adventuring we simplify our lives, including our equipment and gear. We can not haul lots of stuff into the mountains. Wild journeyers reduce total weight and gear to a safe minimum. The elegant journeyer reduces gear primarily to necessities. The practical low limit to what we can carry on our backs helps us to realize how little we actually need, not merely to survive, but to thrive. Wild journeying, with just bare necessities, gives us some of our most rewarding and happy times. We gain valuable perspectives on vital human needs and on how quality of life can be very rich with few things. As a result, we are better able to create ecologically balanced lifestyles in the city.

Well-being and happiness don't require a huge number of possessions. Possessions are often a burden, and attachments can keep us in bondage. We get many other perspectives on the range of possibilities for a satisfying life in relation to material needs and natural limits. The personal and cultural dimensions of the environmental crisis are more directly understood.

Simplifying and reducing possessions consistent with comfort, safety, and a manageable load helps us to compare our desires with real needs. While journeying, satisfying the simplest needs is so enjoyable that we have no desire for the cravings of a jaded palate. Cold mountain water quenches thirst and is more satisfying than exotic cocktails. Breathing clean mountain air is wonderful. We learn in journeying how desires can spawn other desires to become self-perpetuating and insatiable. Wild journeying helps us to appreciate the wisdom in the sacred teachings that fewness of desires is good. We see how to choose and practice voluntary simplicity at home.

Walking on trail teaches us valuable lessons to use in daily life. We learn how to set a sustainable pace, in balanced and rhythmic forms of unified movement of our whole self, our breath, and heart. Our spiritual heart is warm and positive when we walk with enthusiasm. As we learn the art of efficient travel, we are sensitive to achieving balance by adjusting pace, posture, and breathing to the changing terrain. This balance and dynamic harmony puts us in touch with a larger, common life. We learn the wisdom of a slow, steady, sustainable pace, in contrast to making haste with frequent stopping. Passing through the "second wind" barrier, we open to flowing boundless energy (Csikszentmihalyi, 1997). We cultivate mindful pace and careful walking, whether on or off trail. We are ever mindful with each step. Our energy and attention are focused in walking, but we also take in the larger view. The sensuous and visual aspects of wilderness nurture our being. We can put ourselves on "automatic pilot," when the trail is even and well-maintained, and roam without being attached to anything. This is a meditation art or yoga. It is akin to the unifying group movements in Tai Chi and Aikido.

Meditative Awareness and Narrative Communal Connections

Meditation is awareness and total unity with whatever we are doing. We are relaxed, attentive, and aware. Wild walking participates in this enlivening (zen) process. We do not have to think to be. We are aware, intelligent, perceptive, and responsive even without the constant chatter of thought. We sit quietly without fidgeting or fantasizing. Our overly busy lives tend to lose contact with this spontaneous awareness, and yet it is what we are, and it is inexhaustibly rich. Tensions and mental babbling create uneasy divisions within. Saturation in overly stimulating urban print and electronic media separates and abstracts us from this vivid reality of spontaneous, original, primal experience of the world. Meditative walking with pace, balance and mindfulness frees our mind of tensions and thoughts, and we find the universe in this emptiness. During the physical journey we sweat and then drink purifying water; a simple diet cleanses our bodies, and extended total breathing enlivens our spirit. Natural sensations cleanse our senses, while the journey cleanses our minds and feelings. We become whole and know what whole arts are. We have a sense for our place and its story.

Wild journeying increases our understanding in many communal ways. We have more intimate contact with one another than we usually do in daily life, where we can fall into mindless, half-hearted interpersonal relations. We have so many sources of stimulation and so many demands placed on us that we tend to escape into the impersonal and make it a dominant feature of our everyday urban lives. This impersonal manner interferes with sympathy and acting from the heart. In wild journeying we are together twenty-four hours a day in simple, intense, and incredibly beautiful non-distracting situations. We also might spend several hours a day alone with our thoughts and feelings, as our party climbs long alpine ridges or walks through silent forests. This movement, balanced between deep inwardness and intense connection with others and nature, gives rise to nonverbal communion with one another and the natural world. This communion is the mutual feeling side of our journeying community. We enjoy natural serendipity together. We live in a communally conscious space. Conflicts are relatively few and experienced authentically, without the usual manipulations that can characterize the games that urbanites play. Competition strengthens ego, whereas cooperation helps us to forget ourselves by being with others in community.

Thus, we emphasize cooperation, not competition.

As we journey, the physical effort enables us to be more and more relaxed. We have a playful attitude toward our minor aches and pains. Insect bites, skinned legs and elbows, sore muscles, and the cold hard ground are familiar friends. We learn the folly of too much resistance to gravity and other natural forces. Instead of fighting and resisting perceived hardships, we willingly accept and enjoy them as part of the natural contrasts in the whole trip. We have times of intense physical and mental demand, and times of profound relaxation and rest with no demands. We learn to see these not as opposites that are eternally separated, but as complementary aspects of a unified process and activity. They have their sense and significance in their interpenetration, each enhancing the other within a larger narrative journeying context. There can be global and even cosmic narratives implied by and held within each adventure story about a wild journey.

We learn both from hardship and easygoing parts of the journey. We know that just as the rain stops and the sun eventually emerges from the clouds, so too tears of sadness and the clouds of grief eventually dissipate, and lightness and joy return. Just as we need some basic orientation in daily life, so do we in the mountains. As we need meticulous preparation for extended wild journeying, so to for our life work. Our mistakes provide some of our deepest learning experiences, just as they do in daily life in the lowlands. Like life, the whole journey includes highs and lows, heights and valleys. Clearly, the benefits of wild journeying permeate our whole lives, as its practice subtly changes us. Mountains are mountains, but in our stories they are also metaphors and mythic figures. We are wild journeyers in daily life. We are the same at home as we are in the mountains, when we fully internalize the art and walk its way of being in the world.

Connecting with Earth and Other Beings

Wild journeying teaches us about environmental problems and how we can resolve them by working together in harmony with nature. We realize from wild journeying the symmetries between human consciousness, and the principles of ecology that pervade the human and natural world. We see that each of us is an ecosystem in miniature. We learn personal responsibility to our context, and an appreciation for the integrity of the earth's ecosystems, with their many diverse ecological communities, and how they sustain all living beings on the planet. Wild journeying makes us aware, in deep personal ways, of the whole natural world, the ecosphere we inhabit. We come to know it intimately and comprehensively. For balance, modern humans, to the degree that we live in isolation from these rhythms, need more daily contact with them. The less we have to do with natural processes directly, the less we appreciate them, and the more we lose contact with our own deep inner spontaneous nature. But wild journeying reenlivens us and we can take this positive energy home. We return to the city with strength and optimism knowing anything is possible.

Through wild journeying we appreciate all the living beings with whom we share this Earth. We appreciate in the silence of wilderness that we all share and are part of the same creative life force, Ki (Ueshiba, 1985). We sense and are aware of the cycles of life and energy within the ecosphere. We appreciate the interconnectedness of all life and how all things hang together. The natural world is neither hostile nor inimical to us. We are each part of its vast interconnected, ongoing, creative processes. The principles of community, friendship, and human flowering are embedded in the wild wholeness of ocean, sky, wind, flowers, forests, rivers, and mountains. In the Wild Way we share their wisdom.

By practicing the Wild Way we can return to our home, to that vital center in ourselves that is in harmony with the way of Nature and the Universe. Lao Tzu, M. Ueshiba and others in Eastern traditions, learned from Nature and taught this Way, as did teachers in our own wisdom and mystical traditions. These mystical qualities are not occult or weird; they are found at the center of our ordinary daily experiences, once we learn to be aware and receptive. Through wild journeying we know that life sends us many gifts. We take joy in living. We make the most of every moment. With such blessings, we are good citizens of our place on the Earth.

Features of the Wild Way in Systematic Summary

The essential features of wild journeying can be described now using eight overlapping categories: spiritual, physical, narrative-metaphorical, historical, personal-social, ecological, practical, and educational.

1. The *spiritual* include realizing that life and its source are sacred; a growing sense of wonder and awe; a realization that the ecosphere is not hostile but benign; a commitment to a life of increasing awareness and care; a respectful attitude toward life that leads to communion with other persons, life forms and the world as a whole.

2. The *physical* elements include the fitness that results; the skills of balanced movement and the regulation of breath; activities that promote strength, endurance, coordination, flexibility, confidence, and body-mind integration.

3. As adventure *narrative and metaphor,* the Wild Way represents life as a whole. Its narratives have an integrating and unifying power that brings understanding of natural processes to our daily life, whether in human communities, with the complications of modern technology, or in simple rich, natural settings.

4. The *historical backgrounds* of wild journeying reveal its evolution as the art of the Wild Way. The backgrounds to the Wild Way include the spiritual practice of withdrawal from urban society to the wilderness, and the return; the primal vision quests; the tracking skills of the hunter-gatherers; Scandinavian Friluftsliv, that is, life in the free air, the journeys of some mountain men (Dahle, 1994), the skills, values, and spirit of scouting, the craft of modern mountaineering, the survival skills and personal competence of Outward Bound, the healing processes of Wilderness Therapy, and rediscovery. The Wild Way connects the values realized in past tradition and unifies them within our present lives. Some symbolism in wild journeying has affinities with ancient alchemical traditions that focus on unification of body and spirit, the transmutation of base elements of the self to noble forms (e.g., transforming the energy of greed into generosity, indifference to concern, hate into love).

5. The *personal-social:* Solo wilderness treks are intense and yield deep self-knowledge; in the group trip we learn about the nature of the self in its relational interconnections. This learning process gives us the opportunity to go beyond the small ego-self to encounter our larger ecological identification in a community. The practice of this art develops our four elements, spiritual, cognitive, affective and physical, in balanced and integrated ways.

6. The *ecological awareness* of wild journeying is comprehensive and includes deep experiential knowledge of the principles of ecology. The trip as a creative expression is a ceremonial celebration of a unified vision embracing respect for the Earth and the Cosmos.

7. Wild journeying has many *practical* elements central to ongoing daily life, such as learning to pace ourselves in good work, how to create good services and products, to be attentive to detail, to be flexible, to improvise freely, to appreciate quality of relationships and actions, and to see life as a whole.

8. In *education* the Wild Way art can be used to guide undertakings that develop that whole person, in body, feeling, mind and spirit. Its practice unifies our capacities through an expansive, positive spirit. Education, in this sense, is not just job training or professional specialization. It leads to deep self-knowledge and understanding of the interconnected contexts of all life. It brings us back to our sacred wholeness that gets lost in industrial culture. It is practiced with humility, respect, and gratitude which will bless any project or endeavor. The ultimate aim of education is to be complete in ourselves. We can realize this by living in the Wild Way.

The Whole Wild Way Learning System in Outline

The Wild Way is a unified spiritual discipline using ceremonial activities and practices to live in harmony with our place in Nature here and now. The whole learning and practice system is outlined in the remarks below by focusing on the skills and practices that make up the art.

1. Local and ceremonial practices deepen personal knowledge of places, particulars, energy flows, natural signs, and more.

2. Natural and mindful meditations are in rhythms suited to context, party, and self (e.g., as in pace, grade and speed while walking).

3. Skillful means in use and care of equipment (e.g., walking stick, ice-ax, rope, pack, and compass are all used artfully).

4. Elegant actions and powerful techniques use wise forms and patterns of action with least force.

5. Sense of direction, destination, orientation as a sixth sense, route finding and map use, and a sense for being at home while wild journeying.

6. Silence, non-doing, blending in, nonviolence, highly efficient and small energy use, and becoming more alive.

7. Hiking and climbing skills for beautiful cross-country wilderness travel while living outdoors 24 hours a day, as the whole art is practiced.

8. Being ready for anything, weather, hazards, prevention of mishaps, relaxed and always alert.

9. Shifting perspectives, inner and outer journeying, narrative journalizing, centered and being fully in the natural world in tune with the trees, streams and stars.

Concluding as Continuing On

Once we are skilled in wild journeying practice we can continue even in urban parks and gardens. It becomes a daily practice no matter where we are. By dwelling in wilderness places in the Wild Way, we learn how to let the wild come back into daily life. We bring this wild wisdom home. We find the wild way home to spontaneous joy and natural harmony in daily life. This spontaneous creativeness (cosmogenesis) is nature's way. When we are whole, we fully participate in creating meaning and value in our places. We live in a rich meaningful context. Even in urban settings we can visit other levels of reality using such techniques as drumming, dance and ceremony. This rejoins the urban-rural and tame-wild through the Wild Way. From this wholeness, diverse and ecologically wise, place specific communities and cultures emerge.

Through the Wild Way, we complete ourselves and add to the total beauty and value of life on Earth, in our Solar System, in the Milky Way Galaxy. Life flows with deepening satisfaction, appreciation, and joy. There is richness, beauty, and mystery in the wild world. The power of creative energy in spontaneous Nature is manifest in wild places and ourselves. To realize this and share it with others is to fulfill ourselves and reclaim our spiritual life. Our wild adventures become part of our personal and communal stories that are part of a larger and growing mythopoetic narrative context.

Bibliography

Cajete, G. (1994). *Look to the mountain: An ecology of indigenous education*. Durango CO: Kivaki.

Csikszentmihalyi, M. (1997). *Finding flow: The psychology of engagement with Everyday life*. New York: Basic Books.

Dahle, B. (Ed.). (1994). *Nature: The true home of culture*. Oslo: Norges Idrettshogskole.

Dalai Lama. (2001). *Open heart: Practicing compassion in everyday life*. Boston: Little Brown.

Dogen. (1986). *Shobogenzo: Zen essays*. Thomas Cleary, trans. Honolulu: University of Hawaii Press.

Drengson, A. R. (1995). *The practice of technology*. Albany, NY: SUNY Press.

Emerson, R. (1991). *Nature*. Boston: Beacon Press.

Fox, E. (1966). *The sermon on themMount: The key to success in life*. San Francisco: Harper.

Graydon, D. & Hanson, K. (Eds.) (1997). *Mountaineering: The freedom of the hills*. Seattle: The Mountaineers.

Hanh, T. N. (1996). *Walking meditation*. Berkeley: Parallax Press.

Harner, M. (1986). *The way of the shaman*. New York: Bantam.

Hawkins, D. (2002). *Power vs. force: The hidden determinants in human behavior*. Carlsbad, CA: Hay House.

Hunt, V. (1996). *Infinite mind: Science of human vibrations of consciousness*. Malibu, CA: Malibu Books.

Imhoff, D. (2003). *Farming with the wild*. San Francisco: Sierra Books.

Kurtz, R. (1990). *Body-centered psychotherapy: The hikomi method*. Mendocino CA: Life Rhythm.

LaChapelle, D. (1978). *Earth wisdom*. Silverton, CO: Finn Hill Arts.

Lao Tzu. (1971). *Tao te ching*. Baltimore and Middlesex: Penguin.

Laszlo, E. (1996). *The systems view of the world*. Crestkill, NJ: Hampton Press.

Leonard, G. (1999). *The way of aikido: Life lessons from an American sensei*. New York: Dutton.

Leopold, A. (1968). *A Sand county almanac, and sketches from here and there*. London and New York: Oxford University Press.

Liang, T. T. (1977). *T'ai chi chu'an for health and self defense: Philosophy and practice*. New York: Random House.

Marshall, Ian. (2003). *Peak Experiences: Walking meditations on literature, nature, and need*. Charlottesville and London: University of Virginia Press.

Mascaro, J. (Ed.). (1971). *The upanishads.* Baltimore: Penguin.

Muir, J. (1954). *The wilderness world of John Muir.* Boston: Houghton Mifflin.

Naess, A. (2002). *Life's philosophy: Reason and feeling in a deeper world.* Athens: University of Georgia Press.

Osho. (2001). *Awareness: Key to living in balance.* New York: St. Martins Griffin.

Parker, G. (2001). *Aware of the mountain: Mountaineering as yoga.* Victoria, B.C.: Trafford Press.

Ryle, G. (1949). *The concept of mind.* London: Huchinson Home Library.

Shulman, N. (1992). *Zen in the art of climbing mountains.* Boston: Charles Tuttle.

Smith, H. (1991). *The world's religions.* San Francisco: Harper.

Snyder, G. (1990). *The practice of the wild.* San Francisco: North Point Press.

Stevens, J. (1988). *The marathon monks of mount hiei.* Boston: Shambhala.

Streng, F. (1985). *Understanding religious life.* Belmont, CA: Wadsworth.

Sun Bear, Wabun, & Weinstock, B. (1987). *The path of power.* New York: Prentice Hall.

Tagore, R. (1971). *A tagore reader.* A. Chakravarty (Ed.). Boston: Beacon Press.

Thoreau, D. (1991). *Walking.* Boston: Beacon Press.

Toulmin, S. (1990). *Cosmopolis: The hidden agenda of modernity.* Chicago: University of Chicago Press.

Trine, R. W. (1970). *In touch with the infinite.* New York: Bobbs-Merrill.

Trungpa, C. (1984). *Shambhala: The sacred path of the warrior.* Boston: Shambhala.

Twight, M. and Martin, J. (1999). *Extreme alpinism: Climbing light, fast, high.* Seattle: The Mountaineers.

Vivekananda, Swami. (1955). *Karma-yoga & bhakti-yoga.* New York: Ramakrishna-Vivekananda Center.

Ueshiba, K. (1985). *The spirit of aikido.* Tokyo and New York: Kodansha.

Ueshiba, M. (1991). *Bubo: The teachings of the founder of aikido.* Tokyo and New York: Kodansha.

Relevant Websites

www.Aikido-international.org The official website of the International Federation of Aikido.

www.chenbucto.ns.ca/philosophy/taichi/taoism.htm Taoist philosophy and Tai Chi.

www.ecostery.org A website based on respect for place, see articles section for wild way and friluftsliv.

www.ITCCA.org International Tai Chi Chuan Association website.

www.itp.org Website devoted to George Leonard's Integral Transformative Practice.

www.shamanism.org Website featuring Michael Harner's work.

www.bivouac.com Canadian website devoted to all aspects of mountaineering.

www.mountaineers.org Website of the Seattle Mountaineers, rich with information.

Author's Biography

Alan Drengson *is Emeritus Professor of Philosophy and Adjunct Professor of Graduate Studies at the University of Victoria in Canada. He works in Eastern philosophy, comparative religion, environmental philosophy, and cross cultural technology studies. He has taught and practices meditation disciplines related to harmony with Nature. He is the author of many articles and books, including* The Practice of Technology and Beyond Environmental Crisis, *and an unpublished manuscript called* Wild Way Home. *He is the founding editor of* The Trumpeter: Journal of Ecosophy and Ecoforestry.

Correspondence

Contact Alan Drengson at: ecosophy@islandnet.com
For Wild Way workshop information: www.ecostery.org.

Research Directions in Wilderness Therapy

Keith C. Russell

■■■

The purpose of this paper is to: (a) review and evaluate recent research on wilderness therapy process and outcome to identify current research trends; (b) present an overview of key elements of the wilderness therapy treatment model that appears to be supported by empirical research; and (c) to highlight recent studies completed at the Outdoor Behavioral Healthcare Research Cooperative in order to provide an example of how a research program was developed. The goal is to highlight areas for future research and to invite dialogue with other practitioners, academics, and researchers in the international adventure and wilderness therapy community.

■■■

Wilderness therapy evolved from outdoor- and wilderness-based treatment programs that have been in existence for over 50 years, with strong influences found in the Outward Bound wilderness challenge model brought to the U.S. in the early 1960s (Howard, 1984), and therapeutic camping, established in 1946 with programs like the Dallas Salesmanship Club (Loughmiller, 1965). Wilderness therapy has been defined a number of ways in its evolution to its current practice, and is referred to in the literature by numerous terms such as wilderness therapy (Davis-Berman & Berman, 1994), therapeutic wilderness camping (Loughmiller, 1965), adventure therapy (Gass, 1993), wilderness adventure therapy (Bandoroff, 1989), wilderness treatment programs (Kimball, 1983), wilderness experience programs (Winterdyk & Griffiths, 1984), and outdoor behavioral healthcare (OBH) (Russell, 2003). The OBH definition suggested by Russell (2003) was developed by program practitioners who coined the phrase to more accurately describe the manner with which wilderness experiences are being used by contemporary programs to enhance existing behavioral healthcare treatment services. OBH programs utilize elements of wilderness therapy (Gass, 1993; Davis-Berman & Berman, 1994; Russell, 2001) to address the unique needs of adolescents with a variety of emotional, behavioral, psychological, and substance use disorders. Treatment is guided by individual treatment plans implemented by licensed mental health practitioners, with the goal being assessment, and in many (but not all) cases, treatment of presenting client symptoms.

Despite longevity of practice and some reported positive effects from treatment, OBH programs have struggled to gain respect, and are still viewed by the mental health service industry with some trepidation because of well-publicized incidents involving a few programs (Jenkins, 2000; Krakauer, 1995), and because of the perception (whether justified or not) that no empirical evidence exists to support treatment efficacy (Winterdyk & Griffiths, 1984). Although OBH programs are viewed with some suspicion, their numbers continue to grow, prompting state and provincial institutions to determine how best to regulate and provide oversight to program practice. Three-quarters of all OBH programs in the U.S. that responded to a 2000 survey were already in operation by 1990, with the number of new programs steadily rising during the 1990s when many states had begun to establish, or had in place, regulations to standardize the quality of care (Russell, 2003b). Over 85% of all OBH programs are currently licensed by State agencies, making it increasingly difficult for poorly run programs to stay in operation. This increased oversight, along with the establishment of organizations like the Outdoor Behavioral Healthcare Industry Council (OBHIC), the National Association of Therapeutic Wilderness Camps (NATWC) and the National Association of Therapeutic Schools and Programs (NATSAP), has led to increased collaboration amongst programs and well-defined and communicated standards of best practice. Moreover, many programs also pursue national accreditation from well-established agencies such as the Joint Commission on the Accreditation of Healthcare Organizations (JCHAO) and the Council on Accreditation (COA). Despite these positive steps towards identifying and improving best practices in wilderness therapy, there still exists a paucity of research on wilderness therapy practice and outcome. Research has not kept pace with the growth in the number of programs and clients served, leaving many questions unanswered.

Purpose

The purpose of this paper is to review existing research in wilderness therapy, propose a theoretical framework of current wilderness therapy process and practice, and describe longitudinal research effort begun in 1999 at the Outdoor Behavioral Healthcare Research Cooperative, now at the University of New Hampshire. The goal is to provide an illustration to practitioners, academics, and researchers of how this thread of research is in response to specific questions asked by practitioners, and perhaps more importantly, their constituencies, as to what is wilderness therapy and is it beneficial to modern youth in the United States, Canada, and other Western countries. The goal in doing so is to stimulate discussion and debate as to appropriate research designs, data collection, and analysis protocol and to present a model for doing research that is applicable to other mental health and academic systems that are similar to those found in the United States and other Western countries.

Recent Research in Adventure and Wilderness Therapy

To examine recent research interest in wilderness therapy, a broad definition was applied that consisted of: (a) some type of outdoor or adventure intervention, used to (b) help address some type of problem or issue for clients. In no way is this meant to be an exhaustive review of the literature. The focus of the search was to identify those articles that were published over the last five years (1998-2003) that empirically evaluated wilderness therapy process and practice. The search was conducted in Dissertation Abstracts International (DAI), PsychINFO, ERIC, and Academic Premier. Specific journals in the field were also reviewed (*Journal of Experiential Education, Journal of Adventure Education and Outdoor Learning*, and the *Australian Journal of Outdoor Education*). Surprisingly, the journals revealed only a total of six articles that focused on empirically evaluating wilderness or adventure therapy process or practice. These six studies examined the use of wilderness therapy for the treatment of adolescent sex offenders (Lambie et al., 2000), evaluated the effects of a wilderness-enhanced program on behavior disordered adolescents (Brand, 2001) and evaluated process and outcomes of wilderness therapy for adolescents (Russell, 1999; 2000; 2002; 2003). The majority of published material relating to wilderness therapy in outdoor education and related journals consists of discussions and reflections on the intervention and the role it may play in helping a variety of clients. The most active database for current research is the DAI, where a total of 12 dissertations have been written since 1998 focusing on empirical evaluation of the process and practice of wilderness therapy. These publications show refined definitions of the intervention, increasingly sophisticated research methods, and important implications from findings.

For example, Clark (2003) found that wilderness therapy facilitates positive change in adolescents with clinically elevated Millon Adolescent Clinical Inventory (MACI) personality scores, and noted that short-term interventions leading to character change are virtually unheard of in the personality literature. In a study evaluating whether ethnicity could explain variance in self-concept and internalizing and externalizing behaviors, Orren (2003) found that the treatment group did not differ from the control group on self-concept or internalizing/externalizing behaviors, and that African American treatment group participants actually reported lower self-concept scores after the wilderness intervention. Hagan (2003) assessed treatment outcomes using the Youth-Outcome Questionnaire (Y-OQ) and found that adolescent self-reports indicated no significant improvement from wilderness treatment, whereas parents and counselors indicated significant improvement. Winters (1999[b]) utilized an assessment device used to screen for substance use problems and found a large percentage of clients report with significant substance use issues, suggesting that wilderness therapy needs to identify and operationalize substance use treatment protocol as suggested by Winters (1999[b]). Other studies examined self-esteem and locus of control and their relation to group affiliation (Martinez, 2002), a qualitative study of clinicians' perspectives on the treatment process (Chatroux, 2001), a comparison study of a residential and wilderness program (Edgmon, 2002), a case study examining the process and outcomes of an adventure therapy program (Mcnamara, 2002), parents participation in the process and aftercare programs (Webb, 2001), the role nature and wilderness therapy play in women's self-perceptions (Gardner, 2000), and, whether wilderness therapy is culturally appropriate for troubled Navajo youth (Parzen, 2001). Though these studies reflect an increasing interest and sophistication in research design and methods on wilderness therapy, few of these theses have been published in refereed journals. This has been a consistent trend in research on wilderness therapy since the seminal studies on the effects of Outward Bound were first reported in 1960s and 1970s (Burton, 1981; Kelly & Baer, 1968).

Defining Wilderness Therapy Programs and Practice

Wilderness therapy is a treatment approach practiced by OBH programs that utilizes unique dynamics inherent in group living in outdoor environments (Russell, 2003[b]). Most OBH programs subscribe to an eclectic model that incorporates a blend of therapeutic modalities, but do so in the context of wilderness environments and backcountry travel. The therapeutic approach has evolved to incorporate a clinical model which includes client assessment, development of an individual treatment plan, the use of established psychotherapeutic practice, and the development of aftercare plans (Bandoroff & Scherer, 1994; Russell, 2003[a]). Crisp (1997) highlights ways in which wilderness experiences have integrated adolescent psychiatric approaches, and provides a good overview of the ways in which wilderness programs have become more clinical in their approach. OBH programs apply wilderness therapy in the field, which contains the following key elements that distinguish it from other approaches found to be effective in working with adolescents: (a) the promotion of self-efficacy through task accomplishment, (b) a restructuring of the therapist-client relationship through group and communal living facilitated by natural consequences, and (c) the promotion of a therapeutic social group that is inherent in outdoor living arrangements (Davis-Berman & Berman, 1994; Kimball, 1983; Russell, 2001).

Promotion of Self-Efficacy Through Task Accomplishment

Adolescence is a time when a teen begins to form an individual sense of self that becomes increasingly differentiated and which is manifest in a variety of social contexts, including family and peer environments (Harter, 1999). Culture plays a key role in developing an adolescent's sense of self, as identities are assumed and created through dress, music, media, and high-risk behaviors. By removing the adolescent from cultural artifacts that negatively define him or her and may perpetuate substance abusing behaviors, wilderness environments immediately encourage adolescents to develop a sense of self, devoid from cultural influences. Furthermore, treatment approaches that focus on gradual development of self-competence in relation to real-life problems and settings have been shown to have optimal treatment effects (Brown, Stetson, & Beatty, 1989). Based on Bandura's (1977) notion that the relationship between self-efficacy and performance is reciprocal (meaning efficacy expectations influence performance and performance influences efficacy expectations), the gradual development of self-competence in OBH is accomplished through numerous daily living tasks that are real, immediate and concrete, and become increasingly difficult as the process unfolds. Examples of these tasks include setting up a tarp for shelter, successfully packing a backpack, and cooking breakfast over a fire made from a bow-drill set constructed by the adolescent. As adolescents accomplish these daily tasks, participants often forget that they are in treatment, and resistance to the process begins to evaporate as they become simple daily routines. The treatment team directly relates these learned skills to real-life social contexts, facilitating an approach that is concrete and suitable for adolescent's developmental capabilities.

Restructuring of the Therapist-Client Relationship

Many clients enter OBH treatment with a resistance to treatment and authority, and a negative history of involvement in counseling and treatment services. Effective treatment will require an alternative approach to work through this resistance (McCord, 1995). One way that OBH accomplishes this is through "natural" consequences, meaning they are not imposed by authority figures. An example is when staff provide a detailed lesson in how to pack a backpack and the client hastily completes the task, the result is either an arduous day of hiking with an uncomfortable pack or the repacking of the pack. As Bandoroff (1989) states, "...the environment assumes much of the responsibility for reinforcement and punishment, and clients cannot fool mother nature; consequences prescribed by the environment are real, immediate and consistent" (p. 14). The treatment team also engages in the same wilderness experience as the clients, eating the same foods and sleeping under the same tarps, dramatically restructuring the therapist-client relationship that most adolescent clients are accustomed to from previous counseling or therapy. As Gass (1993) states, "...while still maintaining clear and appropriate boundaries, therapists become more approachable and achieve greater interaction with clients" (p. 9). This unique relationship that is built with the treatment team in OBH allows for discussion and discourse to occur without the stigma of traditional therapeutic roles. Russell and Phillips-Miller (2002) found empirical support for this in identifying the relationship established with counselors as a primary reason for client self-improvement.

Promotion of Therapeutic Social Group

Since peer influences are perhaps the most powerful predictor of adolescent anti-social behavior and substance abuse (Winters, Latimer, & Stinchfield, 1997), treatment strategies involving group therapies are appropriate for capitalizing on the considerable influence of peers (Bangert-Drowns, 1988). Drawing on theoretical factors inherent in social learning theory, group living in outdoor environments is facilitated by norms and behavioral patterns that are developed through careful modeling and facilitation by experienced leaders and staff. Within this structure, learning takes place in the field continually through the process of adolescents observing and modeling the behaviors, attitudes, and emotional reactions of others, both students and staff. Bandura (1977, p. 22) states: "... most human behavior is learned observationally through modeling: from observing others one forms an idea of how new behaviors are performed, and on later occasions this coded information serves as a guide for action." OBH facilitates this social learning through: (a) placing experienced and inexperienced group members in the same groups, where pro-social behaviors are modeled; (b) integrating psycho-educational curricula into the treatment process and including metaphoric phases that clients must pass through to "graduate" the program that come with increasing responsibility and reward; and (c) group and communal living that requires constant communication, patience, and trust. Group cohesion and development throughout the experience establish a set of norms and expectations which play key roles in helping participants develop healthy pro-social behaviors and identities (Erikson, 1963). Examples include cooking in teams, leading the group on a hike, and psycho-educational groups which help adolescents address specific issues in their lives with the help of group members and staff. Those who have experienced deep concern about their sense of worth and their ability to relate to others are empowered through these processes.

Review of Wilderness Treatment Outcome Studies

A review of studies was conducted to provide an overview of process factors and outcomes that are typically associated with wilderness therapy programs. Studies that inform wilderness therapy practice also include research on wilderness experience programs like Outward Bound (OB) and the National Outdoor Leadership School (NOLS) because processes inherent in wilderness living and traveling parallel those that occur in wilderness therapy approaches. The crucial difference between wilderness therapy and an OB or NOLS experience is that wilderness therapy programs are specifically designed to address problem behavior in individuals while OB and NOLS are not. This issue highlights a major shortcoming of research in the field: it is difficult to compare and replicate studies from one program or setting to the next. Several reviews were drawn on to examine the outcomes associated with the effects of wilderness programs on participants (Burton, 1981; Cason & Gillis, 1994; Easley, Passineau, & Driver, 1990; Ewert, 1983, 1987; Friese, Pittman, & Hendee, 1995; Gibson, 1979; Gillis, 1992; Gillis & Thomsen, 1996; Hattie, Marsh, Neill, & Richards, 1997; Levitt, 1982; Moote & Wadarski, 1997; Russell, 1999; Vogl, 1990; Winterdyk & Griffiths, 1984). These reviews show that past studies have focused on two primary effects on participants: (a) the development of self-concept, and (b) the development of appropriate and adaptive social skills. Other studies have examined recidivism in criminal behavior and are also reviewed. Unfortunately, there are very few studies related to the effects on substance abuse and dependence, primary outcomes on which current outdoor behavioral healthcare practice is focused. This shortcoming highlights the need for future research in this area.

Studies Related to the Effects on Self-concept

Poor self-concept is considered to be associated with the presence and continuation of delinquent behavior; therefore, much of the research has focused on the degree to which wilderness programs enhance the participant's self-concept. Specific studies on self-concept note that wilderness programs significantly enhance the self-concept of troubled youths by presenting challenges that are attainable and grow in difficulty (Bandoroff & Scherer, 1994; Gibson, 1981; Hazelworth, 1990; Kelly & Baer, 1969; Kimball, 1979; Kleiber, 1993; Pommier, 1994; Porter, 1975; Weeks, 1985; Wright, 1982). However, a meta-analysis conducted by Hattie et al. (1997) suggests that past research in this area has ignored the advances being made in self-concept research and thus earlier studies tended to be simplistic. Recommendations included moving beyond assessing changes in global self-concept and focusing more on specific measures of self-concept, such as the physical, social, and academic dimensions. These earlier studies tended to focus on physical ability, peer relations, general self-concept, physical appearance, academic progress, self-confidence, self-efficacy, and self-understanding (see Hattie et al., p. 48). Marsh, Richards, and Barnes (1984) addressed some of these issues by assessing several dimensions of self-concept in their study of non-delinquent youth and demonstrated that multiple dimensions of self-concept can be changed through a 26-day Outward Bound wilderness challenge program. A more recent study noted that by identifying multiple dimensions of self-concept, identifiable goals of the intervention can be more directly linked to these measures of self-concept (Marsh, 1990). Russell, Hendee, and Cooke (1998) found that increases in sense of self from participation in a wilderness program led to increased student performance in the Federal Job Corps program as well as reduced the likelihood that students would leave the program early before completing their educational and vocational training. Despite reported successes, systematic reviews of self-concept research emphasize the lack of a theoretical basis in most studies, the poor quality of measurement instruments used to assess self-concept, methodological shortcomings, and a general lack of comparable findings (Gillis, 1992; Hattie et al., 1997; Winterdyk & Griffiths, 1984).

Studies Related to the Effects on Social Skills

There is strong evidence that pro-social skill deficiencies are related to disruptive and anti-social behavior and limit abilities to form close interpersonal relationships (Mathur & Rutherford, 1994). Delinquent behavior is often a manifestation of social skill deficits which can be changed by teaching alternate pro-social behaviors. Thus, most OBH and wilderness programs focus on the development of social skills, and research has examined the degree to which participants learn and apply these skills in post-treatment environments. Gibson (1981) determined that interpersonal competence of participants in an Outward Bound program was increased following the experience. Porter (1975) noted a decrease in defensiveness and a large increase in social acceptance. Kraus (1982) concluded that wilderness therapy aids emotionally disturbed adolescents in reaching various therapeutic goals, including a reduction in aggressiveness towards others. Weeks (1985) noted an improvement in participant interpersonal effectiveness in relating to others through learned social skills. In a more recent study, Sachs and Miller (1992) reported that a wilderness experience program had a positive effect on cooperative behavior exhibited in the school setting following completion of the wilderness program. It is notable that this finding was discovered through direct observation of behaviors in a school setting. Although most studies were anecdotal and acknowledged study limitations, the review of the effects of wilderness programs suggest that such programs influence the development of more socially adaptive and cooperative behavior.

Studies Related to the Effects on Substance Abuse

There are few studies reported in the literature on wilderness program effects on clients with histories of drug and alcohol abuse, nor are there many unpublished studies. Three studies report reduced substance abuse from treatment. Gillis and Simpson (1992) noted a positive behavior change and positive effect on relapse from an 8-week residential treatment program with a wilderness component for drug-abusing adolescents. Bennet et al. (1998) found that a therapeutic camping program was more effective at reducing the frequency of negative thoughts and reducing alcohol craving when compared with a residential drug and alcohol treatment model. They also noted a reduction in alcohol use 10 months after the program, with the comparison group reporting 69% abstinence, compared with the control group report of 42% abstinence. Russell and Phillips-Miller (2002) studied 12 case studies four months after completion of a wilderness program and found that three cases (25%) had self-reported that they had relapsed on drugs and alcohol, and which were corroborated with parent interviews, while the other nine (75%) had not relapsed. While these studies report positive results in treatment of substance abuse, the fact that there are only three highlight the lack of research in this area.

Studies Related to the Effects on Recidivism

A review of the criminology literature reveals only a few studies published on the effects of wilderness programs (not boot camps) on adolescent recidivism. A review of studies in the 1970s and 1980s linked wilderness programs with reduced recidivism, reduced frequency of deviant behaviors, and fewer arrests (Winterdyk & Griffiths, 1984). Greenwood and Turner (1987) compared 90 male graduates of the VisionQuest adjudicated program with 257 male juvenile delinquents who had been placed in other probation programs, and found that VisionQuest graduates had fewer arrests. Further evidence in support of VisionQuest's effectiveness is provided in a study by Goodstein and Sonthenhamer (1987) who found an arrest rate for VisionQuest graduates of 37 percent, compared to an arrest rate for control programs of 51 percent. A more recent study by Castellano and Soderstrom (1992) evaluated the effects of the Spectrum Wilderness Program, a 30-day high adventure wilderness program, on the number of post-program arrests. They found reduced arrests among graduates, which lasted for about one year after the program. At this point, the positive program results began to decay to the point where they were no longer apparent.

Motivation to Engage in Treatment

Most adolescents who enter wilderness programs have been coerced into treatment, do not want to be there, and many times are escorted to each facility by parents or a professional service. Consequently, they are extremely resistant to treatment and change. It has been suggested that in general, adolescents appear to exhibit less internal motivation to enter treatment because they have experienced fewer of the negative consequences of their drug and alcohol use (De Leon & Jainchill, 1986; Melnick, De Leon, Hawke, Jainchill, & Kressel, 1997). Therefore, adolescents have often been coerced into entering residential treatment by external influences (Pompi & Resnick, 1987). There are, however, no empirical studies that provide reliable estimates of the extent and type of coercion that occurs in the process (Winters, 1999[a]). Also, research has shown that coercion into treatment and low motivation to change provides a significant barrier to change (Prochaska & DiClemente, 1992). Despite this phenomenon, recent results suggest that OBH treatment appears to be effective at addressing this coercion into treatment and helping clients engage in making changes in their lives Russell, (2003[a]).

Research in the Outdoor Behavioral Healthcare Research Cooperative

The purpose of the Outdoor Behavioral Healthcare Research Cooperative (OBHRC) is to carry out a comprehensive research program to address specific questions asked by the outdoor behavioral healthcare (OBH) industry. OBHRC is a contractual arrangement between the Outdoor Behavioral Healthcare Industry Council (OBHIC) and the University of New Hampshire School of Health and Human Services. The OBHRC plan of work is guided by a "steering committee" of representatives from OBHIC member programs and UNH faculty. A peer review committee of scholars and practicing clinical psychologists review all proposals and publications from OBHRC. In addition to annual risk assessment monitoring for OBHIC programs, and maintaining an on-going database of programs operating in the United States, OBHRC has conducted studies focusing on assessment of treatment outcomes and the role aftercare plays in OBH treatment.

The first major outcome study of OBH treatment effectiveness was launched in May of 2000 and concluded in June 2001 with 1,600 parents and clients participating from eight OBH programs (Russell, 2003). A repeated measure, one-way ANOVA research design was used to assess treatment effectiveness on a census of clients at eight participating programs (Graziano & Raulin, 1997). Participants were surveyed using the Youth- Outcome Questionnaire (Y-OQ) and the Self Report Youth-Outcome Questionnaire (SR Y-OQ) (Burlingame, Wells, & Lambert, 1995) over a discrete time period of June 1, 2000 to December 1, 2000 to track their therapeutic progress in treatment.

The Y-OQ is a parent reported measure of a wide range of behaviors, situations, and moods which commonly apply to troubled teenagers, whereas the SR Y-OQ is the adolescent self-report version. Y-OQ also includes a brief prognosis questionnaire that assesses three primary areas of adolescent risk behaviors to determine the degree to which these factors may effect treatment outcome: (1) existence and severity of family history of mental illness, including both immediate and extended family; (2) current social environment, including integrity and stress on the family structure and socioeconomic status; and (3) the child or adolescent's own medical, developmental, and mental health history (Russell, 2003[a]; Wells, Burlingame, Lambert, Hoag, & Hope, 1996).

There were several implications reported in this study (Russell, 2003[a]). First, adolescent participation in OBH treatment reduced behavioral and emotional symptoms of clients immediately following treatment, as measured by both client self-report and parent assessments using the Y-OQ. Second, scores at 12 months suggested that clients maintained therapeutic progress initiated by treatment, and according to client self-report data, continued to improve. Third, subscale analysis offered insight into specific aspects of behavioral and emotional well-being that are potentially impacted by OBH treatment. Clients and parents showed agreement at discharge in assessing two subscales as being significantly improved: Behavioral Dysfunction (BD) and Critical Items (CI). BD measures a youth's ability to organize tasks, complete assignments, and handle frustration in different settings. The CI subscale measures critical issues such as obsessive-compulsive behavior, suicide, and eating disorder issues. These findings are consistent with the goals of OBH treatment: stabilizing adolescents behaviorally and emotionally and helping them address their patterns of problem behavior. At the 12 month follow-up assessment, Behavioral Dysfunction and Interpersonal Relations subscales were above their cutoff scores (meaning that clients had deteriorated on these issues past a point of normality) for both client self-report and parent assessment. This could reflect the difficulties that parents and adolescent clients have in trying to return to home, school and/or peer environments that, prior to treatment, may have perpetuated problem behaviors.

A subsequent follow-up study (Russell, 2004) contacted parents and adolescents 24 months after the completion of treatment to examine their well-being using a phone interview process. The responses by parents and adolescents suggested that the majority are doing well 24 months after treatment. Also, over 80% of parents and over 90% of youths contacted, believed that OBH treatment was effective two years after the process, offering a unique long-term perspective on evaluating the process. This addresses critiques of studies that conduct evaluations immediately after the program that lend themselves to "post-program-euphoria" and inflated evaluations of program and effects without seeing actual modified behavior or attitude (Hattie et al., 1997). The majority of parents believed that their son or daughter could not have begun their recovery without the initial impact of OBH treatment. This was also corroborated by youth responses, illustrated by this statement from a respondent who was doing "okay" and stated "yes, it opened my eyes to what I was doing from an objective angle and the fact that I needed to turn my life around" (Russell, 2004).

Qualitative assessments and scaled responses also suggested that former participants were doing well in some areas, and not so well in others. In task-oriented areas, like school and participating in appropriate leisure activities, they seemed to be doing relatively better than in staying out of trouble with the law and forming friendships. An important finding was the consistent responses of good to satisfactory communication between parents and youths, suggesting that the OBH process helped facilitate this enhanced communication. In the area of staying out of trouble with the law, respondents suggested youths were not doing as well, with a large number experiencing legal problems (60% of respondents reported some trouble with the law). Parents and youths reported mixed results when asked to evaluate the youth's ability to make friends and form friendships, with almost half citing this as a primary concern. This finding highlights the difficulties faced by youths who have gone through treatment of any kind and their attempts to establish identities, friendships, and lifestyles that are radically different than pretreatment. Many youths spoke of the difficulty of being social and shared a desire to "just blend in" with their peers. During this period following treatment, parents and youths also spoke of many ups and downs, which typify this developmental phase for youth in general. Their stories highlighted how difficult this process is for youth who are also struggling with mental, emotional or psychological disorders, which initiated their need for treatment (Russell, 2004).

Many parents and youths self-reported substance use during the follow-up period. The reality appears to be that most youths are still using substances, even if substance use was a primary focus of treatment (74% of youths in this sample). This is despite the fact that 84% of all youths utilized aftercare services, deemed to be a successful predictor of abstinence in follow-up studies of substance abusing youth (Blanz & Schmidt, 2000; Lash & Blosser, 1999). Though some parents reported that substance use was still a significant concern, they were in the minority. Many comments by parents and youths suggested that using was not perceived to be detrimental to well-being, and that use was more controlled and moderated. One parent stated: "He participates in all these parties, drinking parties, but there is no evidence that he is out of control." A youth, who stated that substance use was a focus of treatment, was asked if he was remaining sober and he replied: "Yes, I am sober, I just drink beer occasionally on weekends but I am careful not to drink too much." This finding highlights the difficulty in gauging appropriate treatment strategies for youths deemed to have substance use issues and how difficult it is to predict in adolescence who will carry substance use issues into adulthood (Winters, 1999[a]). Some researchers in substance use treatment claim a "harm reduction model" may be more appropriate when working with adolescents, reflecting attitudes that the majority of parents and youths in this study seem to have. This approach may be more aligned to OBH treatment philosophy as well. Harm reduction understands that addiction/substance use is a complex phenomenon and recognizes that many, if not most, people do not respond well to traditional models of treatment in which goals are predetermined by the therapist (authority figure). The harm reduction school (or "camp") believes that starting at the client's level (i.e., appreciating what changes he or she might be willing or wanting to make) is the key to alleviating or eradicating addictive behaviors (Tatarsky, 2002).

Aftercare is utilized by most youths in OBH treatment, and many of those who did not participate in aftercare stated that they wished that they had. Aftercare can range from the youth returning home to families and participating in outpatient treatment such as individual or group therapy, to attending a residential program with an educational and clinical focus. Parents and youths cited several reasons for this, including: (a) OBH treatment brought up several issues that still required professional care to resolve, (b) that progress had been made and the parents and OBH staff believed aftercare would facilitate the maintenance of this progress, and (c) that the youth needed an alternative environment so as to not return to old habits and patterns. Many parents believed that the experience was an effective assessment tool and impacted their child to recognize the need for change. This was also corroborated through youth reflection on the process. Youths and parents seem to disagree as to the need for and effectiveness of structured residential aftercare environments. One youth stated: "I hated it, didn't like the program, and all the stuff they made us do." Reflecting a more positive evaluation of residential aftercare placement, one youth stated: "Yes, it impacted me and opened my eyes to who I was and what I was doing." This disconnect between parent and youth evaluations of the need for aftercare is an interesting finding that may challenge OBH program staff to find ways to arrive at a consensus as to what both parties may need and want in aftercare situations. The perception that OBH treatment "fixes adolescents" and delivers from a wilderness experience a youth who is ready to return to peer, family, and school or work environments replete with new-found confidence was simply not supported in this study. Many youths required continued and ongoing treatment in a residential program to address issues raised in wilderness treatment.

Also of note in examining the transition to aftercare was the stated desire for parents to remain connected to OBH programs and staff and to have clearly established aftercare plans. Many parents cited the lack or absence of any plans and felt the programs had more of a responsibility to prepare their families for transition and posttreatment care. Several parents and youths could not recall an aftercare plan, and specifically stated that they had wished they had been able to more easily contact program staff. Parents that did have clear plans and resources for aftercare believed this was crucial for their children. Establishing networks and programs for parents that are affordable and accessible appears to be critical for OBH program effectiveness. This process helps programs to effectively provide primary care and assessment of clients and help families make successful transitions to aftercare situations. Parents identified barriers to placing their children in aftercare services as the excessive costs of many of these services (e.g., therapeutic boarding schools and residential treatment centers), lack of insurance coverage, and lack of knowledge of programs and services available.

Future Directions

OBH treatment is an emerging treatment type with an expanding research interest. Hopefully, future research will facilitate increased understanding of this promising treatment approach. Suggested areas for further research into OBH treatment include a more thorough understanding of the process elements that explain the variance in outcomes previously reported. Future research could also better identify for whom the intervention is most appropriate, using comparison studies between OBH treatment and outpatient, residential and in-home treatment. Because transition and aftercare is such an important factor, future research could also more clearly assess the role aftercare plays in maintaining therapeutic progress. In addition, cost effectiveness studies could be employed to compare the relative cost of OBH treatment to other approaches. It may also be useful to examine how OBH treatment helps families address relationship and communication issues that have been disrupted by previous problem behaviors and the process itself, which typically lasts up to 50 days and includes removing the adolescent from the family. How do programs specifically incorporate the family into treatment? What are the most effective strategies for accomplishing this? It has also been suggested that most clients who enter OBH treatment are resistant to the process (Russell & Phillips-Miller, 2002). Given that coercion into treatment may be a barrier to completing treatment and to embracing change (Prochaska & DiClemente, 1992), future research could more closely examine the degree to which wilderness therapy facilitates the transition from resistance to acceptance of a need for change. There are also no direct studies of the impact of coercion on treatment effects reported in the adolescent literature (Winters, 1999[a]). This would also seem like an important subject for future research.

Bibliography

Bandoroff, S. (1989). *Wilderness therapy for delinquent and pre-delinquent youth: A review of the literature.* (No. ERIC ED377428): University of South Carolina, Columbia.

Bandoroff, S., & Scherer, D. G. (1994). Wilderness family therapy: An innovative treatment approach for problem youth. *Journal of Child and Family Studies, 3*(2), 175-191.

Bandura, A. (1977). Self-efficacy: Toward a unifying theory for behavioral change. *Psychological Review, 84,* 191-215.

Bangert-Drowns, R. L. (1988). The effects of school-based substance abuse education: A meta-analysis. *Journal of Drug Education, 18,* 243-264.

Bennett, L., Cardone, S., & Jarczyk, K. (1998). Effects of a therapeutic camping program on addiction recovery: The Algonquin Haymarket relapse prevention program. *Journal Of Substance Abuse Treatment, 15*(5), 469-474.

Blanz, B., & Schmidt, M. H. (2000). Preconditions and outcome of inpatient treatment in child and adolescent psychiatry. *Journal of Child Psychology & Psychiatry & Allied Disciplines, 41*(6), 703-712.

Brand, D. (2001). A longitudinal study of the effects of a wilderness-enhanced program on behavior-disordered adolescents. *Australian Journal of Outdoor Education, 13*(6).

Brown, S. A., Stetson, B. A., & Beatty, P. A. (1989). Cognitive and behavioral features of adolescent coping in high risk drinking situations. *Journal of Addictive Behaviors, 14*(43-52).

Burlingame, G. M., Wells, M. G., & Lambert, M. J. (1995). *The Youth Outcome Questionnaire.* Stevenson, MD: American Professional Credentialing Services.

Burton, L. M. (1981). A critical analysis and review of the research on Outward Bound and related programs. *Dissertation Abstracts International, 47/04B* (University Microfilms No. AAC812247).

Cason, D. R., & Gillis, H. L. (1994). A meta-analysis of adventure programming with adolescents. *Journal of Experiential Education, 17,* 40-47.

Castellano, T. S., & Soderstrom, I. R. (1992). Therapeutic wilderness programs and juvenile recidivism: A program evaluation. *Journal of Offender Rehabilitation, 17*(3/4), 19-46.

Chatroux, N. C. (2001). *Wilderness therapy: A qualitative study of clinicians' perspectives.* Unpublished doctoral dissertation, California State University, Long Beach.

Clark. (2003). *The effects of wilderness therapy on the perceived psychosocial stressors, defense styles, dysfunctional personality patterns, clinical syndromes, and maladaptive behaviors of troubled adolescents.* Unpublished doctoral dissertation, George Fox University, Newburg, OR.

Crisp, S., & O'Donnell, D. (1997). *Wilderness adventure therapy in adolescent psychiatry.* Paper presented at the International Adventure Therapy Conference, Perth, Australia.

Davis-Berman, J., & Berman, D. S. (1994). Therapeutic wilderness programs: A national survey. *Journal of Experiential Education, 17*(2), 49-53.

De Leon, G., & Jainchill, N. (1986). Circumstance, motivation, readiness and suitability as correlates of treatment tensure. *Journal of Psychoactive Drugs, 18*(3), 203-208.

Easley, A. T., Passineau, J. T., & Driver, B. L. (1990). *The use of wilderness for personal growth, therapy, and education.* (No. General Technical Report RM-193). Fort Collins, CO: Rocky Mountain Forest and Range Experiment Station.

Edgmon, K. J. (2002). Therapeutic benefits of a wilderness therapy program and a therapeutic community program for troubled adolescents. *Dissertation Abstracts International: Section B: The Sciences & Engineering, 62*(10), 4781.

Erikson, E.H. (1963). *Childhood and society.* New York: Norton.

Ewert, A. (1983). *Outdoor adventure and self concept: A research analysis.* Eugene: University of Oregon: Center for Leisure Studies.

Ewert, A. (1987). Research in experiential education: An overview. *Journal of Experiential Education, 10*(2), 4-7.

Friese, G. T., Pittman, J. T., & Hendee, J. C. (1995). *Studies of the use of wilderness for personal growth, therapy, education, and leadership development: An annotation and evaluation.* Moscow, ID: Wilderness Research Center.

Gardner, C. C. (2000). *Woem in body in nature.* Unpublished Masters, California Institute of Integral Studies, San Francisco.

Gass, M. (1993). *Adventure Therapy: Therapeutic applications of adventure programming.* Dubuque, IA: Kendall/Hunt Publishing Co.

Gibson, P. (1981). *The effects of, and the correlates of success in a wilderness therapy program for problem youth.* Unpublished doctoral dissertation, Columbia University, New York.

Gibson, P. M. (1979). Therapeutic aspects of wilderness programs: A comprehensive literature review. *Therapeutic Recreation Journal, 13*(2), 21-33.

Gillis, H. L. (1992, 1992). *Therapeutic uses of adventure-challenge-outdoor-wilderness: Theory and research.* Paper presented at the Coalition for Education in the Outdoors, State University of New York.

Gillis, H. L., & Thomsen, D. (1996, 1997). *Research update of adventure therapy (1992-1995): Challenge activities and ropes courses, wilderness expeditions, and residential camping programs.* Paper presented at the Coalition for Education in the Outdoors, Martinsville, IN.

Goodstein, L., & Sonthenhamer, H. (1987). *A study of the impact of ten Pennsylvania placements on recidivism prepared for the Pennsylvania Juvenile Court Judges Commission.* (No. 7). Shippensburg, PA: Center for Juvenile Training and Research.

Graziano, A., & Raulin, M. (1997). *Research methods: A process of inquiry.* (3rd ed.). New York: Addison Wesley Longman.

Greenwood, P. W., & Turner, S. (1987). *The VisionQuest program: An evaluation* (No. R-3445-OJJDP). Santa Monica, CA: Rand Corporation.

Hagan, J. D. (2003). An alternative therapy for the behaviorally challenged youth: The efficacy of wilderness therapy programs. *Dissertation Abstracts International: Section B: The Sciences & Engineering, 63*(7), 3473.

Harter, S. (1999). *The construction of self.* New York: The Guilford Press.

Hattie, J., Marsh, H. W., Neill, J. T., & Richards, G. E. (1997). Adventure education and Outward Bound: Out-of-class experiences that make a lasting difference. *Review of Educational Research, 67*(1), 43-87.

Hazelworth, M. W., B. (1990). The effects of an outdoor adventure camp experience on self-concept. *Journal of Environmental Education, 21*(4), 33-37.

Howard, T. A. (1984). *Outward Bound in alcohol treatment in mental health. A compilation of literature.* Greenwich, CT: Outward Bound, Inc.

Jenkins, M. (2000). The hard way. *Outside, March,* 45-52.

Kelly, F., & Baer, D. (1968). *Outward Bound: an alternative to institutionalization for adolescent delinquent boys.* Boston: Fandel Press.

Kelly, F., & Baer, D. (1969). Jesness inventory and self-concept measures for delinquents before and after participation in Outward Bound. *Psychological Reports, (25),* 719-724.

Kimball, R. (1979). *Wilderness experience program. Final evaluation report.* (No. ERIC ED179327).

Kimball, R. (1983). The wilderness as therapy. *Journal of Experiential Education, 6*(3), 7-16.

Kleiber, L. C. (1993). *An experiential education program for at-risk youth in the Eagle County School District (CO).* University of Denver, CO.

Krakauer, J. (October 1995). Loving them to death. *Outside, (1)*15.

Kraus, I. W. (1982). *The effectiveness of wilderness therapy with emotionally disturbed adolescents.* Unpublished doctoral dissertation, Georgia State University.

Lambie, I., Hickling, L., Seymour, F., Simmonds, L., Robson, M., & Houlahan, C. (2000). Using wilderness therapy in treating adolescent sexual offenders. *Journal of Sexual Aggression, 5*(2), 99-117.

Lash, S., & Blosser, S. (1999). Increasing adherence to substance abuse aftercare therapy. *Journal of Substance Abuse Treatment, 16*(1), 55-61.

Levitt, L. (1982, July 8-9). *How effective is wilderness therapy: A critical review.* Paper presented at the Third Annual Conference for the Wilderness Psychology Group, Morgantown, WV.

Loughmiller, C. (1965). *Wilderness road.* Austin, TX: Hogg Foundation for Mental Health.

Marsh, H., Richards, G., & Barnes, J. (1984). Multi-dimensional self-concepts: The effects of participation in an Outward Bound program. *Journal of Personality and Social Psychology, 50*(1), 195-204.

Marsh, H. W. R., G. (1990). Self-other agreement and self-other differences on multidimensional self-concept ratings. *Australian Journal of Psychology, 42*(1), 31-45.

Martinez, M. C. (2002). *A wilderness therapy program for a diverse group of at risk adolescent boys. Changes in self esteem and locus of control and their relationship to group affiliation.* Unpublished doctoral dissertation, Alliant International University, San Francisco.

Mathur, S. R., & Rutherford, R. B. (1994). Teaching conversational social skills to delinquent youth. *Behavioral Disorders, (19)*, 294-305.

McCord, D. M. (1995). Toward a typology of wilderness-based residential treatment program participants. *Residential Treatment for Children and Youth, 12*(4), 51-60.

McNamara, D. N. (2002). Adventure-based programming: Analysis of therapeutic benefits with children of abuse and neglect. *Dissertation Abstracts International Section A: Humanities & Social Sciences, 62*(7), 2353.

Melnick, G., De Leon, G., Hawke, J., Jainchill, N., & Kressel, D. (1997). Motivation and readiness for therapeutic community treatment among adolescents and adult substance abusers. *American Journal of Drug and Alcohol Abuse, 23*(4), 485-506.

Moote, G. T., & Wadarski, J. S. (1997). The acquisition of life skills through adventure-based activities and programs: A review of the literature. *Adolescence, 32*(125), 143-167.

Orren, P. M. (2003). *The effects of brief wilderness programs in relation to adolescents participants' ethnicity.*, Alliant International University, San Francisco.

Parzen, M. D. (2001). 'Culturally appropriate' mental health care: Wilderness therapy and Navajo youth. *Dissertation Abstracts International Section A: Humanities & Social Sciences, 62*(1), 226.

Pommier, J. H. (1994). *Experiential education therapy plus family training: Outward Bounds School's efficacy with status offenders.*, Texas A & M, College Station.

Pompi, K. F., & Resnick, J. (1987). Retention in a therapeutic community for court-referred adolescents and young adults. *American Journal of Drug and Alcohol Abuse, 13*(3), 309-325.

Porter, W. (1975). *The development and evaluation of a therapeutic wilderness program for youth.* Unpublished master's thesis, University of Denver, Denver, CO.

Prochaska, J. O., & DiClemente, C. C. (1992). Stages of change in the modification of problem behaviors. In M. Hersen, R. M. Eisler & P. M. Miller (Eds.), *Progress in behavior modification.* (pp. 184-214). Sycamore, IL: Sycamore Press.

Russell, K. C. (1999). *Theoretical basis, process, and reported outcomes of wilderness therapy as an intervention and treatment for problem behavior in adolescents.* Unpublished doctoral dissertation, University of Idaho, Moscow, ID.

Russell, K. C. (2001). What is wilderness therapy? *Journal of Experiential Education, 24*(2), 70-79.

Russell, K. C. (2003[a]). An assessment of outcomes in outdoor behavioral healthcare treatment. *Child and Youth Care Forum, 32*(6), 355-381.

Russell, K. C. (2003[b]). A nation-wide survey of outdoor behavioral healthcare programs for adolescents with problem behaviors. *Journal of Experiential Education, 25*(3), 322-331.

Russell, K. C. (2004). *Two-years later: A qualitative assessment of youth well-being and the role of aftercare in outdoor behavioral healthcare treatment.* (No. 1). Durham, NH: University of New Hampshire School of Health and Human Services.

Russell, K. C., Hendee, J., & Cooke, S. (1998). The potential social and economic contributions of Wilderness Discovery as an adjunct to the Federal Job Corps program. *International Journal of Wilderness, 4*(3), 32-38.

Russell, K. C., & Phillips-Miller, D. (2002). Perspectives on the wilderness therapy process and its relation to outcome. *Child and Youth Care Forum, 31*(6), 415-437.

Sachs, J. J., & Miller, S. R. (1992). The impact of a wilderness experience on the social interactions and social expectations of behaviorally disordered adolescents. *Behavioral Disorders, 17*(2), 89-98.

Tatarsky, A. (2002). *Harm reduction psychotherapy: A new treatment for drug and alcohol problems.* Northvale, NJ: Jason Aronson.

Vogl, R. L. V., S. (1990). *The effectiveness of wilderness education: a review and evaluation.*

Webb, L. (2001). *Therapists' perceptions of wilderness therapy for adolescents.* Unpublished doctoral dissertation, California State University, Long Beach.

Weeks, S. (1985). *The effects of Sierra II, an adventure probation program, upon selected behavioral variables of adolescent juvenile delinquents.* Unpublished doctoral dissertation, University of Colorado, Boulder.

Wells, M., Burlingame, G., Lambert, M., Hoag, M., & Hope, C. (1996). Conceptualization and measurement of patient change during psychotherapy: Development of the outcome questionnaire and the youth outcome questionnaire. *Psychotherapy, 33*(2), 275-283.

Winterdyk, J., & Griffiths, C. (1984). Wilderness experience programs: reforming delinquents or beating around the bush? *Juvenile and Family Court Journal, Fall,* 35-44.

Winters, K. C. (1999a). Treating adolescents with substance use disorders: An overview of practice issues and outcomes. *Substance Abuse, 20*(4), 203-225.

Winters, K. C., Latimer, W.W., & Stinchfield, R. (1997). Examining psychosocial correlates of drug involvement among clinic referred youth. *Journal of Child and Adolescent Substance Abuse, 9*(1), 1-17.

Winters, K. C. L., W. L.; Stinchfield, R. D. (1999b). Adolescent treatment. In R. E. Tarter, R. T. Ammerman & P. Ott (Eds.), *Sourcebook on substance abuse: Etiology, epidemiology, assessment and treatment.* New York: Allyn and Bacon.

Wright, A. (1982). *Therapeutic potential of Outward Bound process: An evaluation of a treatment program for juvenile delinquents.* Unpublished doctoral dissertation, Pennsylvania State University, College Station.

Author's Biography

Keith C. Russell, Ph.D., *is the graduate coordinator of the Outdoor Education program at the University of New Hampshire and the Director of the Outdoor Behavioral Healthcare Research Cooperative (OBHRC) in Durham, New Hampshire USA. Research emphasis includes the design, implementation, and evaluation of wilderness treatment programs, the study of human-nature relationships, the therapeutic values of natural environments, and international protected area management. He teaches courses in statistics, research methods, philosophy and theory of outdoor education, and wilderness leadership for personal growth and therapy. He has been a wilderness educator for more than 15 years in the United States, Mexico, Costa Rica, and New Zealand.*

Correspondence

> *Keith C. Russell, Ph.D.*
> *Assistant Professor in Outdoor Education*
> *Director, Outdoor Behavioral Healthcare Research Cooperative*
> *University of New Hampshire*
> *NH Hall Room 210*
> *Durham, NH 03824 USA*
> *Tel: (603) 862-3047*
> *Fax: (603) 862-0154*
> *Email*: keith.russell@unh.edu

Adventure Development Counselling Research Study: Some "Hows" and "Whys" of Doing Research

Elaine Mossman and Colin Goldthorpe

■■■

Engaging in research to help validate adventure/wilderness therapy (AT/WT) interventions is essential if these services are to be recognized by funders and clients as effective forms of therapy. The aim of this paper is to provide an example of how such research can be conducted, and to show the value of such research to AT/WT programme providers. To achieve this objective, this paper will present the development and findings of the Adventure Development Counselling (ADC) Research Study.

■■■

The ADC Research Study evaluated the outcomes and processes of a community-based multi-modal adolescent mental health programme, known as the "Adventure Development Counselling" programme. This programme integrates individual and family therapy with a 9-day, group wilderness therapy experience. The research methodology adopted combined quantitative and qualitative methods.

The quantitative analysis was able to show that adolescents who participated in an ADC programme achieved statistically and clinically significant improvements in their mental health, and that these improvements were maintained 6 months following completion of the ADC programme. Results are discussed in relation to securing programme funding. Arguments are put forward regarding the value of utilizing widely used instruments with established validity and reliability. The qualitative enquiry provided evidence with which the AT/WT field can promote itself as an effective and (importantly for younger clients) enjoyable alternative to traditional forms of intensive residential therapy.

Background

The Adventure Development Counselling programme has been committed to a programme of research since it first commenced operation over 10 years ago. During this time, programme staff have engaged in an evaluation process that was strongly influenced by the principles of action research. This process consisted of an independent evaluator regularly seeking assistance from the youth, their families, referral agents and other members of the community regarding their perceptions of the value of the programme, and their ideas for improvement. The information gathered was then fed back to programme staff to be incorporated into further programme development, and the cycle was then repeated. This approach has been invaluable in helping to develop and refine the effectiveness of the programme. However, with the current environment of scarce funding and increased accountability, it was recognized that a more formalized type of research was required to demonstrate the clinical effectiveness of the programme. To this end the Adventure Development Counselling Research Study was initiated with the following objectives: (a) To investigate whether ADC clients exhibit statistically and clinically significant improvements in their mental health following programme participation, (b) To identify client characteristics associated with completion of the programme and improved outcomes, and (c) To study effects of the ADC approaches and programme content on individual participants.

In addition to these objectives, the needs of the different stakeholders were also considered. These included, for the funders, providing information on the effectiveness of the programme, in terms of clinical outcomes, measured with established, valid and reliable instruments; for the programme providers, providing information useful for programme development but without intruding onto the operational processes of the programme itself and finally because the principle researcher was to use the research project as the basis of a Ph.D., the study needed to be sufficiently rigorous to meet the academic requirements of the university doctoral research committee.

The Adventure Development Counselling Programme

The programme intervention to be researched was the Adventure Development Counselling programme. ADC has been in operation for over 10 years, and has worked with over 700 young people and their families from a range of ethnic groups. The programme is funded by New Zealand government regional health funding. The young clients are referred from multiple sources for help with alcohol and drug problems and/or other mental health issues. Each programme is on average six months duration. Clients are aged between 13 and 18 years, and typically receive one hour of individual or family therapy each week with a registered psychologist or counsellor, totalling an average of 20 contact hours. In addition, midway through the counselling process, clients participate as a group in a short nine day intensive group wilderness therapy experience in the Southern Alps. Finally, there is a follow-up period of approximately three months involving phone contacts and additional support as required.

The programme uses a systemic-based model to work with the youth, incorporating systems of influence such as family, school, peers, and community. Each programme is individually tailored to the needs and goals of the young person and their family. Within this model ADC counsellors use a range of therapeutic approaches including Multi-Systemic Therapy, Motivational Interviewing, Cognitive Behavioural approaches, Narrative Therapy, Just Therapy, Brief Therapy and Ecopsychology. The focus in most cases is on harm minimization, developing independence through mobilizing the strengths of the young person, and those of their family and other elements of the community. The nine day period of wilderness therapy, known as the "Journey" is strongly focused on achieving therapeutic outcomes. Journey activities include daily goal setting, sessions of group therapy, rock climbing, wilderness tramps, individual reflection times, cooperative group problem solving activities, together with the events arising from day to day living. All are intentionally utilized to achieve individual and group therapeutic goals.

Methodology

A mixed-methods research design incorporating qualitative and quantitative methods was adopted. The quantitative approach entailed a single group investigation of 89 adolescents (mean age=14.5 years). These were the sum of all clients referred to ADC during July 1999 to December 2000. They were assessed using a series of standardized psychometric instruments, immediately prior to, immediately after, and again six months following participation on an ADC programme. The selection of research instruments involved considerable discussion with the ADC counsellors about how to collect valid and reliable data in a way that the counsellors felt would not adversely affect the development of therapeutic relationships with their client. Concern over unnecessary duplication of information collected, and unacceptable delays before counselling could begin were addressed.

The primary measure of treatment outcome was a behavioural symptom checklist known as the Youth Self-Report (YSR; Achenbach, 1991[a]) together with the parallel parent/caregiver version the Child Behaviour Checklist (CBCL; Achenbach, 1991[b]). This instrument was chosen because of its established validity and reliability, availability of norm data, and its wide use internationally, allowing comparisons to be made across studies. Other measures included a test of family functioning (BFAM; Skinner, Steinhauer,

& Santa-Barbara, 1995), counsellor ratings of general functioning (CGAS; Shaffer, Gould, Brasic, Ambrosini, Fisher, Bird, & Aluwahlia, 1983), a DSM-IV based semi-structured diagnostic interview to assess substance abuse/dependency (K-Sads; Kaufman, Birmaher, Brent, Flynn, Moreci, Williamson, & Ryan, 1997), together with current and retrospective self-reports of alcohol and drug consumption, and client ratings of progress on individual treatment goals (these were goals that were personally meaning-ful to the young person, typically around their substance use, anger man-agement, school performance, family or peer relationships). Finally counsel-lors filled out a client characteristic form on demographic and other relevant information. The assessment was able to be spread over the first three coun-selling sessions, so as not to become the major focus of any one session, and resulted in data being collected on multiple indicators of treatment outcome from multiple informants (i.e., youth, parents, and counsellors).

Analyses

The following analyses were carried out on the screened data. Repeated measures analysis of variance (ANOVA) assessed subjects' treat-ment outcome across the three time points. Subject characteristics and con-textual variables were then subjected to direct discriminant functional analysis and standard multiple regression analysis to predict treatment completion and successful outcomes.

To complement the above quantitative analysis, an in depth qualita-tive analysis was also undertaken with clients from one programme. This entailed a combination of participant observation and interviews. The researcher observed a group of clients (n=12) as they progressed through the programme, with particular attention given to their participation on the nine day wilderness-based "Journey." Interviews were conducted with clients and, where possible, their counsellor, parents/caregivers and referral agency. Data generated by this approach was transcribed verbatim and imported into a qualitative data analysis software programme where it was content-analyzed using a general inductive approach. This analysis explored the effect of the different ADC approaches and programme con-tent on this adolescent population.

Results

During the period of data collection, a total of 89 youth were referred onto the ADC programme and pretest data was collected from 92% (n=81). Fifty-three of these clients completed the programme to their counsellors satisfaction. This rate of completion (65%) is similar to other community-based adolescent treatment programmes (Fonagy & Target, 1994; Kazdin & Wassel, 2000). Of the clients who completed the programme, post-test data was collected from 89% (n=47), and 6-month follow-up data was collected from 79% of these clients (n=42). These represent reasonable response rates, especially considering this was a real life community-based intervention, rather than a research trial in a university/laboratory setting.

Descriptive analysis of the data provided a profile of ADC clients and hence, the research sample. This descriptive information was important for several reasons; it provided detailed data on the characteristics of the programme and its clients in a more comprehensive manner than had previously been available. Such information is useful for programme auditing and ensuring services provided meet the needs of the client population being referred. Much of this same data was also used as predictor variables to investigate which populations are best served by the programme. Finally, such data allows appropriate comparisons of this project's results to be made to other programmes. This is particularly important with adventure/wilderness therapy programmes that can vary considerably in the content, style of delivery and target population. A selection of this data describing some of the demographic characteristics of the research sample appears in Table 1.

Table 1
Demographic Information on Clients Accepted on to the ADC Programme (n=89)

Variable		n	%
Gender	Male	61	68.5
	Female	28	31.5
Ethnicity[a]	NZ European	64	71.9
	Maori	20	22.5
	Pacific Island	3	3.4
	Other	2	2.2
Living Situation	Two caregivers (family)	36	40.5
	Single caregiver (family)	44	49.4
	Caregivers (non family)	5	5.6
	Other	4	4.5
Attending School		73	82.0

[a]Ethnicity was based on clients and their families own classification

There were several measures collected that provide a profile of the clinical status of the ADC clients. These included counsellor ratings of global functioning (CGAS), youth and parent reporting of problem behaviour (YSR/CBCL), and DSM-IV diagnosis of substance use disorder (K-Sads). An example of this data appears in Figure 1, which shows YSR/CBCL total problem behaviour, internalizing behaviour (anxiety/depression, withdrawn and somatic complaints) and externalizing behaviour (aggression and delinquency) as reported by the youth and their parents. Also marked on the graphs are what are considered to be the borderline clinical and clinical cut-off points. The authors of the YSR/CBCL derived the cut-off points from analysis of North American normative and clinically referred samples: T-scores falling between 60 and 63 are considered borderline clinical, and those above 63 are considered clinical (Achenbach, 1991[ab]). All YSR raw data was converted to T-Scores to allow for direct comparison across different scales. T-Scores are standardized scores that have a mean of 50 and a standard deviation of 10. As can be seen from the graphs, parents and youth reported more externalizing behaviour than internalizing behaviour. Parents tended to report higher levels of severity across all three measures than did the youth, with the exception of female youth reporting of total problem behaviour. According to the youth and parent reports, the ADC clients would be considered either borderline clinical or clinical on all measures, except for youth reports of internal behaviour which fell just below the borderline clinical cut-off point. The T-Scores of the referred ADC clients suggested that as a group they had more severe symptoms than

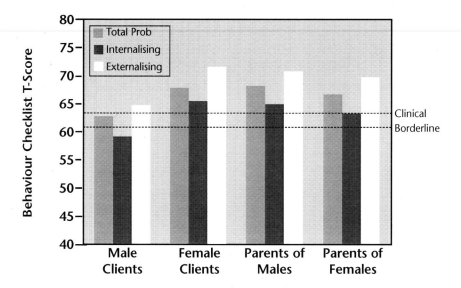

NB: Higher scores represent greater dysfunction

Figure 1. **Pre-Programme Profiles of Total Problem Behaviour, Internalising and Externalising Behaviour Reported by the ADC Clients (n=81) and their Parents (n=63).**

would be found in 90% of adolescents (based on a U.S. adolescent representative sample; Achenbach, 1991[a]). The checklists also provide scores on eight sub-scales of syndromes of behaviour (withdrawn, somatic complaints, anxious/depressed, social problems, attention problems, thought problems, aggression and delinquency); the sub-scale with the highest elevation (greatest degree of severity) for each individual has been referred to as the 'target behaviour' (Weiss, Cartron, Harris, & Phung, 1999). The groups average T-Score for target behaviour was 73.5 (SD=7.9) as reported by the youth, while according to their parents reports it was 76.5 (SD=8.8). These scores suggested that on target behaviour the ADC clients have more extreme symptoms than are found in 98% of adolescents (T-Score of over 70, based on a North American normative sample; Achenbach, 1991[ab]).

Objective one: Do clients show improvement in mental health?

To determine the short- and long-term impact of the ADC programme on its clients, a series of repeated measures ANOVAs were conducted on measures of treatment outcome. It should be noted that the following results reflect the impact of the complete 6-month ADC programme, of which the nine days of the wilderness therapy were just one component.

Figure 2 shows the results of the YSR analysis which shows that there was an improvement (reduction in problem behaviour) from pre to post programme, with further improvements from post programme to follow-up. These improvements were found to be at a statistically significant level across the duration of the programme (total problem behaviour ($F(2,82)=56.8$, $p<0.000$), internalizing behaviour ($F(2,82)=41.7$, $p<0.001$) and externalizing behaviour ($F(2,82)=49.8$, $p<0.001$)). The groups T-scores for total problem behaviour and externalizing behaviour moved from the clinical range to the non-clinical range and internalizing behaviour moved from the borderline clinical range to the non-clinical range (Achenbach, 1991[ab]). Therefore, the results indicated that as well as a statistically significant improvement, there was also a clinically significant improvement.

Post-hoc pair-wise comparisons (with Bonferonni adjustment) showed all pre to post improvements were statistically significant ($p<0.01$). Further improvements post programme to follow-up were also statistically significant for total problem behaviour and internalizing behaviour ($p<0.05$). CBCL (parent reports), although not shown here, mirrored the youth results, also finding statistically and clinically significant improvement following participation on the ADC programme.

Other treatment outcome results are shown in Table 2. All measures of treatment outcome showed statistically significant improvements following participation. There was, however, some degree of relapse observed at 6-month follow-up on two measures, parent ratings of family functioning and

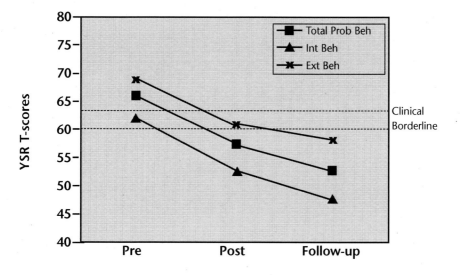

NB: Higher scores represent greater dysfunction.

Figure 2. Youth Self-Report Problem Behaviour (YSR) Following Participation on the ADC Programme (n=42).

client ratings of individual treatment goals.

The final treatment outcome measure was substance use. This proved a difficult measure to assess and analyze. The inclusion of retrospective reporting of pre-programme substance use revealed some interesting results. Youth reported higher levels of pre-programme substance use after they had completed the programme than what they were prepared to report at the start of treatment. Clients and ADC counsellors indicated that an explanation for this was that at the start of the programme, clients lacked a trusting relationship with their counsellor and were, therefore, less likely to be honest about their true levels of consumption. Abnormalities in the distribution of the substance use data meant that non parametric statistical tests were the most appropriate. Analyses of average quantities of alcohol consumption and frequency of cannabis use were carried out using Wilcoxon Matched Pairs tests. When the retrospective reports (post programme ratings) were used, it was found that consumption levels remained significantly lower than pre-programme levels for both alcohol (χ^2=16.87, p<0.05) and cannabis (χ^2 =22.71, p <0.001), although there was some relapse following completion of the programme. It was also noted that immediately following completion only 15.6% still met the criteria for a DSM-IV substance use disorder, compared to 56.5% at the start of the programme.

Table 2.
Treatment Outcome Results Following Participation on ADC Programme

Variable	Pre		Post		Follow-up		Probability
	M	SD	M	SD	M	SD	
CGAS	54.0	7.9	67.4	9.1	–	–	t=8.74 ***
BFAM (youth)	57.8	12.9	52.3	9.6	51.9	9.6	F=12.7***
BFAM (parents)	57.4	12.9	52.0	12.0	56.1	15.2	F=4.5*
Treatment Goals	3.7	1.6	8.0	1.6	7.5	1.8	F=87.95***

*= p<.05; **= p<.01; *** p<.001

Objective two: What client and programme factors are associated with successful outcomes?

To explore what client characteristics might be associated with successful treatment outcomes, two sets of analyses were carried out. First, a direct discriminant function analysis was carried out to investigate what factors could significantly predict whether the clients completed the programme (i.e., predicting whether clients belonged to the group who completed the programme [n=54] or to the group who terminated the programme early [n=35]). Factors that were considered as predictor variables were those individual and contextual factors found by other adolescent counselling research studies, to be associated with programme completion (Kazdin & Mazurick, 1994; Kazdin, Holland & Crowley, 1997; Pelkonen, Marttuenen, Laippala & Lonnqvist, 2000). These included 'individual client characteristics' such as age, gender, number and severity of problem behaviours, age of onset, physical health and criminal behaviour and 'contextual variables' such as family functioning, living situation, status of school attendance, gang involvement, parental history of antisocial behaviour and/or mental health issues, family social economic status, and number of previous interventions.

Results of this study found that programme completion was significantly associated with parental reporting of less serious CBCL total problem behaviour and clients who had participated in a fewer number of previous interventions (DFA=82.3% correct classification; _2=11.87; p<0.01).

The second analysis was a standard multiple regression to explore factors significantly associated with the most successful treatment outcomes of those who completed the ADC programme. The measure of treatment outcome was the difference between pre-test scores and post-test/follow-up scores of YSR total problem behaviour as reported by the youth, with high scores representing the greatest improvements in treatment outcome. To convert these difference scores to standardized z scores, they were divided by the groups pre-programme standard deviation. As with the previous analysis, variables that were considered as independent variables were individual and contextual factors that had been found in other adolescent counselling research studies to be associated with treatment outcome (Fonagy & Target, 1994; Phillips, Hargis, Kramer, Lensing, Taylor, & Burns, 2000; Weisz, Weiss, Han, Granger & Morton, 1995). Predictor variables included 'individual client characteristics' of number and severity of problem behaviours, age of onset, presence of internalizing disorders, level of substance use and number of previous interventions; 'contextual variables' such as family functioning, parental/caregiver support, living situation, status of school attendance, parental history of antisocial behaviour and/or mental health issues, family social economic status and number of concurrent agencies and services involved with the young person; and also 'treatment variables' of total number of counselling sessions, length of treatment, counsellor age and experience.

The multiple regression analysis was able to find significant associations between dependent variables and successful treatment outcome at post programme ($\underline{R}$=.54; $\underline{p}$<0.01) and at follow-up ($\underline{R}$=.70; $\underline{p}$<0.001). Youth who had the greatest improvements in YSR total problem behaviour were those who reported higher levels of severity in pre-programme total problem behaviour, had parents who were involved in post programme assessment and youth who had contact with fewer agencies.

Objective three: What did the participants find most helpful about the ADC programme?

Preliminarily findings from the qualitative data analysis found that ADC clients' talked of three main categories of factors that they felt had been useful in helping them to make positive changes. These were (a) "personal" factors related to their own motivation, expectations and understanding; (b) "counsellor" factors related to the clients feeling like they were able to trust, respect, and have confidence in their counsellor; and (c) "programme" factors related to the content and counselling approaches used in the programme. A particular emphasis was given to the wilderness therapy component, known as the "Journey". As it is beyond the scope of this paper to report on all these factors, the results reported will be limited to the area of most relevance to these proceedings, the wilderness therapy component.

The first point to note is that the Journey generated the most enthusiastic responses from the youth. All the youth interviewed spoke positively about the Journey and how helpful it had been. A common theme that emerged was that it had been a "challenging" but most definitely a "fun" experience. Nearly two thirds of the clients identified the Journey as the single most helpful part of the ADC programme. A common misunderstanding of AT/WT interventions is that they consist simply of participation in outdoor activities providing a recreational experience that is in someway beneficial, not really intentional therapy. However, when asked to describe how the Journey differed from the one-hour-a-week community-based counselling they received, one youth replied: "I wouldn't compare them cause they were just the same."

The ADC participants were asked to describe how the Journey had been helpful to them. The young clients talked of several aspects, including "group factors" such as being able to share similar experiences with other members of the group, and how interactions with other group members had increased their confidence, in particular to be able to speak up in front of people and to be able to make new friends.

"Environment factors" such as the effect of being in a different environment away from everyday distractions and problems, were mentioned by several participants as helping them to think more objectively about things. For a few clients the impact of the natural environment itself was significant. "I felt that I changed partly as a result of just being in such a beautiful place, being in nature, breathing clean air, the pure water, and being surrounded by the mountains."

The "intensity factor" of the wilderness experience was also mentioned by many as being a key factor. They described how the 9-day period was helpful, enabling them to work progressively each day on their therapeutic goals:

> ... cause you've got your hour counselling [community-based coun-
> selling]..., and then you just go back into that environment again and
> you just start it [the problem] all up again, unless you've got major
> will power. But then with the Journey you're there for the whole week
> and then by the end of that, by the end of those nine days you've
> adjusted to it like, you go home and you're still the same [maintained
> changes], that's why it was better...I think it helps doing it everyday
> the way we did.

In regards to the planned activities that make up the Journey, the youth talked about the games and problem solving activities as being "fun," but for achieving therapeutic outcomes, they talked about what the research referred to as "real" activities, as having more of an impact. Real activities included climbing up a rock face and the 3-day walking/camping expedition. Completing these activities appeared to generate strong emotional responses. However, the value of a "fun" experience that the games and problem solving activities contribute to, together with the building of group cohesion, should not be underestimated. Youth spoke of the reason why they would recommend the programme to others was because "it helped you make changes but was fun too". Providing an effective but fun treatment programme may prove to be valuable in addressing concerns over the low-help seeking behaviour among adolescents with mental health concerns (Horwood & Fergusson, 1998).

In summing up how important the Journey component of the ADC programme was, one client used the following metaphor to explain:

> Like on the Journey we talked about carrying around this big heavy pack and how it was good to get rid of the heavy load, and to me [community-based] counselling was like throwing out small stones but on the Journey you got to throw out big stones.

It appeared that the ADC participants experienced the Journey as a more intense form of therapy than their regular counselling, and that although it was challenging, it was definitely a "fun" experience.

Discussion and Conclusions

The findings of this project will be briefly reviewed with particular attention given to the benefit to programme providers of the different types of research methods and their corresponding findings.

The quantitative analysis that used established standardized instruments had several advantages. The profiles achieved through descriptive analysis of such data enabled the ADC programme to reassure funders that the programme worked with the type of clients for whom funding had been prioritized (i.e., youth with serious and complex mental health problems). The New Zealand government's National Mental Health Strategy requires mental health services to be delivered to the 3% of 0-19 year olds who at any given time are most severely affected by mental illness (Mental Health Commission, 1999). However, the number of such services presently provided in New Zealand falls below targeted levels. The ADC programme can, therefore, use these findings as evidence that they are contributing to the supply of services to an identified priority population. This places the programme in a good position to continue to receive funding.

The value of the Achenbach behaviour checklists, the YSR and CBCL, with their published norms and clinical cut-off points that come with the scales had several other advantages. Using these norms and clinical cut-off points, the ADC programme was able to show that there had been 'clinical' as well as 'statistically' significant improvements in their clients' mental health. In terms of clinical significance, Thomson (2002) suggested the ultimate standard is whether the treated individuals as a group are indistinguishable from a normal population. The published norms of the YSR/CBCL allowed for a test of equivalency (Kendall, Gracia, Nath &

Sheldrick, 1999) to be calculated. This revealed that as a group ADC clients were clinically equivalent to normative sample on total problem behaviour post-programme and at follow up. Without the benefit of a control group this was a useful test in estimating the effectiveness of the programme. Further, the wide use of the YSR/CBCL in adolescent psychotherapy research provided the benefit of being able to draw from previous studies in the interpretation of this study's results. The development of new instruments specific to AT/WT programmes has been discussed within the field. However, the points made above support the use of existing standardized instruments. A further benefit of using well-recognized standardized instruments, is they may assist AT/WT programmes to demonstrate that they can produce outcomes on par with other well-established adolescent psychotherapy treatments.

The findings of the treatment outcome evaluation are vital to programme providers. They allow the programme staff to see what they are doing right and what areas, if any, they can improve on. They also provide valuable evidence of effectiveness to prospective clients and funding agencies.

Exploring who the programme is most effective for, enables individuals to be matched to programmes, and allows limited resources for such programmes to be maximized. It can also provide information to programme providers on how they may need to alter their programme to meet the specific needs of certain types of clients. However, the difficulty of determining the type of clients for whom a specific programme may be most effective, was revealed in the multiple regression and discriminant functional analyses. While the variables of problem severity, previous exposure to treatment, parental support and number of agencies involved with the young person significantly predicted either those who completed the ADC programme or who had the greatest outcomes, there was still a large proportion of variance unaccounted for (51-82%). Perhaps some of the more meaningful results to the adventure/wilderness therapy field are in relation to those variables that were not found to predict treatment outcome. Variables such as age, gender and ethnicity did not predict treatment outcome suggesting that this programme was equally effective across these different groups. This is an area of research which is complex and requires further study.

From a methodological point of view the results of this study highlighted the importance of collecting data from multiple informants. There were seemingly contradictory results depending on either youth or parent reporting. In terms of the problem severity, programme completion was associated with clients with less severe total problem behaviour (as reported by parents) whilst the most successful treatment outcomes were associated with the youth with greater problem severity (as reported by the youth). This suggests different results may be found depending on whether parent or youth reports are used, and careful consideration should be given when interpreting results that do not include both types of informants.

The qualitative methods were able to address some of the areas of weaknesses inherent in quantitative analysis. The qualitative analysis was inductive, and allowed for data to be collected on any/all aspects that the participants felt were important, rather than just those preselected by the researcher as in the quantitative analysis. The qualitative analyses were also able to account for individual differences that are typically masked in statistical analysis of the grouped quantitative data. Indeed, results suggested that different elements were significant for different individuals as has been found previously in research on other adventure based programmes (Mossman, 1997). Such methods were also able to explore from the perspective of the participants, the impact of the various programme processes and to compare different programme components.

Findings from the qualitative data analysis suggested that the ADC clients experienced the wilderness therapy as a similar "therapeutic" experience to their regular community-based counselling, but that it was more intensive and challenging, and provided the opportunity for greater therapeutic gains. Aspects of the wilderness therapy that they found helpful, included the interactions among the group, and being in a natural and beautiful environment that was removed from everyday distractions and problems. The games and group problem solving activities were perceived as "fun," while a therapeutic impact was achieved from "real" activities such as rock climbing and the expedition. The results of the qualitative analysis are particularly important in relation to programme development, helping to understand from the perspective of the clients, the relative importance of different elements of the programme.

It is important to recognize several limitations of this study. Without the use of a comparison group and random assignment, the degree to which treatment outcomes can be directly attributed to participation in the ADC programme and generalized to other youth with mental health concerns are limited. Results achieved from this study are only applicable to the specific ADC counsellors who were employed during the period of study, and to the sample of youth who completed the ADC programme during this period. There are also limitations imposed by the validity and reliability issues of self-report measures that were utilized in the study. For example, there were discrepancies found in the youths' reports of alcohol and drug consumption depending on the timing of the data collection. Youth reported higher levels of pre-programme consumption when asked retrospectively (post-programme) about their pre-programme patterns of use. There were also the discrepancies mentioned above according to informants, with differences in parental and youth reports of problem severity. Finally, the norm data of the YSR/CBCL instruments are based on North American samples, and although found to be applicable in many other countries (Achenbach, 1991[b]), have not been evaluated against a New Zealand population.

In conclusion, this paper has shown some of the benefits to programme providers that can be achieved through engaging in evaluative research. Benefits include helping to secure funding, gaining credibility to adventure/wilderness therapy interventions, and assisting programme providers to make decisions in relation to programme development. This paper also provides information on an innovative adventure/wilderness therapy-based programme. It demonstrates that the ADC programme provides a promising alternative to other well-established adolescent mental health programmes, achieving an intensive but fun therapeutic experience.

References

Achenbach, T. (1991)[a]. *Manual for the Youth Self-Report and 1991 Profile.* Burlington, VT: University of Vermont Department of Psychiatry.

Achenbach, T. (1991)[b]. *Manual for the Child Behavior Checklist/4-10 and 1991 Profile.* Burlington, VT: University of Vermont Department of Psychiatry.

Fonagy, P., & Target, M. (1994). The efficacy of psychoanalysis for children with disruptive disorders. *Journal of the American Academy of Child and Adolescent Psychiatry,* 33(1), 45-55.

Horwood, J., & Fergusson, D. (1998). *Psychiatric disorder and treatment seeking in birth cohort of young adults,* Christchurch, New Zealand: Department of Psychological Medicine.

Kazdin, A., & Wassel, G. (2000). Therapeutic changes in children, parents, and families resulting from treatment of children with conduct problems. *Journal American Academy Child Adolescent Psychiatry,* 39(4), 414-420.

Kazdin, A., & Mazurick, J. (1994). Dropping out of child psychotherapy: Distinguishing early and late dropouts over the course of treatment. *Journal of Consulting and Clinical Psychology, 62*(5), 1069-1074.

Kazdin, A., Holland, L., & Crowley, M. (1997). Family experience of barriers to treatment and premature termination from child therapy. *Journal of Consulting and Clinical Psychology, 65*(3), 453-463.

Kaufman, J., Birmaher, B., Brent, D., Flynn, D., Moreci, P., Williamson, D., & Ryan, N. (1997). Schedule for affective disorders and schizophrenia for school-age children— Present and lifetime version (K-SADS-PL): Initial reliability and validity data. *Journal of American Child and Adolescent Psychiatry,* 36(7), 980-988.

Kendall, P., Gracia, A., Nath, S., & Sheldrick, R. (1999). Normative comparisons for the evaluation of clinical significance. *Journal of Consulting and Clinical Psychology, 67*(3), 285-299.

Mental Health Commission. (1999). *Specialist Mental Health Services for Children and Youth.* Wellington, New Zealand: Mental Health Commission.

Mossman, S. E. (1997). An evaluation of an outdoor adventure challenge programme on incarcerated adults. In C. Itin (Ed.), *Proceedings of the First International Conference in Adventure Therapy,* (pp. 293-304). Perth, Australia: AEE/COEAWA.

Pelkonen, M., Marttuenen, M., Laippala, P., & Lonnqvist, J. (2000). Factors associated with early dropout from adolescent psychiatric outpatient treatment. *Journal American Academy Child Adolescent Psychiatry, 39*(3), 329-336.

Phillips, S., Hargis, M., Kramer, T., Lensing, S., Taylor, L., & Burns, B. (2000). Toward a level playing field: Predictive factors for the outcomes of mental health treatment for adolescents. *Journal American Academy Child Adolescent Psychiatry, 39*(12), 1485-1495.

Shaffer, D., Gould, M., Brasic, J., Ambrosini, P., Fisher, P., Bird, H., & Aluwahlia, S. (1983). A Children's Global Assessment Scale (CGAS). *Archives of General Psychiatry*, 40, 1228-1231.

Skinner, H., Steinhauer, P., & Santa-Barbara, J. (1995). *FAM-III Manual.* New York: Multi-Health Systems Inc.

Thompson, A. (2002). "Statistical", "practical", and "clinical": How many kinds of significance do counsellors need to consider? *Journal of Counseling and Development, 80*(Winter), 64-71.

Weiss, B., Cartron, T., Harris, V., & Phung, T. (1999). The effectiveness of traditional child psychotherapy. *Journal of Consulting and Clinical Psychology, 67*(1), 82-94.

Weisz, J., Weiss, B., Han, S., Granger, D., & Morton, T. (1995). Effects of psychotherapy with children and adolescents revisited: A meta-analysis of treatment outcome studies. *Psychological Bulletin, 117*(3), 450-468.

Acknowledgments

This research would not have been possible without the financial support of the Alcohol Advisory Council of New Zealand, the University of Canterbury and the Specialist Education Services (now known as Group Special Education, Ministry of Education). Other important acknowledgements include the ADC counsellors, referral agencies and parents and most importantly the young people who consented to participate in the study and provided invaluable insights into their experience of the ADC programme and its effect on their lives.

Authors' Biographies

Elaine Mossman is a Ph.D. student, enrolled at the University of Canterbury, in New Zealand. She has been involved in research for 13 years, the last seven dedicated to researching AT programmes.

Colin Goldthorpe is a registered psychologist who has worked with young people for 25 years. He is a director of Adventure Developments Ltd. and the clinical director of Adventure Development Counselling programme.

Correspondence

Contact Elaine Mossman at:
e.mossman@clear.net.nz.

Busy Doing Nothing: Exploring the Merits of Inactivity within an Activity-Oriented Wilderness Therapy Program

Val Nicholls

■ ■ ■

The "Doing" of Wilderness Therapy that is generally associated with overt and specific change dominates both the literature and research. The "Being" of Wilderness Therapy associated with stillness, silence, ruminative thinking, and spontaneous and intuitive learning is acknowledged but not generally recognized as an alternate and valid way of knowing, despite recent research findings in the cognitive sciences (Claxton, 1997). This paper outlines the author's doctoral research into participant experiences of "Stillness" within a challenge-based and action-oriented Wilderness Therapy program. The personal experiences that motivated the study and the use of photography as part of the qualitative methodology are described. The paper concludes with extracts from early data collection and analysis.

■ ■ ■

I work in the mountains, on the water, in the caves and off the cliffs of Tasmania, Australia, as a senior facilitator for a Wilderness Adventure Therapy program called Project Hahn. Project Hahn is a not-for-profit community organization whose motto is "Personal Growth Through Challenge and Adventure." Project Hanh runs programs in remote locations throughout Tasmania. Most program participants are between 14 and 25 years old and are considered "at risk" in some respect, either by themselves or others. Participants come to the program voluntarily and have an understanding that Project Hahn is about personal growth and challenging outdoor activities. Participants may refer themselves to a 6-day standard course program; however, most are referred by teachers, counselors, social workers or concerned others. Four-day specialist programs are also run for specific agencies such as the Vietnam Veterans Children's Education Service and a Salvation Army residential drug and alcohol rehabilitation program.

Fundamental to this challenge-based model of Wilderness Therapy is a philosophy about the process of change that is grounded in the development of competence and the confronting of internal limits. Overt, specific, and action-oriented learning, sometimes referred to as first-order change (Gass, 1993) is typical within challenge-based wilderness therapy programs and is regarded as a cornerstone of practice. Change also occurs covertly and spontaneously. This second-order change (Gass, 1993) is often associated with quiet, action free, non-facilitated time, and is also typical within challenge-based Wilderness Therapy programs. However, although journals and texts pay tribute to the healing power of nature and the wilderness (Handley, 1990; 1992), the experience of transcendent or magic moments (Nettleton, 1995), and the inherent spiritual component of Wilderness Therapy (Powch, 1994), there has been little or no systematic attempt to evaluate the potency of these factors for affecting long-term change. These hard-to-define experiences, often associated with physical stillness or inactivity, have, on the one hand, been clustered together as part of the miracle and essential mystery of Wilderness Therapy (Handley, 1990) and, on the other hand, cautioned against as "accidental therapy" (Crisp, 1996).

Personal experience in the field indicates that second-order change is not "B-grade" change. Moments of stillness, whether the bliss of a quiet sit on a mountain top or the frozen "stuckness" of indecision, have often been potent forces for insight and understanding of self that participants have referred to months later as important and instrumental to ongoing change. Typical comments include:

"Time out was a spiritual thing."

" … (sitting there) I felt like I was just me and that's all I had to be, there for here and now."

"Just after (the quiet sit) the penny just dropped. I knew inside myself basically where I stood, which is basically the same place I knew I was, but I felt at ease with it a change in my attitude."

"I still do, I still do take my 10 minutes every night. It's definitely one of the most important tools I've picked up. Just to take time for me, just to take time for me."

"I've taken the quiet times home…it's a really useful tool."

Despite the potency for change contained within these statements, focus in the literature and research sits comfortably on the "mechanistic" components (Powch, 1994) of programming: the "doing" of wilderness therapy that is generally associated with first-order change (e.g., sequencing of activities, the use of narrative, metaphor and non-directive leadership styles, debriefing, etc.). The "being" of wilderness therapy associated with stillness, silence, ruminative thinking, spontaneous, and intuitive learning is acknowledged, but not generally recognized as alternate and valid ways of knowing despite recent research findings in the cognitive sciences (Claxton, 1997).

> We know that the brain is built to linger as well as to rush, and that slow knowing sometimes leads to better answers. We know that knowledge makes itself known through sensations, images, feelings and inklings as well as through clear conscious thoughts. ... To be able to meet the uncertain challenges of the contemporary world, we need to heed the message of this research, and to expand our repertoire of ways of learning and knowing to reclaim the full gamut of cognitive possibilities (Claxton, 1997, p. 201).

Encouraged by Claxton, I embarked on the steep and rugged learning curve of doctoral research. Step one was to determine what I wanted to ask. Trying to find a word or way of getting to what I could feel rather than articulate was tricky. "Busy Doing Nothing" easily came to mind, and was catchy as a title that could help keep me focused, but I needed to get narrower, to isolate what it was I was going to study. I opted for the word stillness and decided that in the research, it would be used broadly to encompass the nuance of interpretation suggested by the Macquarie Thesaurus. Stillness is defined as "free from bubbles, at rest, stuck, silence, no movement." All Project Hahn programs are underpinned by a course plan that outlines projected activities for the trip such as kayaking, bushwalking, abseiling, and debriefing. The focus of this research is on the interludes between and during these active components of the journey. Thus, Stillness in this context, as the starting point for the study, is used broadly to describe a physical rather than an emotional state.

It took me a year to write my first sentence: The aim of this study is to use grounded theory methodology to develop an understanding about the impact of Stillness within an activity-oriented wilderness adventure therapy program.

It took longer to isolate the questions that could guide the study and data gathering process:

- What do participants identify as experiences of 'stillness' within a challenge-based Wilderness Therapy program?
- How do participants describe these experiences?
- What are the characteristics of these experiences?
- What are the causal conditions of these experiences?
- What meaning do participants attach to the varying experiences of 'stillness'?
- How do participants attach value to the 'stillness' experience?
- What factors influence the nature of 'stillness' experiences?
- How do participants describe the consequences of the experience in the short and long term?

Research Methods

Participants

Participants for the pilot study on which this paper is based were drawn from two Bridge Specialist programs. The Bridge Specialist Program evolved out of a partnership established between Project Hahn and the Salvation Army Bridge Program. The Salvation Army Bridge Program is modeled after Bridge Programs operated by the Salvation Army in other states around Australia and is comprised of a 12-week course for people with drug, alcohol, or gambling addictions. The Project Hahn Bridge Specialist Program is offered as an adjunctive intervention opportunity for clients in the last six weeks of their residential program. It consists of an orientation day on Mount Wellington followed by a 3-day bushwalk and a day of abseilling. The 4-day journey is regarded as an adjunct to the rehabilitation occurring at the Bridge Program. It aims to provide an opportunity for participants to experiment with new behaviours in an alternative environment beyond the support structure of the Bridge Program. The course is underpinned by the same ethos and bush counselling approach as all other Project Hahn programs.

Methodology

It was clear that a research method was needed that could provide for the interpretation of actions and events, as well as reflect the multiple perspectives of the research participants. It was important to be able to delve beneath description to look for themes, connections, concepts, and processes at work. Qualitative research and Grounded Theory appeared to meet this need.

Strauss and Corbin (1998) succinctly describe qualitative research in terms of the type of research that produces findings not arrived at by statistical procedures or other means of quantification. Qualitative data is in the form of words rather than numbers and is typically obtained through interviews, observations and focus groups rather than surveys and questionnaires. Hence, qualitative research is particularly appropriate in research that seeks to understand meanings, processes, contexts, and causal relationships.

Grounded Theory is not a theory at all. It is an overall strategy, or method for doing research, and as such, has its own particular set of techniques and procedures. The method provides for both thick description of participant experiences and a set of concepts and linking propositions that will provide theory and explanation about the research phenomena (May, 1986, p. 178). "Grounded" infers that theory will generate from, and therefore be grounded in, data (Strauss & Corbin, 1998). Research participants are engaged as critical members of the research team. Throughout the data analysis, participants engage in verifying the data and emerging theory. This role of participant as co-researcher sits comfortably with the mutual respect and neutral power relations engendered in Wilderness Therapy programs. Grounded Theory methodology dictates that data collection and analysis are linked from the beginning of the research and interact continuously, becoming increasingly focused and specific as the research develops.

One of the initial concerns about the study and the interview process was that it was heavily dependent on verbal language, a communication skill that many Project Hahn participants struggle with. This challenge was met in part by harnessing the power of photography to clarify assumptions (Collier & Collier, 1986) and facilitate the exploration of personal values, beliefs, attitudes, and meaning making (Prosser & Schwartz, 1998), as well as its ability to function as a visual narrative and aide memoir (Harper, 1987; Gass & Mackey, 2000).

Participants were invited to make a visual and written, or drawn, diary of their experience. They were each given a disposable camera for their private use and access to the Project Hahn camera for more general snapshots. One of the facilitators also created a detailed photographic journal of the trip. An interview was conducted within 10 days of completion of the program. The semi-structured format of the interview incorporated Stimulated Recall methodology (Marland, 1977; Tuckwell & King, 1980) and Photo Elicitation techniques (Bogden & Biklen, 1992). The interview was constructed around the participants viewing of their personal photographic diary, the Project Hahn snapshots and photographs taken by the assigned facilitator. Participants were encouraged to select photographs that connected with their personal experiences of the program and talk aloud about the thoughts, feelings, reactions and perceptions that the photographs evoked. With the participants' permission, the interview was tape-recorded and later transcribed for analysis.

Preliminary Findings

Participants responded enthusiastically to the review of their own and the facilitators' photographs. The photographs evoked memories and emotions and paved the way for fruitful dialogue:

> "That's it, he's got it right there, that says it all."

> "That's not me in the photograph but that's exactly how I felt…"

> "Just looking at it now brings it all back, makes me tingle."

> "That one says it all, I can't put it into words but that says it all."

It is also interesting to note that some participants deliberately staged photographs in order to better convey their experience.

> "That's a good photo, it just sums it up, we were all just sitting there having a laugh and a smoke, and feeling real. Actually we didn't smoke inside we just did that for the photo, we took it outside."

Any concern that the camera might interfere with facilitator and participant rapport (Bogden & Biklen, 1992) has been dissipated by participants' extraordinary interest in the project and enthusiasm about viewing and securing copies of the photographs. "It's really nice to know that someone is interested in my experience."

Bogden & Biklen (1992) liken the process of data organization and analysis to the "piling" and "sorting" of masses of toys strewn across a gymnasium floor. The initial piling and sorting of data from the pilot study began with the garnering of occurrences of stillness identified within the semi-structured interviews and by participants as a direct response to the invitation to talk about the "doing nothing times, the quiet times when nothing much was going on." "Watching," "a quiet sit" and "sitting around the fire" emerged as dominant themes.

Watching.

"Watching others" was always described in specific relation to the watching of others physically struggle. Disbelief, development of empathy, and a reenvisioning of self and other characterized the experiences described below.

> Mike: "I was just elated, I couldn't believe she did it because I had a bit of animosity towards her, well not her personally, just differences in character. Like she's a really out going person and she's got a bit of a rough tone to her voice and um, added to that, um, she sits down to breakfast and she wants her knife and fork and says to me pass me that or give me that, she makes no real effort to do much for herself

and wanted us to put the tents up for her and that. I kind of didn't say much but that did start to get under my skin and started rubbing me up the wrong way but um, the only thing that saved her from me totally thinking she's just a walking catastrophe was the willpower and strength with which she did everything and I sort of realized that I was being too hard on her. That she's been just as hard on herself with expectations of things, and I should over look all that because behind all that, it's just like a façade that would upset people unless they knew about her, behind that façade was actually a person who was very capable and against all odds, physical or mental whatever, was able to achieve all these goals and go down this rock and everything...But when she got down to the bottom, I just yelled out and ran over and gave her a big hug, I just couldn't believe it. She said she was starting to cry and that and I just had water in my eyes and I said 'Look at my eyes!' and I was just really stoked for her and that was it, that was the seal in the coffin for me, I had great respect and extra time for Sally after she did the abseil because she just done everything. It spun me, there wouldn't be many, I felt privileged because there wouldn't be many, I don't think a lot of girls would go on that trip and do the abseil like Sally."

John: "...once again it was seeing people achieve and seeing that sense of joy in their face I guess it just lifted the whole group up to another level...I got a bit of compassion back, which you tend to loose in addiction, compassion for others, compassion for yourself."

A quiet sit.

Participants spontaneously used the phrase "a quiet sit" to refer times when they intentionally separated themselves from the group to spend an amount of time sitting in silence and for occasions when the facilitator initiated an invitation to the group to briefly sit in silence. Whether the facilitator or participant initiated the opportunity to sit quietly in one's own space, the potential for a transformational relationship with stillness emerged. Participants expressed the experience in existential terms such as, "I felt free," "I felt truly alive."

Some sits provided the opportunity to relax and think through issues; others were described as free from thought, indescribable and "a direct source." Immediately following the latter experiences, some participants described a shift in consciousness, an embodied knowing, intuition, and relief.

John: "Yes, I went down on the rocks...I didn't come up with any answers, not any answers at all, but, it was clear thinking and after coming away from there, I knew inside myself, basically, where I stood, which is basically the same place I knew I was but I felt at ease with it, if that makes any sense... a change in my attitude and the way I see the problem....to get relief in that, like I said, was part of the emotional side of the journey for me, and it's probably one of the most brilliant things I have ever experienced in my life, relief in knowing, knowing inside myself, not just thinking, actually knowing inside myself that that is the way it is. Just to accept it. It's just the way it is."

Participants identified a choice to participate, the absence of distraction and drugs, enough trust to be left alone and a slow enough pace to allow for the opportunity to arise as essential to a positive "quiet time" experience.

Sitting around the fire.

The fire is often used as the focus point for facilitator-led debriefs at the end of the day. Other sharing and discussion (e.g., beyond the debrief) that occurred around the fire was regarded in this study as unscheduled activity and therefore within the focus of the research. The fire provided a safe venue for the sharing of personal history, thoughts, feelings and the nurturing of friendships, self-awareness, and confidence. Underpinning these positive sharing experiences was a stated sense of trust, acceptance, and absence of drugs.

Pete: "I wouldn't be doing that at home with certain people or friends. I don't think I'd have that trust."

John: "I stayed up on two of the nights, after everyone had gone to bed, with the campfire. I actually went to bed one night then jumped back up, and just sat around the campfire, and I didn't think, I just took some time out and I just stared...that came as a relief to me."

Mitch: "In the quiet time (alone) you are yourself, you already know who you are really, you know what I mean? But around the campfire you can actually, um, tell other people how you really feel and think with no judgement on it...like I felt I wanted to tell people how I felt and what I got out of it with no wall and no guard and all that sort of thing. Um, I think, just to get that feedback from people, do you know what I mean?"

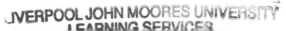

Summary

At this most fundamental level of inquiry into the data, it was clear that stillness had the potential to function as a vehicle for personal, interpersonal, and transpersonal growth. There are also indications of prerequisite conditions for this kind of learning. Signaling potential significance is the explicit and implicit negotiation of trust and power. Similarly a qualitative difference is intimated between "magical" moments that enhance the participants' sense of well being at the time and those that play a part in the long-term positive transformation of thinking and behavior.

From here, the way forward is via the ongoing cycle of data collection and analysis and the detailed line by line coding of transcripts in order to delve beneath the words, to ask "What is going on here?" and to think in terms of concepts and categories and their properties and dimensions.

There is a long way to go but I am learning. I am learning a lot about myself. I have learned that it is a privilege to sit and listen to participants' stories. I am learning restraint. I want to rush in and elicit connections, theories, and solutions. I am learning to come to terms with overwhelm. Like being in the mountains, I am trusting that the steady plod will get me there and leave me breath to look around for depth, detail, and nuance, the extraordinary in the ordinary.

References

Bloom, B.S. (1953). Thought processes in lectures and discussions. *Journal of General Thought, 7*(3), 160-169.

Bogden, R. & Biklen, S. K. (1992). *Qualitative research for education: An introduction to theory and methods.* Boston: Allyn and Bacon.

Claxton, G. (1997). *Hare brain tortoise mind: Why intelligence increases when you think less.* Fourth Estate Ltd.

Collier, J. & Collier, M. (1986). *Visual anthropology: Photography as a research method* (Rev. ed). Albuquerque: University of New Mexico Press.

Crisp, S. (1996). When does wilderness become therapeutic? The need for broader frameworks: Experiential reconstruction of developmental foundations. *The Australian Journal of Outdoor Education 2*(1), 9-18.

Gass, M. (1993). *Adventure therapy: Therapeutic applications of adventure programming.* Association for Experiential Education. Dubuque, IA: Kendall/Hunt Publishing Co.

Handley, R. (1990). *The wilderness therapist: Leaving it all to nature.* National Symposium of wilderness outdoor programs for offenders. Canberra, Australia.

Handley, R. (1992). *The wildreness within: Wilderness enhanced programs for behaviour disordered adolescents. A cybernetics systems model.* Fourth National Conference on children with emotional or behaviour problems.

Harper, D. (1987) The visual ethnographic narrative. *Visual Anthropology 1*(1), 1-19.

Marland, P. W. (1977). *A study of teacher's interactive thoughts.* Doctoral dissertation, University of Alberta.

May, K. A. (1986). Writing and evaluating the grounded theory research report. In W. C. Chenitz & J. M. Swanson (Eds.), *From practice to grounded theory* (pp. 146-154). Menlo Park, CA: Addison-Wesley.

Mulvey, E., Arthur, M., & Repucci, N. (1993). The preventment and treatment of juvenile delinquency: A review of the research. *Clinical Psychology Review*, 13, 133-167.

Nettleton, B. (1995). *Transformational moments in outdoor education. Australian Journal of Outdoor Education* 1(1), 8-14.

Powch, I. G. (1994). *Wilderness therapy: What makes it empowering for women? Wilderness therapy for women: The power of adventure.* Hawthorn Press.

Prosser, J. & Schwartz, D. (1998). *Photographs with sociological research process in image-based research: A source book for qualitative research.* London: Falmer Press.

Strauss, A. & Corbin, J. (1998). *Basics of qualitative research* (2nd ed.). Thousand Oaks, CA: Sage.

Tuckwell, N. & King, L. (1980). Stimulated recall methodology. *Issues in educational Research*, IX W.A. Institute for Educational Research.

Author's Biography

Melding skills derived from an eclectic career as a speech pathologist, potter and outdoor educator, **Val Nicholls** *has worked as a facilitator of Wilderness Adventure Therapy for eight years with Project Hahn in Tasmania, Australia. Val is currently enrolled as a doctoral student exploring the merits of inactivity within action-oriented Wilderness Adventure Therapy programs.*

Correspondence

Valerie Nicholls
Project Hahn
P.O. Box 296
Rosny Park
Tasmania 7018
Australia
ven56@uow.edu.au.

The Adventure of Engaging Traumatic Brain-Injured Patients in a Therapeutic Challenge Course Program

Guy Lorent, Luk Peeters, Thomas Debaenst

■■■

A Challenge Course Program for Traumatic Brain-Injured (TBI) patients of a psychiatric hospital was organized. The authors focused on the high frequency of anosognosia (lack of awareness due to TBI) and its different behavioral symptoms such as refusal to participate in revalidation, incapability to learn from feedback, communication problems about relevant functionality issues, and difficulties dealing with confrontation. These symptoms are evaluated in view of the patients' participation in an Experiential Outdoor Learning Program. The complex clinical picture of anosognosia is analyzed, and a program that was developed to address this challenging condition is reviewed. Working principles of the program are described, and program findings are presented along with recommendations for future efforts to treat this population through experiential programming.

■■■

The Problem

In the field of mental health, motivation is a prerequisite to initiate therapeutic engagement. If a patient is not motivated toward change, the vast majority of therapists or therapeutic communities will renounce treatment. Several reasons account for the lack of motivation toward change. A patient may not recognize a behaviour or feeling as inappropriate or harmful, or may not acknowledge his or her own responsibility in the occurrence of disruptive situations. This is a problem concerning many groups of patients in need of care/cure including our target group: patients with traumatic brain injury (TBI).

TBI patients suffer from a combination of neurological and psychological defects that often lead to a lack of awareness of their own possibilities or disabilities (Prigatano, 1991). This can lead to difficulties in recognizing a need for change. Due to the lack of awareness, the patient may verbally deny that a certain behaviour poses a problem, but his behaviour, indirect speech, and emotions may in fact be causing significant difficulties for primary caregivers and others with whom he or she interacts on a regular basis (Weinstein & Kahn, 1955). Therefore, change may be necessary due to the disruptive effect of the behaviour (Wallace & Bogner, 2000). The contradiction often seen between verbal and nonverbal communication may suggest some possibilities for treatment since it demonstrates that this phenomenon is not an entirely untouchable neurological process. Instead, it implies that there are underlying psychological processes that may be amenable to treatment.

Based on observations within the structured setting of a psychiatric hospital, the authors concluded that adventure activities might function as an effective catalyst towards behavioural change with TBI patients. The observation of such patients in a 5-day challenge course program allowed them to identify a number of important issues that have to be taken into account when working with this client group. These will be discussed later in this paper.

Traumatic Brain Injury

TBI patients suffer from a variety of problems including neuropsychological, locomotor, and emotional problems. These problems include memory distortions, attention problems, hemiplegia, balance problems, disinhibition, loss of speech, aggression, depression, an unrealistic and non-adapted body image, seizures, and psychotic episodes. Other debilitating symptoms may include a reduced or vanished capability to formulate goals, solve problems, carry out a plan, and exert fine locomotor control. However, it is the lack of self-awareness that most clearly impedes the chances of successful revalidation and poses a major stress on caregivers (Wallace & Bogner, 2000).

Problem of Lack of Awareness

Anosognosia refers to the lack of knowledge, awareness, or recognition of disease. The terms "lack of insight" or "lack of awareness" are also encountered frequently and stress the importance of reduced awareness of neuropsychological deficits. This lack of self-awareness on the part of the TBI patient is by far the most difficult symptom that families must deal with. It results in the absence of motivation to get treatment, as the patient is unaware of the inappropriate nature of their behaviour (McGlynn & Schacter, 1989). There is a failure to implement compensation strategies, and difficulty maintaining realistic goals for rehabilitation. TBI patients often do not benefit from therapy, and social exclusion and breaking of family ties is common. Anosognosia also limits vocational possibilities.

The Complex Clinical Picture of Anosognosia

The diagnosis of anosognosia is the result of an interaction in which the observer compares the patient's responses to questions about his disability with his behaviour in situations in which his capacities are tested. Thus, anosognosia takes many forms and is expressed in various spheres of function (McGlynn & Schacter, 1989). A hemiplegic patient for example, may claim that he is perfectly well and not partially paralyzed; or he may admit some weakness and assign it to a trivial cause. He may not deny the paralysis explicitly but express delusions about the affected member, disowning it or referring to it as a foreign body. A patient may deny all his disabilities, part of his disabilities, or use different forms of denial for each disability. Anosognosia is thus a concept that provides unity to phenomena that might otherwise be regarded as discrete disturbances in cognition, perception, attention, or affect.

Importantly, the term anosognosia in its literal meaning of "lack of knowledge of disease" is not accurate for many anosognosia patients. Many patients display implicit knowledge of the extent of their difficulties. They may deny a disability verbally, but not in their behaviour (Weinstein & Kahn, 1955). For example, although a patient may claim that he or she is fine, he or she does accept the role of patient. Another example might be a patient who denies symptoms, yet takes medication, submits to procedures, and does not ask or attempt to leave the hospital. For example, most hemiplegic patients who deny that they are partially paralyzed do not try to walk on their own.

Implicit awareness of disability is also indicated in the selectivity and content of delusions and confabulations. Patients may be delusional or confabulatory only about the body part whose function is impaired, or they may deny one disability but not another because of the personal meaning attached to the dysfunction. This implicit awareness shows the involvement of psychological mechanisms, namely coping behaviours. Denial, in particular, being the most relevant coping behaviour in the context of anosognosia. Thus, the symptom picture of anosognosia reflects the direct neurological and indirect psychological effects of brain injury.

Certainly, premorbid personality characteristics are considered important determinants of ways in which the individual handles the struggle. As mentioned, denial syndromes are a common way to cope with this struggle. Premorbid experiences are determinants of the existence and form of denial and other symbolic representations of incapacity, as well as the content of delusions and confabulations. The types of disability that are denied include neurological symptoms directly attributable to brain injury such as blindness, left and right hemiplegia, left and right hemianopia, aphasia, alexia, deafness, involuntary movements and paraplegia.

Denial may also arise from premorbid experiences that influence the type of adaptation to a non-neurologic loss of function, such as denial of the loss of an amputated limb, the scars and contractures following severe burns with associated encephalopathy, incontinence, a craniotomy or head injury, and the illness itself. For many patients who develop explicit verbal denial, their illness is seen as a kind of personal failure or weakness involving a loss of prestige and integrity (Lewis, 1991). Thus the deficit the patient denies is not necessarily the direct result of a brain lesion, but rather premorbid experiences influence the type of adaptation to the loss of function following brain injury.

We consider the anosognosia and its resulting behaviour as a combination of neurological damage and a psychological defense mechanism. If a person is not fully aware of his possibilities after an injury or after the onset of a disease, he will experience the corrections, or feedback, of others as threatening to his sense of self. This compels him to react strongly to this feedback and to hold firmly to the distorted image he has of himself. We observed that many brain-injured people hold onto the identity, goals, values, behaviours, and abilities that they had before the injury. Each confrontation with their anosognosia strengthens their defensive walls.

Another aspect of this entrenchment is the threat of disintegration, which Goldstein calls "catastrophic reaction" (cited in Prigatano, 1999). Anosognosia patients cannot accept the circumstances of their medical condition because the reality of their present condition is not acceptable since it represents a threat to their identity. Thus, the important function of denial serves as a form of protection. Therapy to treat anosognosia must take this identity issue into account.

There are important clinical considerations related to these phenomena. Patients who use denial as a coping mechanism are not conscious of this process. If the therapist tries to make the patient acknowledge the denied aspect of his illness by sheer willpower and motivated self-control, both he and the patient will be frustrated. Many proposed therapies for anosognosia provide patients with massive feedback training (Schlund, 1999; Fordyce & Roueche, 1986). The goal of this form of therapy is to teach the patient the consequences of his brain damage by repetition. Although some investigations do find some improvement of the anosognosia, this approach is considered questionable, because the confrontation technique that the therapist uses can cause patients to retreat even further into denial.

An Alternative Approach

We do not believe that anosognosia should be considered an obstruction to treatment that must be resolved before treatment can progress. Instead, it is at least partially a motivated process with an adaptive value and meaning. Through the mechanism of denial, the patient tries to avoid aspects of reality that would cause more damage than he or she can cope with. This behaviour is a meaningful reaction of a person to a meaningful situation. The specific danger that arises when denial is eliminated has to be investigated by the therapist (Lewis, 1991) and the adaptive capability of this behaviour must be understood in order to treat it effectively. This behaviour serves a goal and it is the treatment providers' task to discover its meaning for the patient and how it helps that person to avoid, solve, or approach his or her problems. Therefore, the mechanism of denial is important to the patient and in the process of trying to reduce its occurrence, we should consider alternative ways of reaching the pursued goal.

The Experiential Outdoor Learning Program

The approach proposed here is not only to work toward socially appropriate behaviour but also to work on the patient's new identity in a non-threatening way. While the goal of therapy could be the heightening of self-awareness, ultimately it is geared towards the promotion of socially accepted behaviour.

The Experiential Outdoor Learning Program consisted of five separate days where a group of patients were invited to participate in adventure activities. The interval between sessions was approximately one month. The only selection criterion was that the participants had to be responsive to the instructions given by the facilitator. The staff during the outing included a nurse, a neuropsychologist, an occupational therapist, and a psychomotor therapist.

The different activities were selected to provide the possibility of utilizing the strengths of each participant. This provides the opportunity to get positive feedback from the group and from the successful completion of the activities themselves. In working with physically and psychologically challenged patients, this kind of feedback is most valuable. We observed many situations where the power from these accomplishments gave participants enough strength to shed their maladaptive coping system.

When considering the choice of activities, major modifications were made to fit the broad range of physical abilities and limitations within the target group. Examples of such modified activities included: Spider's Web, Whole in Space, Mohawk Walk, High Balance Beam, Obstacle Course, Gutter Ball, Bullring, Orientation Circuit, Flying Fox, and Adapted Low Ropes Course Elements. Some of the activities were already adapted to universal (e.g., wheelchair and limited physical abilities) use. The Spider's Web, for example, was set up to accommodate wheelchairs. The climbing wall was equipped with a counterweight system so that limited strength was needed. The Balance Beam could also be used with a wheelchair. The introductions, interventions, and debriefs had to be modified to meet the special memory and speech features typical for some of the participants.

Taking the above mentioned issues into account, we will summarize some principles of an approach (Bieman-Copland & Dywan, 2000) that expanded our therapeutic thinking and that were operationalized and into an outdoor setting.

"Mind the Gap": No Comparison with Former Life

An important issue in working with TBI patients is the interaction between their life prior to and after the injury. Their existing self-conception is based on their pre-TBI period. Where a lack of awareness poses difficulties in their proper assessment of the situation at hand, it is important to remember that they are viewing the situation from the perspective of their pre-TBI period.

Brain injury can damage one's capabilities to process information in an efficient and comprehensive manner. In a complex situation with many stimuli, it is a difficult task to regain control. In a situation where the whole of the stimuli and demands cannot be integrated, the individual tends to return to one's pre-TBI self-image. Due to this phenomena, it might be impossible for the patient to correct his self-image, or the patient might refuse to accept the limitations encountered. Regardless, an evolution towards an awareness (implicit or explicit) of the present physical and cognitive capacities must be pursued. Therefore, a goal of the program is to not engage in a discussion of someone's abilities before the injury, but rather to encourage reflection on one's capabilities here and now; helping to build the patient's self-esteem based on his current achievements.

It is important to understand each patient's pre-TBI characteristics, including how one used to be, how one reacted to stress, how one coped with difficulties, and how one related to others. However, the primary emphasis of our approach is how the client evaluates oneself today, recognizing what are the person's strengths, weaknesses, perspectives, and goals in life. We work with the abilities that the TBI patient sees in him or herself and refrain from imposing our own assessment of a patient's capacities and limitations.

Specific Ways to Process the Activities

We choose to always frontload the activity by asking the participants how they thought that they would perform in the upcoming action and videotape this explicit statement. During the review that followed the activity, the patients were asked to compare their pre-activity statements with their actual accomplishments. By applying this structure, the patients were able to bridge expectations and estimations with actual outcomes, without having to deal with his or hers own memory problem or being dependent on a caregivers memory. It is often observed that caregivers become scapegoats for encountered failures.

We also asked what the participants thought that they needed to perform the given task. Examples that the participants came up with included: the use of both arms, intelligence, ability to orientate, and the help of others. This helps the patients to focus on the reality of the situation and their capabilities and limitations. It is important at this point not to judge if the answers are adequate, only to facilitate the thinking about the questions. It is up to the patients to determine the adequacy. After each task or activity, we asked them if their "toolbox" was sufficient or if there were too many "tools" in it. In order to avoid confrontation in these early developmental stages of the program, we asked them what they thought that they would need when reengaging in the same activity if they wanted to improve their performance.

At this point we often observed that patients started to explicitly verbalize their physical disability and proposed alternative ways to deal with it. They could state the things that were difficult or impossible for them, often accompanied with some emotion. Importantly, at this point delusional thoughts may be more likely to manifest themselves in more psychotic patients. A confrontation with their abilities as well as their limitations can cause a psychotic reaction. This happened to a patient (who previously lost an arm in a car accident) when he reached the top of a 40-foot climbing wall. His eyes shifted which was a sign that his achievement was too overwhelming to integrate into his reality. The days following, back in the hospital, he was very delusional and aggressive. This reaction occurred during each of the following outdoor trips. The patient achieved something that he thought was not possible with his disability and decompensated afterwards. However, each time the strength of his reaction decreased, and eventually it disappeared.

Getting Connected

Getting connected is another crucial aspect of the working alliance in two different ways. First, it is important to build a trusting therapeutic relationship. Second, we have to find an issue to work with that a patient is able to acknowledge. Patients with anosognosia often propose issues unrelated to their injury or irrelevant to their problem. For example, they may suggest goals such as "do powertraining," "smoke more cigarettes" and so on. In order to develop trust and rapport, we engage in their proposed goals as a first step towards our goal.

Iceberg Politics

Although the therapeutic actions are limited to the issues agreed upon, this does not prevent the therapists from working simultaneously on other themes. Here a comparison can be made to an iceberg, only a small part of which is visible while the main part is beneath the surface of the sea. By addressing the minor issues first, the patient is sometimes able to build a necessary trusting relationship that provides the necessary basis to challenge more difficult problems. In the meantime the therapists try to rehabilitate the other problems as well, but without making them the subject of conversation. This may mean creating a stimulating environment in which other problems can be addressed (e.g., physical revalidation). A patient who does not want to engage in physical therapy to regain his ability to walk, can nonetheless be challenged to walk over a wooden girder in order to reach the group on the other side. A patient with equilibrium problems is not interested in therapy, because he does not acknowledge it is a problem. However, we can challenge him to walk the Mohawk Walk, which at the same time addresses this revalidation issue.

In contrast to the situation in the hospital during revalidation where patients have to practice certain movements as an end in itself, the experiential outdoor activities provide attractive goals that divert the focus away from the actual behaviour. The confrontation is thus decreased because the focus tends to be on succeeding in the activity. This provides a unique possibility for the patient with anosognosia to experience movements, situations, and interactions that one would normally avoid, as well as a unique learning opportunity and a chance to discover one's present abilities.

Do Not Judge, but Elicit Thinking

Because of the obvious unfeasibility of many proposed goals, the therapist is often compelled to react in a restrictive or disapproving way. The repeated communication of this judgement can be experienced by the patients as a disapproval of their self-determination, personality, or values, and may push them further into a defensive state of being. Therefore, it is important that the patient's proposals are questioned with authentic interest instead of being dismissed immediately. The therapists will ask questions, some out of genuine curiosity, some within the framework of designing an action plan. They will even risk putting words in the patients' mouths if this helps the latter to uphold their existing self-image. However, in an effort to stimulate more critical thought, the therapists also challenge the patients' choices.

To illustrate, a 25-year old male patient with memory problems, lack of awareness, delusions, and auto-destructive behaviour as a result of a motor vehicle accident, chose a difficult path to go up a 40-foot climbing wall. We (the therapists) knew that he was not capable of achieving this goal. We also knew that if he did not succeed, he would get angry and he would withdraw and flee into delusions or self-destructive behaviour.

Given this, we encouraged his choice but at the same time proposed to develop a step-by-step climbing program with his ambitious wall route as the final step. He refused and tried the difficult path, giving up after nine feet. We first congratulated him for these nine feet, acknowledging that he knew that it would be difficult and that it took courage to attempt it. Next, we encouraged him to go on with "his" first plan; take the easy wall first and then gradually move to the more difficult levels. The purpose of this intervention was to try to support his self-esteem as much as possible, avoiding embarrassment and providing him with a valid alternative. Believing that he himself was the author of that plan provided him with the necessary motivation to take it along. He first practiced at the easier levels and when he then finally tried the difficult path, hereby limiting his own goal to 20 feet, he succeeded.

The Good, the Bad, and the Ugly

Rules are necessary when people live together. TBI patients often challenge these rules. In our program set-up, the "the good, the bad, and the ugly" paradigm was used to make a discussion of these rules possible. The "ugly" is the caretaker who creates the rules; that person is referred to by the rest of the team as the one responsible for the existence of the rule. He or she is to be addressed by the patient who wants to change the rule. The "bad" is the therapist who repeats the rules and implements them. This one has to confront the patient repeatedly when the rules are violated. This creates space for the "good," who can avoid these confrontations by referring to the "ugly" and the "bad" and engage in a collaborative relationship with the patient (Bieman-Copland & Dywan, 2000). He depicts himself as not being a full member of the group that makes the rules and can, together with the patient, take an objective view of the situation and look for alternative solutions.

As is common in traditional clinical settings, rules are often challenged in outdoor settings as well. At least one of the staff members in our program assumes the role of the "bad." He points out the restrictions and imposes them. The facilitator in charge is responsible for the collaborative relationship; he acts as the "good" guy. Together with the patients, he can look for a way to make the assignment work by discussing how to deal with the restrictions and how they can find their way between the established boundaries.

The Truth Lies Within: No Reference to Brain Damage

As mentioned previously, we do not confront the patients with their brain damage and the consequences of it when they show signs of a lack of awareness. The way that they see the world and the problems that they are experiencing is where we begin the work.

To refer to their brain damage has several disadvantages. The responsibility for behaviour, emotion and cognition is then no longer their own and any communication about difficulties can be discarded. Furthermore, the matter of brain damage is highly sensitive and the patient may easily lose confidence and trust in the therapeutic relationship. Only when the patient her or himself brings up the matter, should information be given.

Program Findings

The main goal of this program was to explore the possibilities and limitations of an adventure therapy approach in addressing the lack of awareness issue. It is evident that we wanted to improve the patient's awareness, but we also wanted to provide an opportunity to give necessary therapy to patients that were not motivated because of their anosognosia. Pre- and post-test measurements of the patients' self-awareness were taken in order to evaluate the impact of the program. However, because of the small number of participants in this program, the findings were not statistically significant and will not be reported here. Instead, we will comment on some of our observations.

Behavioural Changes

We observed an astonishing change in motor activity and responsiveness of certain participants over the different sessions and even during the course of one day. For example, one of the participants was known in the hospital as an apathetic, almost mute patient. After half a day outdoors, he actively walked behind the group and helped them to reach the goal, paid attention to everything that happened and even gave an elaborate explanation of his thinking and actions after one specific activity. The mere fact of changing the environment also seemed to provoke a change in behaviour for many of the patients. It is rather difficult to create a challenging environment in a psychiatric hospital with its daily routines. Living together with many mentally and physically challenged patients creates an environment that is sometimes too tolerant of deviant behaviour and sometimes too restrictive to permit creativity. Going outdoors can be enough to create a stimulating climate.

The Issue of Trust in the Therapeutic Relationship

It appeared that the adventure experience had a positive impact on the patient's trust in the therapeutic relationship which transferred to other situations, even on hospital grounds. To promote this transfer even more, we videotaped each activity and we watched the tapes with the whole group on a regular basis. By reviewing the videotaped activities and referring to their accomplishments throughout the day, the positive and trusting relationships developed during the outdoor activities are brought into the hospital. Not only was the patients' trust influenced, it was also noticeable that caregivers demonstrated growing trust in the autonomy and therapeutic abilities of their patients.

Moving Toward a Greater Awareness

Some patients, previously denying that anything was wrong with them and therefore, not wanting therapy, were now able to explicitly state their limitations. This evolution towards awareness is remarkable, but unfortunately was only witnessed during the outdoor activities and did not seem to transfer to hospital grounds.

How to Motivate this Client-group Effectively

The art of motivating was important in framing each activity. We achieved the best results if we vaguely addressed the day's plan. "We go out, dress warm!" was often sufficient. If we gave them more information, patients would hesitate or even drop out. A description of the planned activities gave rise to uncertainty, fear of failure, and/or fear of confrontation. This was not verbally expressed but was clear from the patients' refusal to engage in the program. Notably however, while this appeared to be an important element in successfully implementing the day's activities, we recognize that this practice gives rise to ethical considerations regarding the issue of "informed consent." This is something to be considered in the future.

Important Considerations for Program Development

TBI patients have various neuropsychological problems that can affect the reflection phases of an adventure program and create a real challenge for the outdoor therapist. The therapist will have to surmount difficulties in verbiage and pronunciation, concentration and amnesia, and impulsivity and apathy. In our program we tried to approach this by repeating the same pattern of reflection throughout the total program sequence and by making these reflections immediately after the activities while the participants still remembered them. During activities we sometimes assigned a mentor to each patient, to guide them through the activities and to be able to react to events as they happened.

Another important problem was the lack of continuity over the different sessions because of memory problems. Often participants did not have an explicit recollection of the activities of the previous session. One patient even denied having met the outdoor therapist previously, although non-verbally she was showing signs of closeness and recollection. In our opinion outdoor trainers should be prepared to accept apparently strange behaviours and be guided more by the communicative aspect of that behaviour than by language.

We found it important to make the participants feel comfortable each time that we left for an outdoor activity. Due to memory problems the facts are often forgotten, but the emotional evaluation stays. Thus, if we wanted to motivate the patients to participate in the next session of the program, it was crucial that they felt positive about the previous activity. This was a dangerous issue, because it influenced our therapeutic attitude. We noticed that in order to have the group achieve success, we were, at times, too directive in our facilitation. Consequently, we noticed a tendency to move away from our experiential therapeutic practice and towards a therapist-centered approach. Facilitators should be aware of this tendency and guard against it.

We are still debating whether an individual or a group approach is better for TBI patients. We have the impression that individual activities seem to be a better entre for personal development than group challenges. In an individual activity, success (and failure) can only be attributed to the client's own actions. At least at the beginning of a series of activities, an individual program can address the specific individual problematic issues and build confidence towards more complex (group) challenges.

Conclusion

Overall, we noticed increased compliance, higher motivation, more cooperation, and sometimes an astonishing change in behaviour. Based on our observations, this type of Adventure Therapy program offers a well-designed intervention that avoids many of the problems encountered in standard therapies typically used to address anosognosia. In this program we only began to explore the possibilities of Adventure Therapy with the adaptations implemented for our target group. The next step is to design new programs to broaden our therapeutic outdoor experience with this target group; to refine our processing methods, including how to introduce activities and motivate the client system in an ethical way; and to integrate measurements that will allow a more objective evaluation of our present findings. We also want to provide more attention to the role and function of the primary caregivers in the rehabilitation process of the TBI patient.

References

Bieman-Copland, S., & Dywan, J. (2000). Achieving rehabilitative gains in anosognosia after TBI. *Brain and Cognition, 44,* 1-18.

Fordyce, D. J., & Roueche, J. R. (1986). Changes in perspectives of disability among patients, staff, and relatives during rehabilitation of brain injury. *Rehabilitation Psychology, 31*(4), 217-229.

Gass, M. A. (1993). *Adventure therapy: Therapeutic applications of adventure programming.* Dubuque, IA: Kendall/Hunt Publishing Co.

Goldberg, E., & Barr, W. B. (1991). Three possible mechanisms of awareness of deficit. In Prigatano, G.P., & Schacter, D.L., *Awareness of Deficit After Brain Injury* (pp. 152-175). New York: Oxford University Press.

Heilman, K. M., Barrett, A. M., Adair, J. C. (1998). Possible mechanisms of anosognosia: a defect in self-awareness. *Phil.Trans.R.Soc.Lond.* 353, 1903-1909.

Lafosse, C. (1998). *Zakboek Neuropsychologische Symptomatologie.* Leuven: Acco.

Lewis, L. (1991). A framework for developing a psychotherapy treatment plan with brain-injured patients. *Journal of Head Trauma Rehabilitation,* 6(4), 22-9.

McGlynn, S. M., & Schacter, D. L. (1989). Unawareness of deficits in neuropsychological syndromes. *Journal of Clinical and Experimental Neuropsychology,* 11, 143-205.

Prigatano, G. P. (1991). Disturbances of self-awareness of deficit after traumatic brain injury. In Prigatano, G. P., & Schacter, D. L., *Awareness of Deficit After Brain Injury* (pp. 111-126). New York: Oxford University Press.

Prigatano, G. P. (1999). *Principles in Neuropsychological Rehabilitation.* New York: Oxford University Press.

Schlund, M. W. (1999). Self awareness: effects of feedback and review on verbal self reports and remembering following brain injury. *Brain Injury,* 13, 375-380.

Wallace, C. A., & Bogner, J. (2000). Awareness of deficits: emotional implications for persons with brain injury and their significant others. *Brain Injury,* 14, 549-562.

Weinstein, E. A., & Kahn, R. L. (1955). *Denial of illness: Symbolic and physiological aspects.* Springfield, IL: Charles C. Thomas Publishing Co.

Authors' Biographies

Guy Lorent has a master's degree in Clinical Psychology and is working in the Psychiatric Centrum Caritas in Gent, Belgium. He has more than 10 years experience in managing the behavioural consequences of traumatic brain injury. The past several years he has been focusing on an approach for the management of anosognosia.

Luk Peeters has a master's degree in Educational Sciences and is a licensed Gestalt Psychotherapist. He has been working in the experiential outdoors since 1985 with several target groups and in several countries. He co-manages Exponent, a European Ropes Course construction and training company and works as an independent trainer for several Train-the-Trainer Institutes.

Thomas Debaenst has an M.D. in Clinical Psychology. His dissertation focussed on the neuropsychological and neuropsychoanalytical aspects of anosognosia, and he has been specializing in the phenomenon of unawareness of deficits ever since. He has been working in the Psychiatric Centrum Caritas in Gent, Belgium.

Correspondence

Contact Guy Lorent at: guy.lorent@pccaritas.zvl.org
Contact Luk Peeters at: training@exponent-cts.com

Adventure Therapy or Therapeutic Adventure?

Ian Williams

■■■

Controversy and debate continues with respect to the appropriate naming of practices that make use of adventure activities in therapeutic settings. Implications for the use of two alternative terms are discussed: adventure therapy and therapeutic adventure. Results from a study involving a large-scale, community-based sample of Australian adolescents are presented. Findings support the argument for distinguishing between these two descriptive terms.

■■■

Despite recent and ongoing advances in the practice, theory and research of adventure therapy, a fundamental issue remains unresolved. The term used to describe what has become a somewhat eclectic field (Doherty, 1996) is as problematic today as it has ever been. Practitioners representing a diversity of philosophies, programs and practices ranging from brief, stand-alone guided adventure activities to extended, multi-systemic psychotherapy in the outdoors are describing their programs as "adventure therapy" (Gillis, 1992). While diversity itself does not present a problem, these approaches are poles apart and render it difficult to identify a common thread linking them together under the one banner. What is the essence of these programs? What characteristics uniquely identify them as different from other types of programs? And what descriptive label best encapsulates these characteristics? While it is beyond the scope of the present paper to answer these questions, attention will be directed towards the last of these in exploring the validity of the use of the term "adventure therapy" to describe the range of practices currently labeled as such.

In one of the few comprehensive publications within the field, Gass (1993) described adventure therapy as being used typically to enhance other therapeutic interventions rather than replacing them. An important distinction was made then between providing treatment and enhancing treatment. During the 10 years since this was written, adventure therapy seems to have taken on a new life and has gradually come to be presented as the therapy itself. While this may simply reflect the natural evolution and development of the field, it seems to have occurred without sufficient critical reflection. What was once therapy enhancement has become therapy.

Around the same time, discussion was appearing in the literature on the suitability of the term adventure therapy in describing such programs. Itin (1993) described therapy as a process of applying a specific approach to addressing a specific problem. Accordingly, he suggested that most of the work in the field was better labeled therapeutic, rather than therapy – just because something has a positive outcome does not therefore make it therapy. Itin correctly identified the intent of a practitioner to treat as an important characteristic of therapy, but seemed to suggest that this by itself was sufficient to legitimately describe one's work as therapy. Others have also highlighted the importance of practitioner intent. Berman and Davis-Berman (2000) noted that while participants of many adventure-based programs experience positive outcomes, these outcomes are often incidental rather than intentional. Such programs may be better described as therapeutic rather than therapy, by virtue of the fact that practitioner intent for specific positive outcomes is absent.

In a subsequent paper contrasting differences between adventure therapy and therapeutic adventure, Itin (2000) attempted to distinguish the two based on the "level at which the change process is addressed" (p. 177). More specifically, it was claimed that therapeutic work focuses on concrete behavioural change, while therapy is aimed at modifying meta-level behaviours. While limited support for this particular view can be found in the literature, others agree that not only are intentions to treat important in therapy (Alvarez & Stauffer, 2001), but so too are the specific outcomes being addressed (Hans, 2000). Additional factors identified as important in conceptualizing adventure therapy include the presence of a theoretical framework (Amesberger, 1998), the use of participant assessments and treatment plans (Crisp, 1998), and evaluations of participant progress and outcomes (Russell, 2001).

This conceptualization of therapy is consistent with that described in the influential Belmont Report (1979), which states that the practice of accepted therapy typically refers to "interventions that are designed solely to enhance the wellbeing of an individual patient or client and that have a reasonable expectation of success" (p. 4). While this report was targeted at biomedical research, its description of therapy is equally valid to the field of adventure therapy. This position is echoed by Davis-Berman and Berman (1994) who suggest that programs whose primary focus is on the planned and purposeful facilitation of emotional growth in participants are accurately described as therapy.

It should be noted at the outset that the focus in this paper is on the field of adventure therapy, however, the arguments presented herein apply equally to related practices known variously as wilderness therapy, wilderness adventure therapy, adventure-based therapy, adventure-based counselling, and others. Indeed, the debate surrounding definitions and distinctions between therapy and therapeutic is not unique to the domain of adventure therapy. In a comprehensive review detailing the development of the more established field of recreation therapy, James (1998) makes constant reference to therapy as a purposive intervention, involving deliberate use of activities through conscious effort. Early practitioners in this field were criticized for their lack of specificity in treatment, as well as failing to delineate between activity as therapy and activity as entertainment. Today however, following many years of discussion, one of the dominant positions held within the field posits that the primary purpose of such services is to provide experiences and opportunities to help change, restore, treat, remediate, or rehabilitate in order to improve functioning and reduce or ameliorate the effects of illness or disability (Idyll Arbor, 2003).

While some have questioned the utility of spending time attempting to reach consensus about naming (e.g., Gillis, 1992), it is the contention of the present paper that not only is this a worthwhile pursuit, but one of fundamental importance with substantive implications. Before embarking on a discussion about the relative merits of current naming protocols, it is prudent to take a moment to consider the value of such an endeavour.

What's in a Name?

Adventure therapy or therapeutic adventure? Does it really matter what we call it? As long as outdoor programs are producing positive outcomes, then perhaps it is academic as to what label we give to it. Is it just a question of semantics and personal preference as to what name one uses? Four arguments are proposed in an effort to present a clear rationale for the importance of making considered decisions about naming and labeling in this field.

Reflecting Practice

The terms used to describe programs offered should correctly and accurately reflect their practice. If the descriptor used is to have any meaning at all, then it should be congruent with the nature of that which it describes. For example, hormone replacement therapy (HRT) describes a specific therapy in which depleted levels of naturally occurring hormones are replaced, or supplemented, with natural or synthetic hormones. Cognitive behaviour therapy (CBT) is a specific form of psychotherapy which focuses on the gradual modification of dysfunctional thoughts and behaviours. In contrast, what can one say is the focus of adventure therapy? And how is it different from outdoor education or adventure recreation? It seems fairly self-evident to suggest that the label should reflect the practice, until we take a closer look at unpacking the "adventure" and the "therapy" in "adventure therapy." What is adventure? What is therapy? Does the term adventure therapy accurately reflect the work carried out under this banner? Further discussion of these questions continues below.

Informing Clients

In the provision of services to clients, we are bound to ensure that they are truthfully informed about the nature of these services. The labels we use to describe our programs are particularly important in this respect. Describing a program as adventure therapy carries with it certain meaning to prospective participants. Clients rely on the accuracy of any descriptive terms used to represent the service (or product) they are contemplating using. This is no different from retail consumers relying on product labels to accurately reflect the nature of their purchase. A tin of baked beans with a label reading "Cooked Legumes" would be considered somewhat uninformative. A light-weight, synthetic sleeping bag called the "Arctic Snow Haven" would be considered misleading. And an adventure company describing its outdoor recreation trips as "therapy" would be tantamount to false advertising. The point to note is that it matters to prospective clients what label we give to our programs in order to assist them in making informed decisions.

Ethical Implications

Closely related to our obligation to accurately inform clients as to the true nature of our programs, is an ethical imperative to do what we say we will do. If we offer a program of therapy, this is what should be delivered with all that this entails. It is unethical to claim a program offering therapy, but deliver instead a program of recreation, of adventure education, or even of personal development. Clients come to us with needs, and rightly expect to have these needs met.

Furthermore, just as practitioners not trained in leading and facilitating adventure activities may well put their clients at risk, so too do those not trained in providing therapy. Few would question the importance of proper training to competently set up a safe rock climbing activity, but what of therapy? To offer a program of therapy ethically requires that its practitioners are adequately trained to do so. In the absence of such training, a program and its practitioners misrepresent themselves by claiming to offer therapy, and potentially place their participants at serious risk of physical, emotional and psychological harm. If a program describes itself as adventure therapy, then it is ethically bound to provide just that.

Professional Identity

The consistent use of a meaningful term to describe the work undertaken in this field helps in establishing a professional identity. In this way practitioners may be seen by others as being part of a larger, unified collective, while those within the field may develop a greater sense of belonging to a community of practitioners. It is difficult to readily identify with others engaged in similar types of work without an overarching identity or shared vision with which to relate. In this way, the term adventure therapy represents not just a label, but also suggests some commonality in purpose, in philosophy, and in practice. Furthermore, it has implications for establishing and developing other aspects of a professional body, such as theory building, research and evaluation, training, and codes of conduct.

Despite the continued discussion and debate around distinctions between adventure therapy and therapeutic adventure, the arguments presented above underline the clear importance of persisting with this issue and in making considered decisions about naming in this field.

What is Adventure Therapy?

The term adventure therapy comprises two concepts, each with fairly well-defined meanings.

Typical definitions of adventure mention novelty, excitement, danger, risk, hazard, challenge, and thrill. When we talk of outdoor adventure pursuits, we often think of activities such as abseiling, rock climbing, high ropes courses, white water rafting, sailing, snow skiing and even bushwalking. Most, though not all, adventure therapy programs make use of such activities. Few would argue about the validity of "adventure" in adventure therapy, after all, this is one of the hallmarks of such programs. However, on consideration of the "therapy" in adventure therapy, there seems to be some contention.

Given that it is the therapy rather than the adventure which is of primary focus ("adventure" is a descriptor of the type of therapy being provided), some consideration is justified regarding the nature of therapy. So in asking "What is adventure therapy?", it is necessary to first consider "What is therapy?" While there is some debate as to what constitutes therapy, the general theme across various writings and definitional sources suggests that the term therapy refers specifically to a treatment designed to relieve or cure an illness, disability, or other bodily, mental, or behavioural disorder. Therapy has a curative or remedial focus, with consequential improvements and positive changes intended in recipients.

Does this accurately describe the range of programs falling under the banner of adventure therapy? Further elaboration of this question is warranted. Five guidelines are proposed below to assist in identifying appropriate use of the term therapy in adventure therapy. In the section that follows, it should be noted that the use of medically oriented language here is not intended to reduce adventure therapy to a sterile mode of clinical intervention, but rather to make use of well-established concepts and draw on relevant fields of expertise. Other terms could be used equally instead (e.g., rehabilitation instead of treatment; problem identification instead of diagnosis).

Diagnosis.

A logical precursor to the commencement of any form of therapy is the identification of the condition to address in prospective program participants. If a program sets out to relieve or treat a particular condition, then one must first be clear that the condition is present in the target group; a problem condition must first be identified (diagnosed) in order for it to be treated through the application of the therapy. A program targeting depression reduction, for example, might involve selection of suitable participants based on some form of diagnosis of depression. In other words, problem identification must precede the instigation of therapy. What is the problem this program is aiming to address? If you are not clear about what you are treating, then how can you possibly treat it?

Programs which have as their generalized goal the improvement of participant functioning (or health and well being) are better described as personal development programs rather than therapy. A key point to note is that in the absence of diagnosis, a program may still be therapeutic. Positive program outcomes are not contingent upon problem diagnosis, though these may be more serendipitous than those achieved through therapy. An important distinction is made here between therapy and therapeutic, a theme that will be explored in further detail in later sections.

Treatment.

A program or activity described as therapy must have, as its primary intent, a specific curative or remedial goal. If there is no intent, there can be no therapy. If we accept that therapy is about treatment (in the broadest sense), then it follows that intention to rehabilitate, to cure, to improve participant functioning is required. Therapy does not happen by chance or accident; it is a planned activity with specific intent. This intent of remedial outcome is a necessary, but not sufficient, condition for therapy to take place. In other words, it must be present for a program to be a therapy, but by itself it is not enough to establish that program as a therapy; intent alone does not create therapy. Conversely, in the absence of specific remedial intent, a program may still be therapeutic (e.g., participants may feel better following the program), but it is not therapy. Positive outcomes may still emerge for participants of adventure programs, even if no specific intention of such outcomes is planned.

Specificity.

With diagnosis (guideline 1) comes problem identification and the intention to address that problem (guideline 2) within the program structure. Hence, a third guideline for a therapy program is specificity. A program of therapy is specifically designed to target and address the particular characteristics and needs of the client group. There is a direct correspondence between the condition diagnosed and the program implemented. In this way, a program of therapy should be designed in response to the problem identified. This is in contrast to a program that looks the same regardless of the problem condition or client group being served. Therapy targets specific problem conditions, whereas "non-therapy" may simply have a broad therapeutic outcome (e.g., participant's mood is temporarily elevated). As previously mentioned, programs with generalized outcome goals are better thought of and described as development programs rather than therapy programs.

Framework.

The capacity to design a therapy program which specifically targets the identified needs of a client group relies heavily on the presence of adequate practitioner knowledge of underlying theory. An established body of knowledge (science) forms the basis of more recognized therapies (e.g., behaviour therapy, gene therapy, speech therapy), and adventure therapy should be no exception. This body of knowledge, or conceptual framework, guides the practitioner in designing an intervention tailored to their client needs. Practitioners with formal training in this knowledge are called therapists. While the science of adventure therapy is still in its infancy, practitioners have a wealth of resources to draw upon from allied professions such as psychology and education.

Efficacy.

Describing a program as therapy presumes that the outcomes of such an intervention can reasonably be expected to be positive and efficacious, that participants are somehow better off for having taken part in the process. If a program does no good, then it is difficult to justify the label therapy. If a program does harm, then it is clearly neither therapy nor therapeutic. Only those activities generally shown to make a positive contribution to the functioning of participants can sensibly be considered as therapy. The question remains then as to how one knows if their program has indeed achieved positive outcomes? Determination of the efficacy of a program requires systematic research and evaluation of processes and outcomes. Were the goals of the program met? Was a meaningful positive change observed in clients as a result of their participation in the program? What aspects of the program contributed to these changes? Practitioners who fail to evaluate their work and thereby monitor its efficacy are falling short of the standards required for the ethical delivery of a program of therapy.

In summary, therapy describes quite a tightly defined area of practice. Not only are these guidelines proposed here as principal characteristics of therapy, but they also form a logical sequence of steps in the planning and execution of such therapy.

1. Diagnosis: what is the problem?

2. Treatment: embark on a process that addresses the problem.

3. Specificity: develop a program specifically designed to remedy the problem.

4. Framework: base the program design on sound principles.

5. Efficacy: did the program do what it was intended to do?

From this perspective, it can be seen that the description above does not encompass the gamut of programs currently falling rather loosely under the banner of adventure therapy. In many instances, programs would be more accurately described as therapeutic adventure rather than adventure therapy, and it is to this notion that we now turn.

Therapy vs. Therapeutic

It is suggested then that adventure therapy involves a combination of diagnosis, treatment intention, specificity, theoretical frameworks, facilitation by trained therapists, and systematic research and evaluation. Additional elements characterized by the setting and process (adventure and/or wilderness) render this type of intervention "adventure therapy."

The term therapeutic is less constrained and restrictive than therapy. The Cambridge International Dictionary of English (Procter, 1995) gives the following definition of therapeutic: "causing someone to feel happier and more relaxed or to be more healthy." Therapeutic thereby describes an effect or outcome on participants. In contrast, therapy describes a process: "a treatment which helps someone feel better, grow stronger, etc., especially after an illness" (Procter, 1995). To illustrate this distinction, watching a funny movie when you are feeling low can be therapeutic because it makes you feel good; however watching funny movies is not a therapy, per se. Therapeutic still implies some form of curative action—a change to a healthier state of functioning. However its use in everyday language renders it somewhat more appropriate, and less misleading, in describing much of the work in this field than does the term therapy.

Not only is there an important conceptual distinction between therapy and therapeutic, but there is also a relevant linguistic difference (Berman & Davis-Berman, 2000). As a noun, therapy describes what is done; it encapsulates a process outlined by the five guidelines above. In contrast, therapeutic is an adjective, which describes an outcome. It is clear therefore, that the process of therapy leads to therapeutic outcomes by definition; however therapeutic outcomes are not necessarily preceded by therapy.

Therapeutic adventure programs do not call for diagnosis, need not have particular outcomes specified, may be generalized in nature, need not rely on an existing body of knowledge, may be run by facilitators trained in adventure activities only, and do not rely so heavily on research and evaluation (see Table 1).

Table 1
Key Differences Between "Therapy" and "Therapeutic"

Therapy	Therapeutic
requires problem identification	no diagnosis required
specific remedial outcomes are intended	non-specific or serendipitous outcomes
involves targeted intervention that treats the identified problem	more generalised in nature
program design and decision-making based on a body of theoretical knowledge	need not rely on guiding framework
systematic research and evaluation of both process and outcomes	does not rely so heavily on research
facilitation by trained therapists	specialist therapy training not needed
describes a process	describes an outcome

Empirical Support

In an effort to begin to empirically explore some of these questions, data from a large longitudinal research project were analyzed. The Australian Temperament Project (ATP) commenced in 1983 with the recruitment of 2,443 infants, aged 4-8 months old. The sample was selected to be representative of the Australian state of Victoria. In 12 waves of data collection to the year 2000, parents, maternal and child health nurses, teachers, and in recent years the children themselves, have provided information on domains including temperament, behaviour problems, health, school achievement, social skills, peer relationships, depressive symptoms, and substance use. A complete methodological reporting of the overall study is beyond the scope of this paper. For further details, the reader is referred to Prior, Sanson, Smart, and Oberklaid (2000).

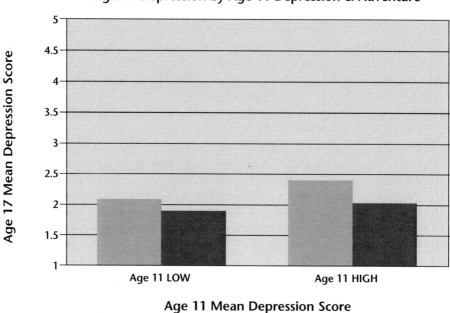

Age 17 Depression by Age 11 Depression & Adventure

Figure 1. Mean depression scores at age 17 comparing non-adventure group with adventure group for those low on depressive symptoms at age 11, and for those high on depressive symptoms at age 11.

The analyses reported investigate participants' responses at age 15 to a self-reported measure of outdoor adventure involvement ("I am involved in outdoor adventure activities") using a 5-point scale (never, rarely, sometimes, often, very often). Of 1,294 adolescents who completed the adventure item, 399 described being involved in adventure activities either "often" or "very often" (adventure group), while 895 adolescents participated in adventure activities "never," "rarely," or "sometimes" (non-adventure group).

Responses on this measure were compared with earlier (age 11) and later (age 17) measures of depressive symptoms and anxiety. No differences were found between the adventure group and the non-adventure group in earlier (age 11) levels of anxiousness or depressive symptoms. However, the adventure group demonstrated significantly lower levels both of anxious symptoms, $F(1, 1117) = 31.20$, $p < 0.001$ and of depressive symptoms, $F(1, 1116) = 30.28$, $p < 0.001$ at age 17, compared with the non-adventure group.

Subsequent analyses across both groups showed that for those low on depressive symptoms at age 11, depressive symptoms at age 17 were significantly higher for those in the non-adventure group compared with those in the adventure group, $F(1, 794) = 18.14$, $p < 0.001$). Similarly, for those high on depressive symptoms at age 11, depressive symptoms at age 17 were significantly higher for those in the non-adventure group compared with those in the adventure group, $F(1, 227) = 9.33$, $p < 0.01$ (see Figure 1). Similar patterns were also observed in the relationship between age 11 and age 17 anxious symptoms (see Figure 2).

Taken together, these findings suggest preliminary empirical support for the protective effect of frequent participation in outdoor adventure activities against experiencing depressive and/or anxiety symptoms. Those who regularly participate in outdoor adventure activities seem to experience lower levels of subsequent depressive symptoms and anxiousness than those who do not participate in such activities. However, while these data are promising, it would be premature to conclude a simple causal relationship between participation in outdoor adventure activities and levels of depressive and/or anxiety symptoms. Further studies are required to explore the nature of these relationships. Additional details of the present

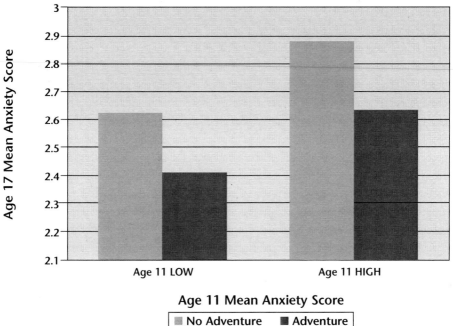

Figure 2. Mean anxiety scores at age 17 comparing non-adventure group with adventure group for those low on anxiety symptoms at age 11, and for those high on anxiety symptoms at age 11.

analyses are due to appear in a forthcoming research paper. The author may be contacted for further information.

It is important to note that this is not a study about adventure therapy. No therapy, per se, has taken place. These adolescents have not enrolled in a program specifically designed to target some form of psychopathology. Rather, they have self-selected to participate in recreational adventure activities. And yet there appears to be a significant therapeutic outcome experienced. This is what we might reasonably describe as therapeutic adventure.

The distinction between adventure therapy and therapeutic adventure is an important one. The data presented suggests that young people participating recreationally in outdoor adventure activities may be gaining something psychologically meaningful from their experiences. Given that these gains are apparent in the absence of a program of adventure therapy, one can reasonably expect that adventure therapists should be able to facilitate even greater gains through their legitimate adventure therapy practices. How can practitioners in their work distinguish between this form of unguided outcome and the planned outcomes of adventure therapy? Unless practitioners in their work are substantively adding to these gains through their involvement, then one must wonder whether in fact adventure therapy is taking place. In such cases where additional gains are not evident, perhaps the program on offer is better described as therapeutic adventure, with practitioners accompanying participants on their own respective journeys of therapeutic change. Practitioners are encouraged to critically reflect on and evaluate their programs in light of these considerations.

Conclusion

The present article has attempted to contribute to the ongoing debate around terminology in the developing field of adventure therapy, by explicating the differences between what can reasonably be presented as therapy, and what is more accurately described as therapeutic. Empirical findings from a large-scale community study have been presented which provide support for the contention that adventure therapy and therapeutic adventure should be considered distinct endeavours. Rather than intending to be prescriptive in its discussion of adventure therapy, this paper aims to promote considered reflection about the appropriateness of language and labels used in this field. Practitioners are encouraged to think more critically about the manner in which they describe and represent the work that they do. Those programs utilizing adventure experiences and principles that are congruent with the five guidelines outlined above may be more accurately described as adventure therapy than those programs that do not. Practitioners running adventure programs falling into the latter category should consider adopting the term therapeutic adventure to describe their work.

Further attention and contributions are required to add to the growing body of literature, in order to more clearly articulate the defining characteristics of the particular mode of therapy labeled adventure therapy. Such contributions must inevitably focus in part on other important aspects of the development of a profession including: continuing participation in and production of research and evaluation activities; ongoing refinement and expansion of theory development; the establishment of regional, national, and international governing bodies; the formulation of a code of conduct; and development of professional training and accreditation programs. As the field continues to develop and struggle to establish a clear sense of identity, it is timely for us to stop and consider critically what we are doing: Adventure Therapy or Therapeutic Adventure?

References

Alvarez, A. G. & Stauffer, G. A. (2001). Musings on adventure therapy. *The Journal of Experiential Education, 24*(2), 85-91.

Amesberger, G. (1998). Theoretical considerations of therapeutic concepts in adventure therapy. In C. Itin (Ed.), *Exploring the boundaries of adventure therapy: International perspectives, proceedings of the First International Adventure Therapy Conference*, Perth, Australia, July 1997. Association for Experiential Education.

Berman, D. S. & Davis-Berman, J. (2000). *Therapeutic uses of outdoor education. ERIC Digest.* ERIC Clearinghouse on Rural Education and Small Schools. Charleston, W.V. (ERIC Document Reproduction Service No. ED448011) Retrieved December 15, 2003, from the ERIC database.

Crisp, S. (1998). International models of best practice in wilderness and adventure therapy. In C. Itin (Ed.), *Exploring the boundaries of adventure therapy: International perspectives, Proceedings of the First International Adventure Therapy Conference*, Perth, Australia, July 1997. Association for Experiential Education.

Davis-Berman, J.L. & Berman, D. (1994). *Wilderness therapy: Foundations, theory and research.* Dubuque, IA: Kendall/Hunt Publishing Co.

Doherty, T. (1996). Clinically focused wilderness therapy expeditions. *Insight, 4*(3), 1.

Gass, M. A. (1993). Foundations of adventure therapy. In M. A. Gass, (1993). *Adventure therapy: Therapeutic applications of adventure programming.* Dubuque, IA: Kendall/Hunt Publishing Co.

Gillis, H. L. (1992). *Therapeutic uses of adventure-challenge-outdoor-wilderness: Theory and research.* Paper presented at the Coalition for Education in the Outdoors Research Symposium Proceedings, Bradford Woods, Indiana. Retrieved from http://fdsa.gcsu.edu:6060/lgillis/AT/Content/CEO92.htm

Hans, T. A. (2000). A meta-analysis of the effects of adventure programming on locus of control. *Journal of Contemporary Psychotherapy, 30*(1), 33-60.

Idyll Arbor (2003). *Professions.* Retrieved from http://www.idyllarbor.com/cgi-bin/SoftCart.exe/professions.htm?E+scstore

Itin, C. (1993). A common understanding: Therapy vs. therapeutic. *Insight, 1*(2), 2.

Itin, C. M. (2000). Adventure therapy vs. therapeutic adventure: Critical differences and appropriate training. In K. B. Richards (Ed.). (2003) *Therapy within adventure: Proceedings of the Second International Adventure Therapy Conference*, University of Augsburg. Germany: Ziel.

James, A. (1998). The conceptual development of recreational therapy. In F. Brasile, T. Skalko, & J. Burlingame, (Eds.), *Perspectives in recreational therapy: Issues of a dynamic profession.*

Prior, M., Sanson, A., Smart, D. & Oberklaid, F. (2000). *Pathways from infancy to adolescence: Australian Temperament Project 1983-2000.* Melbourne, Australian Institute of Family Studies.

Procter, P. (Ed.). (1995). *Cambridge International Dictionary of English,* Cambridge University Press.

Richards, K. (2002). *Adventure therapy: Exploring the healing potential of the outdoors.* www.brathay.org.uk/academy/adventure_therapy_seminar.pdf

Russell, K. (2001) What is wilderness therapy? *The Journal of Experiential Education, 24*(2), 70-79.

U.S. Department of Health, Education and Welfare. (1979). *The belmont report: Ethical principles and guidelines for the protection of human subjects of research.* Washington, D.C.

Author's Acknowledgments

The author would like to thank the contributions made by Professor John Toumbourou in assistance with the preparation of this manuscript. Acknowledgment is also extended to the Institute of Family Studies in Melbourne, Australia, for access to data from the Australian Temperament Project.

Author's Biography

Ian Williams *currently works as a Research Officer at the Centre for Adolescent Health in Melbourne, Australia. He has undergraduate training in Outdoor Education and Psychology, and is presently completing postgraduate study in Clinical Psychology. Over the last 15 years, Ian has worked with a wide range of groups in the outdoors in settings including recreation, education, corporate training and therapy.*

Correspondence

Ian Williams
Centre for Adolescent Health
Gatehouse St.
Parkville, Victoria
Australia, 3052
ian.williams@mcri.edu.au

Envisioning the Birth of a Profession: A Blueprint of Evidence-Based, Ethical, Best Practice

Simon Crisp

■■■

The field of Adventure Therapy faces a potentially new and exciting era. We are poised, ready to embark on the final leg of a journey toward becoming a profession. Any foundations for a profession need to be the values and ideals that foster consensus, unity and guide the profession's direction. Of perhaps even greater importance, these principles should ensure the realization of the full value of Adventure Therapy to society, which is to provide the most effective and humane reduction of human suffering and the promotion of well-being as possible. This paper outlines a proposed vision for the professionalization of Adventure Therapy and discusses some of the obstacles that may impede the realization of such a vision.

■■■

The field of Adventure Therapy has made considerable progress toward the development and refinement of intervention methods over the last two decades. However, our attentions now need to turn to examining elements of what this future profession of Adventure Therapy will hold as core principles — a blueprint that will define it and shape its growth forward. Importantly, such principles should guide us toward universals in practice, while allowing diversity, and provide the core pillars, or keystone foundations of a profession. The endeavor of adventure-based interventions used for therapeutic purposes has a genesis from many influences and directions (Davis-Berman & Berman, 1994; Miles & Priest, 1990). These unique contributing perspectives have enabled the formation of exciting and highly innovative approaches and methodologies (Gass, 1993; Itin, 1998; Richards, 2003). This developmental strength, however, now itself poses a challenge to a unified and coherent professional discipline with clear objectives and direction. If a viable profession is to be born, the very many, and sometimes disparate viewpoints need to be unified into a single paradigm. Many of the concepts that could contribute to this paradigm have already been well developed. What will be important to guide its final creation, is a blueprint of core values, that will allow all parts to integrate into a meaningful whole.

Any future profession will be best served if the following three keystone principles in this blueprint are embraced. First is the notion of evidence-based practice. That is, all practices should be based on empirical evidence where possible, and that significant efforts should be put into generating such evidence. Second is the notion of ethics-based practice. That is, all our profession's activities should be subject to a comprehensive and relevant ethical code. Finally, drawing these two principles together, the final keystone principle is best practice. That is, methods and procedures employed should be based on documented models that incorporate the highest standards of care with approaches that are supported by research, or related therapeutic approaches known to be the most effective with the client in question. What is considered best practice should be continually explored, debated, and updated by the field.

This paper discusses the three keystone principles and then follows with a sketch of a vision for an Adventure Therapy profession. Following this, obstacles and alternatives to this vision will be considered, and finally, the question of whether the vision is achievable is explored. However, before proposing any vision, it would be timely to consider three critical questions: (1) Does a united vision currently exist? (2) How will those in the field know when the status of a profession has been achieved? (3) How will those outside of the field know when the status of a profession has been achieved?

Critical Questions

How will the field know if it has reached the status of a profession?

The field faces some unavoidable issues on the path to professionalization. First and foremost, the field needs to achieve a healthy and respectful "marriage" between the clinical professions and the field of adventure learning. Indeed, Bunce (1997) called for this in 1997 at the first International Adventure Therapy Conference. By marriage, I believe there needs to be a clear understanding of, and respect for, the origins and history of both fields, a commitment to ongoing education about the other, and a partnership based on equal commitment to mutual benefit through the relationship. Valuing those assets in the other that each party lacks provides fertile ground for continued growth. Ultimately, both fields must combine together to form an optimal single entity sited on common ground. To do this requires an appreciation of the other's strengths, and a differentiation of roles. This, in turn, is likely to require a sharing of power in the relationship, where one party may hold greater power than the other at different times and in different ways. Put another way, both parties need to be prepared to relinquish power at times. However, with any gains made by either side, there must also be losses. When we see this sort of relationship between the two fields, we will be seeing the foundation of a profession.

Further, a united profession would require that divergent theoretical and practice issues find some integration, providing a coherent whole. That is, theoretical and applied aspects of each field that have the potential for conflict and difference, are brought together in some way. This integration need not be static, but in fact, may create an important tension and dynamic that drives the growth of new paradigms and continued theoretical and methodological evolution.

Finally, forming an identity is the third essential task for Adventure Therapy to know that it has achieved the status of a profession. Therefore, some form of professional body would seem to be critical to achieve this. When there is identity with, and visible membership of, a single group that is unambiguous and strong, then practitioners will see themselves, and will begin to function as a profession.

How will those outside the field know when Adventure Therapy has achieved the status of a profession?

Having a clear identity that is visible in the form of a professional body will be central to outsiders seeing the field becoming a profession. However, there are two more important requirements that come before this. First, and most importantly, the field needs to have accumulated a convincing body of evidence that Adventure Therapy: (a) is effective—that is, it can treat disorders and/or enhance people's functioning and well-being; (b) is safe, that is, it does no harm (psychologically as well as physically); and (c) is comparable—that is, it is as good as, or better than other alternatives (such as other psychotherapies or drug treatments). Second, some mechanism of accountability must be in place and be perceived to be effective in protecting the public from harm. If the field promotes the idea that Adventure Therapy is a powerful intervention for therapeutic change, then the field must concede that it has equal potential to do harm. Every beneficial treatment has side effects, and history has shown that Adventure Therapy certainly has, at least, the potential to physically maim or kill. The public will only view the field as a profession if it has a visible mechanism in place to police unethical or dangerous practices, and is therefore accountable to the community. A professional body or association with a regulated membership, articulated standards of practice, a code of ethics and the means and will to expel practitioners who do not practice within minimum, safe standards is critical for this.

Does a united vision currently exist, and is the field to become a profession?

The three conditions needed to achieve the status of a profession are highly interrelated. The field of Adventure Therapy will only properly integrate divergent theoretical and practice issues, and form as a single, unambiguous and strong group when it has managed to marry the fields of adventure leadership together with the therapeutic professions. To gauge this readiness, and the reality of a true marriage, one can look to what supposedly aims to unite the two fields: The International Adventure Therapy Conferences (IATC). It is interesting to consider the third IATC, as well as the previous two, in terms of what has been presented and by whom. These two viewpoints can provide some objective perspective about the state of the relationship. In particular, it can tell us much about (a) whose ideas the field is being exposed to the most, and (b) what type of information is valued and promoted most. Also important is the converse of this. That is, whose ideas are being heard the least, and what topics are valued least.

The theme of the third IATC was "Quality and Ethical Practice". However, despite this supposed emphasis, a breakdown of all the presentations shows that over half of the major topics presented were program descriptions (21, or 30%) and facilitation and methods (16, or 22%). One third of presentations covered theory/culture (13, or 18%) or networking/ miscellaneous topics (10, or 14%). Ironically, the least presented topics were the ones most central to the conference theme: Research had 7 papers (10%) and ethical/professional/risk-management had 4 papers (5%), of which this paper was one. The keynote addresses concerned themselves most with theory/culture issues (4 of 10), followed by program descriptions (2) and networking/miscellaneous (2). No keynote presentations addressed the themes of quality or ethical practice. It is likely that those outside of the field would be surprised to see such a minimal emphasis on attempts to accumulate a body of evidence that might justify this practice, and even less interest in ways to establish a means to protect the public from harm. This would suggest to others that the field is a long way from achieving the status of a profession.

When the backgrounds of the presenters are considered, and therefore the emphasis of perspective, the clear majority are from an adventure or non-therapy background (48, or 63%), and only 1 in 3 (28, or 36%) had a therapy background (using a very broad criteria). The most important perspective, people who actually have actually married the two disciplines— dual-trained practitioners—were featured in just over 1 in 5 presentations (16, or 21%). This pattern continues in the keynote addresses: Adventure or non-therapy backgrounds comprised 8 of the 10 speakers, and only 2 had a therapy background. Only one speaker had dual training. These statistics are a rough gauge of what the field seems most concerned with and what perspectives are being promoted the most. This data does seem to suggest that as a field, there is little evidence of much of a marriage, and very little interest in showing the public that Adventure Therapy is an integrated profession with the requisite balance of perspectives, or indeed deserves to be seen that way.

The following sections outline three keystone principles critical to advancing the field beyond this particularly underwhelming position.

Evidence-Based Practice

The concept of evidence-based practice has its origins in medical research that aims to determine the optimal treatment approach for any given disorder. At the very least, practice decisions are based on what is known about any given problem and the appropriateness of any, and all, available treatment options. Ultimately, an evidence-based approach aims to answer the question "what treatment approach is best for which clients, and with which disorders?" Obviously, such an approach requires a concerted and combined effort on the part of researchers and practitioners to be as systematic as possible in their approach so that such information may be accumulated. Newes (2001) argues the need for this well. This approach behooves practitioners to base their interventions on what is known to be the most effective and suitable approach for any client, and not simply to guess what might work, or to limit the client's options to those approaches that suit the practitioner to provide. Importantly, evidence-based practice is client-centered rather than practitioner-centered.

When applied to Adventure Therapy, this approach would seek to determine if, and when, Adventure Therapy is effective with various types of clients and problems. Other questions can also be examined. How do practitioners maximize gains, and how do they guard against negative outcomes? What are the most important elements of an Adventure Therapy intervention, and do these change with different clients and different problems? What activities, methods and levels of risk are required to be effective? How do clients of Adventure Therapy experience the process? What would make Adventure Therapy more appealing, and more accessible for clients? How do Adventure Therapy interventions compare to other treatment methods? There are many effective and very well-documented treatments for different problems, so how does Adventure Therapy compare to these? These are the sorts of questions that any member of the public, potential client or funding body would rightly ask. Without any convincing answers currently, the field appears very amateurish. It will be a momentous day when the field can confidently state, with documented specifications, which Adventure Therapy intervention for which client at which time is the most effective and economical.

Ethics-Based Practice

A profession should see its primary objective to serve society before its own interests. All therapeutic disciplines have a well-developed set of ethical guidelines as a defining pillar of the profession. Importantly, such ethical guidelines are specific to their discipline's practices. Indeed, the term "discipline," in part, refers to these ethical principles that determine how that profession conducts itself in a disciplined way. For this field to become a discipline, we need to articulate a set of ethical guidelines that are specifically developed for the unique issues that arise in the practice of Adventure Therapy. The Therapeutic Adventure Professionals Group (TAPG) of the Association for Experiential Education in the United States must be applauded for developing a brief set of ethical principles. These have existed for over a decade, but unfortunately appear to be seldom referred to. Ethical practice will only become standard practice when practitioners are educated about how to apply ethical principles in their work. For this reason, the field needs to enter into discussions about ethical practices and develop detailed ethical guidelines for specific circumstances, or client issues. Indeed, many therapeutic professions have done this to give greater practical clarity to the ethical dimensions of their practice. For instance, simply an awareness of the existence of a set of principles is no guarantee that practitioners will bring ethical thinking and decision making to their work. A profession that holds ethical practice as central to its work will be active in viewing all of its activities from an ethical perspective. An ability to apply ethical principles to practice needs to be central and foremost to any training of a professional Adventure Therapy practitioner.

Finally, as with any reputable profession, there needs to be some mechanism of accountability. This usually takes the form of structures set in place to establish and monitor standards, as well as being a means for the public to have some recourse for substandard or unethical practice. This, of course, gives credence for the establishment of a professional association or a government regulating body. Having strict criteria for membership of an association is one of the most accountable means to sanction unprofessional or unethical practices. It is through expulsion or other disciplinary action that the public can gain confidence that standards are being set, monitored, and upheld.

Best Practice

Best practice, or best known practice is just that. It is what the existing knowledge base identifies as being the optimal way of practicing. Having clear guidelines of how best to practice provides a reference for practitioners, researchers, and the public for what are important procedures that most likely to lead to therapeutic outcomes for clients, while minimizing the potential for negative outcomes. Principles for best practice should be able to be applied to any setting, client group or program type. Obviously, best practice incorporates, and should be reflective of, both evidence- and ethics-based practice. The guidelines should be atheoretical, and applicable within any cultural or philosophical framework.

In an international study tour in 1996, the author attempted to glean from 14 different programs, what practitioners viewed as essential best practices in Adventure Therapy (Crisp, 1997). While just a starting point, these principles still stand as useful and practical guidelines for optimal Adventure Therapy practice. In brief, these principles are:

1. Systemic framework—interventions take account of the client's system (e.g., family).

2. Assessment process—before treatment, there is a comprehensive assessment of client needs.

3. Treatment planning—meaningful treatment goals are established based on a formulation of the client's needs.

4. Flexibility of approach—interventions are tailored or adapted to best meet the needs of the client.

5. Integration—the intervention is linked during or after to other therapy and case-management.

6. Monitoring of client outcomes—therapeutic progress and effects of the intervention are monitored.

7. Theoretical paradigm—the intervention is based on a theoretical rationale that is defensible and not likely to be dangerous.

8. Therapist skills—the intervention is administered by staff with a sufficient level of training in therapy and adventure leadership that is commensurate with the therapeutic needs of the client.

9. Risk management—procedures are in place to safeguard the physical and psychological safety of clients.

10. Ethical issues—all direct-care staff have a practical and working knowledge of pertinent ethical issues.

11. Research—the intervention is informed by current research or involves ongoing, evaluative research that contributes to a knowledge base.

12. Training—field staff maintain their skills and update knowledge regularly.

The author is not aware of any other attempts to formally discuss or define best practices. This is unfortunate as the field needs to vigorously discuss, debate and articulate the critical elements that define best practice within it.

A Vision for a Profession: Setting the Agenda

These principles are attainable and will ensure that society achieves the maximum benefit from the use of resources devoted to Adventure Therapy programs. However, if we do adopt these principles, then important questions arise. For instance: Where do we look for evidence and how do we generate it in ways that are applicable and relevant? What are the ethical issues that are unique to Adventure Therapy? What really are the universals of best practice in Adventure Therapy, and how do we keep our notion of best practice current? How do we demonstrate and communicate these keystone principles of our profession to the community? To advance this field towards a profession—to give it birth—then we must set an agenda with these tasks and questions as priorities.

Fulfilling such an agenda will require substantial effort and commitment. However, it will allow the field of Adventure Therapy to build something of great value and worth for clients. It will be helpful to imagine what this vision might look like so that a tangible picture of the profession can be constructed:

- Dual-trained practitioners will be common, and Adventure Therapy teams will always have a staff member comprehensively "triple-trained" in therapy, adventure leadership and the specialized discipline of Adventure Therapy.

- Adventure Therapists (triple-trained professionals) will be the most prolific and substantive contributors to the professional knowledge-base, theoretically in terms of practices, and in the production of research.

- Conferences and professional meetings will see regular discussion and increased material on ethical issues.

- There will be an active and resourced commitment to building an evidence-derived knowledge base.

- There will be active and vital local professional bodies (i.e., associations), and less importantly, an international association.

- There will be accessible and comprehensive training schemes that highlight ethical and psychological risk management practitioner competencies.

- The profession will be valued highly by the community such that any client who is likely to respond best to Adventure Therapy will be supported to access it.

- Adventure Therapy will sit alongside well-established therapies such as group therapy, psychotherapy, family therapy, and medication therapies as an equally legitimate treatment.

- Adventure Therapy will not be considered "alternative" to other treatments but a "frontline" intervention, or treatment of choice, for certain clients and problems.

This vision is desirable, achievable, and worthy. The three core principles of ethical, evidence-based and best practice are essential as foundations. It is now worth considering what obstacles lie on the path to this outcome, and further, what alternatives might eventuate if this direction is not taken.

Obstacles to the Vision

While there are likely to be may factors that could impede progress toward the vision outlined above, some of the more obvious or difficult issues that currently face the field will be considered.

First, and most centrally, a full marriage between the fields of adventure leadership and therapy does not exist, or if it does, it is currently substantially unbalanced and, or dysfunctional. Using this metaphor, there are a number of problems that inhibit this relationship. One issue lies in terms of communication. Both fields have very different cultures. Each field has a preferred language that is often esoteric, and both fields have different rules and approaches to how they communicate. There seems to be little shared understanding here, and this appears to be a major stumbling block for effective dialogue. Of critical importance, there are few bilingual voices (those dual-trained), and few people who are visible enough to effectively role-model an integrated understanding of both fields. Given the dominance of adventure leadership voices (as evidenced at the third IATC), this means there is little theoretically, conceptually or in practice that appears familiar, or understandable to mainstream therapy professions. With a predominance of non-therapy language and conceptualization of the field, it is difficult for mainstream therapists and academics to contribute, or find commonality. Lastly, there is a very strong "tribal loyalty" operating in both fields. It appears that there is concern that standards may be, or are being, compromised by the other. However, at this point, it appears that the therapy tribe is well outnumbered by the adventure, or at least adventure *and* non-therapy tribe.

Second, there is a vacuum of expertise to drive the field forward. There are very few broadly experienced dual-trained practitioners. In addition, and as discussed earlier, the field appears to be dominated by the adventure, and, or non-therapy field. The lack of dual-trained expertise means that the establishment of a comprehensive and meaningful knowledge base will take considerable time to develop, and there will always remain a risk that issues and needs of the adventure leadership field will dominate the agenda.

Dialogue in conference forums and the like tend to value process over *content* (doing over thinking), *art* over *science* (creativity over analysis) and *philosophy* over *psychology*. This imbalance is due largely to the predominance of the adventure leadership field. Professional dialogue tends to philosophizing rather than critical analysis and development of theory drawn from research data or mainstream therapy literature. Additionally, and again due to the drive predominantly from adventure leadership, the field appears preoccupied with techniques—the ubiquitous "bag of tricks"—and not with more important skills, from a therapy perspective, of client assessment and screening, treatment planning, psychological risk-management, managing staff team dynamics, and defining minimum competencies.

In terms of research, there are often calls for the need to establish a convincing body of evidence about the efficacy of Adventure Therapy. However, action to this end, and resources allocated to it, has, with few exceptions (Berman & Anton, 1988; Crisp & Hinch, 2003; Davis-Berman & Berman, 1989; Cason & Gillis, 1994; Russell, 2002), not occurred (Newes, 2001). The limited number of quality program evaluations are likely due to a combination of factors. One of those is a lack of understanding about the benefits of research, as well as the lack of expertise in clinical (or applied) research, as opposed to academic research. Questions of program efficacy are not well-answered by academic research methodologies. The field urgently requires experienced clinical researchers to expand the empirical research knowledge base.

Another obstacle to marrying the adventure leadership and therapy fields are feelings of possessiveness to what is assumed to be the essence of Adventure Therapy. Differences in renumeration and professional status between these two fields leads to considerable unease, where practitioners from the better renumerated and higher status therapy field may be envied, and then resented for what is felt like "moving into the territory" of the adventure leadership field. Frequently, the content of conference papers by those with an adventure leadership background support the view that all activities, including therapy, undertaken within adventure or wilderness contexts fall exclusively under the jurisdiction and expertise of the adventure leadership field. It could be hypothesized that this issue is based on a number of factors including resentment or fear and an ignorance of, and, or disregard for what is involved in the practice of therapy. Understandably, therapists may resent and justifiably hold serious ethical concerns about adventure leaders with little or no relevant or equivalent training, referring to themselves as "therapists" or providing therapy services.

In the experience of the author, those trained in therapy are generally very willing to acknowledge the specialized skills of the adventure leader, but the reverse is less common. While there are easily demonstrated and tangible skills required for expert adventure leadership, the skills required for expert therapeutic practice are often less tangible and not acknowledged, dismissed as being "politically incorrect," or seen as being able to be gained from life experience by anyone. In particular, this extends to a lack of understanding of the history and existing knowledge base of mainstream therapies, conventional clinical and therapeutic practices such as diagnostic or client case formulation, treatment planning case management, and so on. Also misinformed, is the view that unmodified, conventional outdoor education philosophy and practice alone is sufficient in and of itself as a therapy, and so is often promoted as a superior, more ideologically acceptable, alternative form of therapy—the "essential" Adventure Therapy.

Adventure leaders are experts in exposing psychologically healthy clients to physical risk, and *may* have learned how to effectively manage the psychological results of this practice in their clients. However, for many uninformed adventure leaders, they may not be aware of any reasons why they cannot simply transfer these sorts of skills to special populations, and then undertake what they have the promoted or relabeled as adventure therapy. In practice this entails exposing psychologically *vulnerable* clients to risk, both physical and psychological, and then intuitively managing the client's reactions by attempting to guide them to "learn something from the experience." So, in this paradigm, conducting therapy and therefore being a therapist would appear to be a natural progression for those with an outdoor leadership background. However, these adventure leaders need to: (a) be reminded of the need to practice within limits of their expertise, and (b) acknowledge that there are highly trained professionals who hold expertise well above theirs in terms of psychological safety and therapeutic processes, including assessing the appropriateness of exposure to risk both psychological and physical. If these adventure leaders understand how critical these two points are to ethical practice, then they are more likely to be willing to participate in the marriage that will ultimately protect, and far more reliably enhance, clients' well-being.

Additionally, there seems to be an understandable resistance toward acknowledging the high level of education and intensity of training required to practice as a therapist, and the years of supervised experience required to become skilled in undertaking therapy with a range of clients and problems. Also, there is a concerning lack of understanding of professional ethics by adventure leaders who have received no formal education in the ethical issues of therapy. The potential danger of this problem was highlighted at the first IATC where many conference presenters and delegates with adventure leadership background arbitrarily adopted the title of "Adventure Therapist" and, or described any, and all, adventure programs as "Adventure Therapy." As the majority of adventure leaders lack this training in the application of ethical principles to therapeutic practice, it is understandable that they struggle to appreciate the importance of this fundamental ethical issue. Finally, those from therapeutic professions have personally been through the process of becoming a professional sanctioned in the eyes of society, for example through registration or licensing. They are members of well-established and thriving professions and professional bodies. It is this expertise that therapists also bring to the marriage. Adventure leaders need to acknowledge, and be guided by this most valuable expertise, no matter how tempting it might be to discover the journey for oneself, or in fact, reinvent the wheel as it were.

These obstacles are challenging ones, but must be overcome if the field is to progress. Most importantly, a difficult, but essential step in overcoming these obstacles is rectifying the imbalance in representation and presence between the adventure leadership and therapy fields in common forums such as conference (e.g., keynote presentations), publications, and the like. Role models and programs that highlight progressive best practice, should be given the greatest prominence. This will be achieved most effectively if dual-trained practitioners who, quite rightly, epitomize the marriage that is sought, are given maximum voice.

Why Accept the Vision?

Of course, the vision presented here is only one, and a beginning point at that. However, the field needs to be cognizant of the risks that continue to exist in alternatives to this vision. The potential for negative scenarios are real, and should be held in mind. This helps to weigh up the benefits for progress on professionalism against the costs of a lack of progress, and the potential detrimental consequences that could eventuate should the field fail to achieve professionalism as outlined in this paper.

The most likely scenario involves the continuation of what could be argued to exist currently. That is, that the field continues to fail to show much more than a very few quality or convincing studies demonstrating any evidence for the benefit of Adventure Therapy. In addition, unethical practices are not uncommon, and practices are highly variable in their standard as no evidence-based guidelines exist. In this scenario, Adventure Therapy continues to be perceived as a risky experimental intervention. This situation leaves the field marginalized and overlooked by funding bodies. As a therapeutic modality, it would not be included within mainstream therapeutic services that are offered to clients who could benefit. It could be expected that with a lack of adequate resourcing, the field would struggle on the periphery and would have difficulty attracting high quality dual-trained practitioners, researchers, and influential advocates in the community. In this scenario, the field of Adventure Therapy continues to be at risk of being widely perceived as Adventure *Quackery*. Practitioners with insufficient, or no consistent training would practice maverick and untested approaches, producing poor, or potentially detrimental outcomes for clients. This would give little confidence to the public of the field holding much value, and would likely lead to a vicious cycle where poor standards and practices repel resources and expertise that could improve training and standards.

Most importantly, this alternative outcome would also be disastrous for our clients. First, there would be very few real, adequately resourced Adventure Therapy programs on offer because the field was generally not supported. This would mean two things. First, that many marginalized clients who may only become engaged in an Adventure Therapy or a similar program, remain at risk and suffer. This would have obvious individual, social, and economic costs. Second, those clients who were able to access those few programs that did exist may be exposed to poor standards or ignorant practices. This would likely be damaging to them and worsen their situation, and they might lose hope of receiving assistance from any form of therapy. Besides being a waste of valuable resources, the entire concept of Adventure Therapy would be at risk of being rejected entirely by society.

Is the Vision Achievable?

Despite the sizable obstacles the field faces, currently a number of developments in the Australian and New Zealand context suggest the vision outlined here can be realized. A working group is currently developing a proposal document on the viability of the formation of an Australian and New Zealand professional association of adventure and wilderness therapy practitioners (PAAWTP Working Group). In addition, the Australian Wilderness Adventure Therapy Accreditation Scheme has been established (Crisp, 2003). This scheme provides a comprehensive and universal training pathway leading to accreditation for practitioners with adventure leadership, therapy, and dual-trained backgrounds. One key aim of this scheme is to provide a common training experience for practitioners regardless of background so they become exposed to each other's practices, skills, and conceptual frameworks. At the time of writing, over 50 trainees have completed the first stage of accreditation. They have come from the majority of Australian states and overseas, and components of the scheme are being considered for incorporation into university courses in different states in Australia. The scheme appears to be accessible and holds potential to be established widely, possibly in other countries. Importantly, a balanced number of trainees from adventure and therapy professional backgrounds are participating (65% adventure leadership), and many trainees are pursuing, or come with, dual-trained professional backgrounds.

Finally, in terms of practice standards, Crisp and Noblet (2003) have recently documented detailed practice guidelines for a range of client types and service settings that are based on principles of international best practice (Crisp, 1997). Finally, there appears to be an increased focus on quality treatment outcome research using meaningful outcome measures (Crisp & Hinch, 2003; Mossman, 2004; Russell, 2002).

Conclusion

It has been proposed that a blueprint for a profession requires three keystone foundations. It has been argued that the field needs to be evidence-based, ethics-based and focused on best practice. A thorough understanding of the ethical issues in all the field's activities is critical to ensure the best for our clients, the profession, and society. In particular, outcome-based evaluation of programs, in combination with best practice guidelines are critical to clarify complex ethical problems that are part of daily adventure therapy practice. It is the application of this process that can assure us, and our clients, that they are most likely to have the optimal therapeutic experience, and this will therefore define us individually as professionals, and as a group, a profession.

References

Berman, D. S. & Anton, M. T. (1988). A wilderness therapy program as an alternative to adolescent psychiatric hospitalization. *Residential Treatment for Children and Youth, 5*(3), 41-53.

Bunce, J. (1997). A question of identity. In C. M. Itin (Ed.), *Exploring the boundaries of adventure therapy: International perspectives—Proceedings of the First International Adventure Therapy Conference.* Boulder, CO: Association for Experiential Education.

Crisp, S. J. R. (2002). *The Australian wilderness adventure therapy accreditation scheme,* NeoPsychology—*Youth*Psych Consulting, Melbourne. www.neopsychology.com.au

Crisp, S. J. R. (1997). International models of best practice in wilderness and adventure therapy. In C. Itin (Ed.), *Exploring the boundaries of adventure therapy: International perspectives-Proceedings of the First International Adventure Therapy Conference.* Boulder, CO: Association for Experiential Education.

Crisp, S. J. R. & Noblet, M. L. (2003). *Guidelines for the practice of wilderness adventure therapy.* NeoPsychology Publications, Melbourne. www.neopsychology.com.au

Crisp, S. J .R. & Hinch, C. (2003). *Evaluation of the benefits of wilderness adventure therapy: Findings from the systemic wilderness adventure therapy research and development (SWA-TRAD) project.* NeoPsychology Publications, Melbourne. www.neopsychology.com.au

Davis-Berman, J. & Berman, D. (1994). *Wilderness therapy: Foundations, theory & research.* Dubuque, IA: Kendall/Hunt Publishing Co.

Davis-Berman, J. & Berman, D. S. (1989). The wilderness therapy program: An empirical study of its effects with adolescents in an outpatient setting. *Journal of Contemporary Psychotherapy, 19*(4) 271-281.

Davis-Berman, J. & Berman, D. S. (1994). Two-year follow-up for the wilderness therapy program, *Journal of Experiential Education 17*(1), 48-50.

Gass, M. (Ed.). (1993). *Adventure therapy—Therapeutic applications of adventure programming.* Dubuque, IA: Kendall/Hunt Publishing Co.

Cason, D. & Gillis, H. L. (1994). A meta-analysis of outdoor adventure programming with adolescents. *Journal of Experiential Education 17*(1) 40-47.

Itin, C. (1998) (Ed.), *Exploring the boundaries of adventure therapy: International perspectives—Proceedings of the First International Adventure Therapy Conference.* Boulder, CO: Association for Experiential Education.

Miles, J. C. & Priest, S. (1990). *Adventure education.* Pennsylvania: Venture Publishing Inc.

Mossman, E. (2004). *An evaluation of short & long-term outcomes and factors associated with success in the Adventure Development Counselling Programme.* Unpublished doctoral thesis. University of Canterbury, New Zealand.

Newes, S. L. (2001). Future directions in adventure-based therapy research: Methodological considerations and design suggestions, *Journal of Experiential Education, 24*(2), 92-99.

Richards, K. (with Smith, B.) (Eds.). (2003). *Therapy within adventure: Proceedings of the Second International Adventure Therapy Conference,* Zeil Publishing, Augsburg, Germany.

Russell, K. C. (2002). *Longitudinal assessment of treatment outcomes in outdoor behavioural healthcare,* Technical Report. University of Idaho.

Russell, K. C. & Hendee, J. C. (2000). *Outdoor behavioural healthcare: Definitions, common practice, expected outcomes and a nationwide survey of programs.* Technical Report. University of Idaho.

Author's Biography

Dr. Simon Crisp, *a Clinical Child, Adolescent & Family Psychologist is founder and director of Neo Psychology. He has been facilitating outdoor programs for over two decades, and pioneered the development, practice and research of Wilderness Adventure Therapy programs in Australia for the last 12 years. He established the Australian Wilderness Adventure Therapy Accreditation Scheme in 2002, has supervised, trained and lectured on Adventure Therapy to hundreds of people for over a decade, and has been a passionate clinical researcher of adventure therapy interventions during this time.*

Correspondence

Dr. Simon J.R. Crisp
Director, Neo Psychology
P.O. Box 86 Clifton Hill
3068 AUSTRALIA
Tel: +61-(0)3-8430-2208
Email: simon@neopsychology.com.au
Website: www.neopsychology.com.au

A Confluence of Cultures: Wilderness Adventure Therapy Practice in Australia and New Zealand

Cathryn Carpenter and Anita Pryor

■■■

In exploring where profession meets passion, practitioners in Australia and New Zealand identified that relationships, culture, land, healing, and journeys lie at the heart of our work. This paper presents significant aspects of the discussions held with 76 practitioners working in the field of wilderness adventure therapy that attended the South Pacific Regional gathering near Melbourne, Australia in 2002.

Histories, landscapes, and cultural factors have influenced the evolution of wilderness and Adventure Therapy programs in New Zealand and Australia. Practice is different in each country, yet over the course of four days—with place, space, and sufficient time, practitioners from either end of the Tasman Sea experienced a confluence in practice, where commonalities were found, uncomfortable clashes were explored, and agreement reached on certain personal, professional and cultural implications for the field of Wilderness Adventure Therapy in this region.

This paper offers a summary of selected passionate conversations, a collation of shared elements of practice, and presents the strategies and recommendations for further consolidation of the field in this region. The structure of the paper follows a merging of practice:

I. *Being in the Land—understanding the contexts in which these discussions occurred, including the importance of place, land, culture and spirit.*

II. *Making Connections with people and place—exploring the what, how, and why of wilderness and adventure therapy programs in this region.*

III. The Journey Ahead—identifying impediments, future directions, and possibilities as we contemplate the "where to" next.

■ ■ ■

Being in the Land

In a world where our vision becomes ever more blinkered by the dominance of a single cultural way and where such dominance threatens the survival of other ways of thinking and being, there is an urgent need for more stories (Taylor, cited in Neidje, 1989, p. v).

At the second International Adventure Therapy Conference in Germany in 2000, delegates attending the South Pacific Regional meeting agreed that while the content of presentations and issues being debated were stimulating and relevant, in some cases it didn't necessarily reflect the heart of practice in our region. Amongst other elements, access to "people-free" places, with relative freedom to explore and innovate, were seen as opportunities peculiar to our contexts. As Bunce had articulated, "In the case of New Zealand, we are increasingly aware of our unique cultural identity, and are finding that some imported theories and models of practice do not fit for us" (Bunce, 1997, p. 46). These experiences provided the impetus for the South Pacific Forum.

In April 2002, 76 people from all states and territories of Australia, and from both islands of New Zealand gathered for a South Pacific Regional Wilderness Adventure Therapy Forum in Victoria, Australia. The invitation was directed toward practitioners and others using activities and adventures in the outdoors for specific therapeutic purposes. Primary aims for the forum were to share practice, to plan for a consolidated regional approach, to increase our understanding of the heart of practice in this region, and to disseminate outcomes at the third International Adventure Therapy Conference.

A preforum questionnaire helped to shape the 4-day event, facilitated by a professional from outside the field. Questions posed in community sessions led to smaller, self-facilitating discussion groups, which in turn fed back to the larger community. A practitioner from Europe assisted us to critique our own conversations through "fishbowl debates." In this way, the forum was made up of "shared conversations" rather than formal presentations, enabling delegates to attend as both practitioners sharing their expertise, and as participants engaged in learning. Emergent "areas of interest," "hot topics" and the "heart of our work" are ultimately what guided the experience. All discussions were documented and compiled by forum organizers as *Shared Conversations* (Pryor & Carpenter, 2002). A database of practitioners, and an interactive website for the field in this region were further outcomes. www.therapeuticadventure.com.au

In examining the heart of practice, delegates were asked what they saw as significant in shaping the work, practice, programs, and experiences for participants in this region. A summary of answers includes:

- Ready access to national, state, and regional parks
- Provision of a non-judgmental and supportive environment within programs
- "Time, Place and Space" to explore new coping mechanisms, relationships, and definitions of self within programs (especially in wild places)
- Essential elements: Relationships (self, others, and environment), Process/Processing, Choice, Risk, Experience/Experiential, Personal Responsibility, Reflection, and Healing/Growth

These elements individually are not necessarily unique to the South Pacific Region. When practitioners explored how these elements interact within the heart of their practice, we were further able to gain insight into the unique approaches within the South Pacific experience of wilderness adventure therapy.

During our shared conversations, Land, Culture and Spirit emerged as major undercurrents in our practice. These themes at times caused small ripples that seemed to slide by with little notice then suddenly reverberate within the group, forcing participants to reexamine their own practice in the light of these issues. Threading their way throughout the course of the forum, whatever the topic or question raised, these same themes bubbled to the surface of conversation across the community. Obviously, the forum provided an opportunity for many to remember these aspects in our work, and it became clear that as we further our attempt to understand how practitioners see their field or profession, we must continue to explore themes of land, culture and spirit.

Land

The first significant theme included discussions on the words we use (or don't use) to describe wild places we access for our work. The use of the word *wilderness,* could be interpreted as ignoring the traditional habitation and spiritual connections of the Maori and Aboriginal people. Talk of "people-free places" was discussed as implying "culturally free," thereby again ignoring traditional heritage. During the course of the forum, the words *land, country* and *bush* became more commonly used by many to describe the wild places accessed for the work. As an indigenous participant at the forum explained, "you just need to say land and it brings up so much" (Pryor & Carpenter, 2002, p. 51). In fact, some believe land, country, bush, are at the heart of their practice. Small groups of delegates defined their practice in the following ways:

- "Using the Earth's gifts and its magic to help heal people. All with a big dose of human compassion and awareness." (p. 26).
- "Bush Change Experiences." (p. 27).
- "Listen to the land—learn and know. Build this. Be honest with program experiences. Grow something authentic. Rituals are of the land." (p. 33).
- "Reconnecting people to the land in which we live." (p. 33).

(Pryor & Carpenter, 2002).

Cultural Presence

The second significant theme was acknowledgement (or lack of acknowledgement) of the cultural presence inherent in the Australian and New Zealand landscapes, as well as the traditional custodians of the land we access for our programs. Adopting indigenous "rites of passage" experiences and "telling traditional stories" emerged as ethical dilemmas for those practitioners seeking to respect the traditions, cultures, languages, and rich indigenous histories associated with the land. This issue is of international concern for some. As Wilson-Schaef (1995), of mixed North American heritage, stated, "white minds tend to seek out ceremonies, rituals or magic as a fix... when this knowledge is not deeply grounded in the worldview of its own culture it looses all meaning and power." (p. 6). As one participant of the forum suggested, "don't take our rituals, create your own." (Pryor & Carpenter, 2002, p. 34) One practitioner from New Zealand (NZ), stated, "How I work and operate in wilderness and outdoors areas is based on the treaty of Waitangi, a cornerstone of practice and belief, and a wonderful vehicle for how NZ people work." (Pryor & Carpenter, 2002, p. 33). Whilst it appears that "seeking permission" from cultural custodians is embedded within practice in at least northern New Zealand and the Northern Territory in Australia, during the course of the forum more practitioners came to understand this as an ethical and moral imperative in their work.

Spirit

The third significant theme that emerged within various discussion groups was that of the importance of spiritual connection with the land for participants and staff within programs. There was some talk of the need to agree that this concept has different meaning for people from different cultures, but spirit is central to the heart of practice for a significant number of practitioners. "Land is not real estate...land is part of the essence of who indigenous people are. It needs to be understood within the context of their spirituality and their holistic sense of creation and humanity"

(Wilson-Schaef, 1995, Feb. 16). For a small group of practitioners their practice was defined as, "Cleansing of the spirit and soul with excitement." (Pryor & Carpenter, 2002, p. 25).

In examining where land, culture, and spirit meet, we must somehow include the dynamic processes surrounding an experience where intuition, feelings, history, and trust play a part. Perhaps honouring of culture and land, creation of space and time, and trust in the natural processes at work, all within an experience of country, is a way of connecting these themes. Along with an examination of our behaviours and use of language, these elements become important in shaping a cultural identity of practice for any region. If we seek to gain broader understanding of wilderness adventure therapy, developing a shared language over time will be critical to a sense of collective identity. As Brookes (1994) states, "the language we use does not merely convey our thoughts; it shapes our thinking." (p. 25). During the forum, Gilsdorf also reflected, "Reconciliation is a deep process. The essence of what you are doing is about reconciliation—from an outsider's perspective this might be fundamental [to understanding the heart of practice]." (Pryor & Carpenter, 2002, p. 35).

Making Connections with People and Place

"If you have come to help me, you are wasting your time. But if you have come to help me because your liberation is bound up with mine, then let us work together" (Aboriginal Activist Sister, cited in Loynes, 2002, p. 123).

This section summarizes current practice in the region, including how and why programs operate, an overview of participants and providers, and also typical programmatic experiences. A summary of essential elements of practice is also presented. It needs to be acknowledged that this provides only a general representation of programs within the region, as the information is limited to only those programs and organizations that participated and those practitioners who elected to attend the forum independently.

Program Settings

Programs represented at the forum operated as small businesses or not-for-profit organizations. This has several possible implications. First, the relatively small size of organizations may make programs more vulnerable to changes in political and social climate. Second, economies of scale would suggests that smaller organizations may be relatively resource-intense, whereas larger programs may find greater efficiency in operating structures thereby making their programs cheaper to run overall. In addition, without collaboration, smaller programs and organizations may be less likely to have models and practices incorporated into broader social service structures (e.g., in health and education) and may therefore remain reliant on shorter-term financial support.

Program Staff

Programs represented at the forum generally employ 2 to 4 full-time staff and 2 to 6 part-time staff. Diverse educational and training pathways for staff were identified, with over 40 different qualifications listed by practitioners. The fact that practitioners undertook so many educational or training pathways to reach their current positions speaks of certain conditions and implications worthy of consideration. It has the potential to create rich diversity within staff teams, leading to diversity in practice styles and/or approaches. (Carpenter, Cherednichenko, & Price, 2000). This factor may also reflect greater employment mobility, which may be due to job opportunities or the move toward short-term funding in the social services. On the other hand, broad ranging educational and training pathways for staff may reflect a relative lack of education and/or training options specific to our field, and may lead to inconsistency in practice standards (Crisp, 1997). These ideas have yet to be rigorously tested within the region.

Program Clients

Programs represented at the forum provide services for 50 to 80 clients each year (including pre- and post-experience services). Where programs involve wilderness/outdoors/bush experiences, groups are made up of 8 to 10 participants, with 2 to 4 staff in attendance. Clients are drawn from both urban and rural environments. From those programs represented, it appears that programs in the South Pacific recruit clients experiencing a broad range of health and life issues. Practitioners identified the following client issues:

- "Adolescence," including health and well-being
- Self-esteem and other issues related to sense of self
- Behavioral issues
- Personal management, including personal, social and living skills
- Substance misuse and abuse, and related health risks and issues
- "At risk" indicators, including personal, social, environmental, emotional, legal
- Grief and loss
- Unemployment
- Social, family and educational system breakdown
- Poverty, disadvantage, lack of supporting services and opportunities
- Loss of culture, identity, discrimination, and racism
- Confusion over "place in the world," including sense of belonging

A closer examination of the reasons participants engage with services provided insight into the issues faced by community members within this Region. As Handley (cited in Reddrop, 1997) stated:

> Two important aspects of Australia enable outdoor programs a high probability of success. These are: the abundance of rugged wilderness environments, and the perception of a need for programs that address issues such as juvenile justice, homelessness and increasing crime (p. 167).

These issues are generally seen as common across wide-ranging communities in many contexts, including for indigenous and non-indigenous members. Some see these as problems associated with the deficit of an individual, and therefore interventions seek to "treat" the individual. Others would argue that these issues are symptoms of a breakdown in community structures that traditionally gave members a sense of connectedness, belonging, and a role within economic and social structures. Interventions from this perspective seek to build healthy communities, which therefore promote resilient individuals who have meaning, purpose and sense of belonging. "It is not the individual who needs healing; it is the social and societal arrangements" (Brookes, 1994, p. 27). Perhaps these different approaches can be envisaged as falling along a continuum, with individual treatment at one end, and community building at the other.

Program Aims

In attempting to understand the ways in which organizations in this region prepare for and attend to the needs of participants/clients, delegates were asked: "What are the values that guide your practice?" and "What leads you to develop programs in the ways you have described?" Delegates were asked to share the philosophical approach, rationale or mission statements of their programs. The following list was developed from program documentation and illustrates the wide diversity in aims for programs in this region.

- "To provide a safe but challenging environment that encourages young people to make changes that will enhance their life chances."
- "All journeys are made, by and for young people, to get the self respect, trust, courage and skill to have a good life because grog, sniffing, violence and crime are no good."
- "To respect people, self, and land."
- "To experience a journey about challenge and choice."
- "To enable individuals to recognize their personal worth and to support and encourage them in working toward realizing their full potential in life, as identified by them."

- "High quality, safe, challenging wilderness and adventure experiences can provide 'at risk' young people with an opportunity to learn and discover, and experience themselves, others and their environment in new and positive ways."
- "We will be holistic in our attitudes and universal in our approach, and provide as many facilities, options and stratagems as possible. We will ensure that not one aspect or one single basis for change will dominate the whole."

(Pryor & Carpenter, 2002, p. 69).

There are numerous challenges apparent when reading this list. How do we collate such aims and approaches without "watering down" individual approaches? How do we articulate the unspoken idealism apparent within the South Pacific Forum? "Enhancing young people's lives" might be seen as a dominant assumption, rationale or mission for these organizations and also as a worthy social service. Perhaps the "challenging experience," or the "journey through land" are seen as generally "empowering processes," through which individuals are enabled to "value themselves more" or "find greater satisfaction in life." These statements also resound with moral and/or ethical value imperatives. To synthesize these philosophies might be to say that some programs consciously and unconsciously assist individuals to reconnect with the land, culture and spirit as integral to enhancing connections for people. Very important to a synthesis of common practice is to follow Brookes (1994) line of questioning, "What are our tacit assumptions? What is the background hum of social change and stability at work within these words?" (p. 26).

Program Processes

The aims of organizations in this region are generally closely related to the identified needs of participants. Although a reasonable percentage of practitioners (more than half) were recorded as having training in therapeutic techniques or recognized clinical therapist qualifications, noted was a lack of use of the terms therapy and therapeutic for describing the work. Practitioners in this region described the processes and methods of their work in the following ways:

- Interventions—for change
- Support—to reintegrate into schools and society
- Improving—the participants' self-management skills
- Focusing—on participant successes, finding solutions
- Assisting—the process of change and personal growth
- Strengthening—connections to others and community

It is interesting to note that these processes may as well imply educational or social change experiences as therapeutic experiences or a conscious intentional process of therapy. Perhaps, as Crisp (1997) identified, "while the authority of a therapist is a relative 'given' in the United Kingdom and United States, this is often a source of tension with Australian clients." (p. 64). Whilst requiring further investigation, this tension may also describe a cultural characteristic for people/clients in this region as being less willing, less able, or less interested in accessing or paying for "therapy". For a small group of delegates practice was defined as "to facilitate healthy change and personal growth rather than 'therapy'" (Pryor & Carpenter, 2002, p. 38).

Program Venues

All of the programs represented at the forum used outdoors, remote or isolated bush environments, yet only one emphasized the "wilderness." Discussions explored how the modern understanding of wilderness may more closely represent a remote conceptual space rather than an area of land, or physical location. As mentioned earlier, delegates experienced turmoil over the terminology used for places accessed by their programs (i.e., is it wilderness, land, country or bush?). One group chose to explore this theme more closely, and explored why programs use land, how programs related to land, and what participants gained by experiencing land. The following list explores the significance of the natural landscape, as described by practitioners during the forum:

- "We operate in remote locations in order to foster disequilibria, group dynamics, a sense of connectedness to the earth and each other."
- "Provides a great dimension to challenge clients in physical and emotional ways."
- "Connection with the land inspires and teaches."
- "Journeying through remote, natural environments lies at the heart of our programs, the relationships that emerge, evolve beyond the duration of the experience."
- "The outdoor environment is the learning medium for the journey, exploring the cycle of land, self and others."
- "Bush/land/wilderness permeates all aspects of the experience in conscious and unconscious ways."

(Pryor & Carpenter, 2002, p. 70).

North American practitioners describe one of the main uses of wilderness for therapy as fostering disequilibria through a use of unfamiliar environments (Davis-Berman & Berman, 1994; Gass, 1993; Luckner &

Nadler, 1997). Clearly this is also a factor in the South Pacific; however, the Australian and New Zealand practitioners appear to emphasize natural places as not merely unfamiliar, but at the heart of the therapy itself.

Essential Elements of Practice

In an attempt to understand what practitioners felt were critical components in program development and delivery, a group brainstorming process brought out wide-ranging essential elements within our collective practice. These elements were refined through further group processes, until the following conceptual components emerged:

- Relationships—self, others, and environment
- Process/Processing
- Choice
- Risk
- Experience/Experiential
- Personal Responsibility
- Reflection
- Healing/Growth

Each element was expanded to connect with stories of practice, key words of meaning and current theoretical frameworks. These words obviously contain multilayered meanings, as well as diverse definitions. At the risk of oversimplifying or undermining complex program processes or in-depth discussions, one initial way of interpreting this collection of essential elements into a general statement about collective practice in this region follows. Within programs, individuals are readied to accept responsibility, make choices, take risks, reflect on their relationship with themselves, others, and the environment, thereby allowing healing or growth to occur. The practitioner may be said to support individuals by encouraging opportunities for transition to occur, within the experiential process they are providing. In order to more closely examine the heart of practice in this region, these elements are clearly worthy of further investigation.

The Journey Ahead

"We need the knowledge the pakeha [white people] brings from all over the world as well as the sense of belonging and the whakapapa [genealogy/history/culture] of the Maori. The separate paths our people have trod can unite in a highway to the future that is built on the best of both."

Dame Whinia Maori elder (Wilson-Schaef, 1995, Feb. 22).

In addition to exploring the "heart of the practice," the South Pacific community of practitioners examined challenges and future directions for the field here. Together, delegates explored the question "What holds us back in our work?" and examined areas for attention and action. These conversations led to "Community Decisions," (made by the entire community of practitioners attending the forum) towards further consolidation of the field in this region.

Impediments to Practice

Delegate experiences at the first International Adventure Therapy Conference in Perth, Australia in 1997, and more recent local experiences, have shown that practitioners in this field find it difficult to move forward with a shared approach. Delegates of this forum were asked: "What are the obstacles, problems, impediments and systemic issues that get in the way or bog us down?" Program concerns included the typical effects of working in the outdoors (employment conditions, fatigue, stress, isolation, time away from home, lack of a union to tackle these issues); the challenges of working with "sometimes difficult people" (including difficult personal feelings); emotional safety; setting aside personal judgements; and reconnecting back with "normal life" after programs.

The South Pacific region is currently determining whether we are a professional entity, or a collection of people working within various professions, but sharing this field of work. For those who called this a "profession," concerns included: program isolation; a lack of clear professional identity and credibility; a lack of clear educational pathways for employment; a lack of national guidelines and standards; a lack of ethical guidelines; a lack of accountability (except to the coroner's court!); a lack of effective evaluation and research relevant for this region; the "ego" of some practitioners; and the "dodgy-ness" of other practitioners. For those who described this as a "field" concerns included: a lack of shared language about the work; different cultural perspectives; a lack of good descriptions for promoting the work to others (including participants); a lack of knowledge/options about program evaluations; the difficulty of dispelling myths and assumptions in the community about the work; the difficulty of defining the field; and the frustrations of having others define the field for us.

From a social or political perspective, various problems were identified including inflexible education systems; labeling and stigmatizing of participants; the breakdown of families; the creation of welfare-dependent citizens; lack of adventurous options for older people; community perceptions of wilderness adventure therapy; a conservative political climate; and short-term, tightly targeted, competitive tendering for funding. These were seen as impediments or difficulties affecting work. Regarding the natural environment, concerns about sustainable land management, high use of natural resources, increased regulation of public land, and growing lack of space were seen as particular obstacles for this region. From these problems came passionate discussion about what was needed in order to consolidate and move the field forward in Australia and New Zealand.

Areas for Attention and Action

Delegates agreed on issues of greatest concern, and were invited to participate in small working groups of interest. Each group brought their recommendations back to the whole community. Working groups explored issues of:

- Ethics—standards, lack of a professional association, boundaries, responsibilities, core values, principles, best practice
- Research and Evaluation—development of shared resources, research database, evaluation tools, establishment of a working party
- Land—"respect," "permission," belonging, roots/family, balance, connection, conservation, reconciliation
- Cross-cultural Practice—understanding, respect, listening, relationships, recognition of traditional cultures, beliefs, uncomfortable issues, processes for cross-cultural practice
- Staff Skills—core competencies, "therapist," skills, accreditation, quality control, educational pathways to wilderness adventure therapy, the need for teams, Australian standards, collective identity

While groups met and focused their discussion on the above topics, common themes for the development of the field surfaced. Emerging themes for attention and action included: training, qualifications, standards in practice, research, literature, evaluation, ethical practice, cross-cultural practice, words/definitions (including a shared language), management issues, staff exchanges, community networks and links, and funding submissions. These themes were determined to be priorities for the field, across a range of practitioner positions, experience and interest.

Community Decisions

On the last morning of the forum, delegates considered current needs and future directions, asking, "How will we further consolidate practice in this region?" Although no timelines were set, delegates agreed to work toward the following goals in small action groups:

- To develop a research resource
- To form a group to gain funds for collaborative research, including for a review of evaluation tools
- To embed cross-cultural practice in our work now, including

respect, permission, and invitation

- To develop a set of ethical guidelines for the field, and investigate the process of becoming a professional association

- To continue to work on the following significant issues:
  - (a) Clarifying who we are and what we do (identity, collective body)
  - (b) Australian standards for practice
  - (c) Opportunities for staff exchange and peer supervision
  - (d) Developing beyond this forum

Future Pathways

Now, more than a year since the South Pacific Forum, some movement towards these aims has taken place. The upcoming second South Pacific Forum will no doubt illuminate outcomes towards a clearer identity for the field here. The following list comes from later discussions particularly within the Bush Adventure Therapy Network of Victoria, and incorporates practitioners' hopes for action yet to be taken:

- A collection of the histories of practice in this region

- A study of current programs and current models of practice in this region

- Development of efficient dissemination strategies, enabling open sharing of information in this region. Includes development and maintenance of website (www.therapeuticadventure.com.au.) for information, dissemination, efficiency and interactive educational purposes

- Encouragement of local, regional, and national networks

- A meta-analysis of research already undertaken in the field in this region

- A survey of current evaluation tools for practice and programs in this region (including culturally specific tools, tools for process evaluation as well as outcomes, and tools that assist programs maintain the integrity of program processes within evaluation processes)

- Development of a professional association of wilderness adventure therapy practitioners to support good practice and nurture high standards

- Sharing of practice between others and ourselves

Conclusion: Journeys to the Heart of Practice

Wilderness and Adventure Programs are gaining worldwide recognition as an effective approach to engaging people struggling with a variety of difficult life circumstances in a participatory process of change. At the second International Adventure Therapy Conference, approximately 20 Australian and New Zealand delegates agreed that an apparent lack of emphasis on wilderness within international Adventure Therapy practice might reflect an inherent cultural or regional difference for practice in the South Pacific. In order to encompass this possible regional difference, the forum upon which this paper reports invited those from within the field of Wilderness Adventure Therapy to participate. Discussions reflected rich reasons for why natural environments are important to the heart of practice in Australia and New Zealand, leading to deep debate around issues of Land, Culture, and Spirit.

Practitioners discussed, argued, shared, and challenged understandings of their own practice and the practice of others. Along the way, delegates "teased-out" and somehow "got at" the characteristics of practice occurring within this region, across the breadth and range of practitioner experiences and programs represented.

For some practitioners living in Australia and New Zealand, practice could be summarized as an organic merging of:

- Programs *to consciously and unconsciously assist individuals to reconnect with the land, culture and spirit, integral to enhancing connections for people and their communities.*

- Practice *where individuals are readied to accept responsibility, make choices, take risks, reflect on their relationship with self, others, and the environment, allowing healing and growth to occur.*

- And Practitioners *who support individuals by encouraging opportunities for transition to occur, within a shared experiential and/or therapeutic process.*

The terminology remains contentious: Are we therapists, practitioners or workers? Are we working in wilderness, nature, the land or bush? Are we a profession or a field? However, it seems practitioners in this region are committed to working toward a shared understanding of similarities and differences. This summary of shared conversations provides an early attempt to describe the essential elements of practice occurring within this region. From these conversations it would seem that practice in this region rests on foundations broader than the terms wilderness, adventure, and therapy, and must include terms such as healing, journeys, and relationships in attempting to articulate the means, methods and aims of practice in this region. It is critical that we identify a name for our profession that is inclusive of all these aspects of our work.

Confluence of Culture goes beyond the South Pacific region. These findings have implications for international practice, networking and research. It appears important, for example, that we attempt to value the unique evolutions of programs spawned in diverse cultural contexts, and seek to understand the differences. As this field continues to develop and grow, questions of theory and practice need to be explored alongside questions of land, culture and spirit. Appropriate evaluation methods and tools need to be developed in order to define and describe the different cultural contexts and their implications for program development, delivery and outcomes. Ultimately, to examine practice without an understanding of the contextual conditions from which practice evolves may be to ignore the heart of practice.

References

Brookes, A. (1994). Is cyberspace the next frontier for adventure-based counselling? *The Outdoor Educator*. Journal of Victorian Outdoor Education Association, July 1994. p. 21–28.

Bunce, J. (1997). A question of identity. In C. Itin. (Ed.), Proceedings of 1st International Adventure Therapy Conference: *Exploring the Boundaries*. Perth, Australia: COEAWA 1997, p. 46–55.

Carpenter, C., Cherednichenko, B. & Price, M. (2000). *Wilderness experiential learning*. Unpublished manuscript. Victoria University: Melbourne, Australia.

Crisp, S. (1997). International models of best practice in wilderness and adventure therapy. In C. Itin. (Ed.), Proceedings of 1st International Adventure Therapy Conference: *Exploring the Boundaries*. Perth, Australia: COEAWA 1997, p. 56–74.

Davis-Berman, J., & Berman, D.S. (1994). *Wilderness therapy: Foundations, theory and research*. Dubuque, IA: Kendall/Hunt Publishing Co.

Gass, M. (Ed.), (1993). *Adventure therapy: Therapeutic application of adventure programming*. Dubuque, IA: Kendall/Hunt Publishing Co.

Loynes, C. (2002). The generative paradigm. *Journal of Adventure Education and Outdoor Learning*. 2(2), 113-125.

Luckner, J., & Nadler, R. (1997). *Processing the experience: Strategies to enhance and generalize learning*. Dubuque, IA: Kendall/Hunt Publishing Co.

Neidje, B. (1989). *Story about feeling*. Broome, Western Australia: Magabala Books. Aboriginal Corporation.

Pryor, A. & Carpenter, C. (2002). *South Pacific Forum for Wilderness Adventure Therapy: Shared conversations*. (Available from School of Education, Victoria University, P.O. Box 14428, MC Vic 8001, Australia).

Reddrop, S. (1997). *Outdoor programs for young offenders in detention. An overview*. Hobart, Tasmania: National Clearinghouse for youth studies.

Wilson-Schaef, A. (1995). *Native wisdom for white minds: Daily reflections inspired by the native peoples of the world*. New York: Random House/Ballantine Books.

Authors' Acknowledgments

To the participants who brought their energy and passion to the South Pacific gathering, thank you! These stories represent your experience and expertise in the field of Wilderness Adventure Therapy in Australia and New Zealand. We hope you will use your shared stories for better understanding of your own work and the work of others. We look forward to continuing this work at future gatherings.

Authors' Biographies

Anita Pryor *currently coordinates The Outdoor Experience Program (of Jesuit Social Services), an alternative program for young people experiencing difficulties associated with drugs/alcohol. Within this role, she supervises delivery of a therapeutic wilderness program and development of community-based adventure and wilderness programs, co-facilitated with a range of youth services in Melbourne, Australia.*

Cathryn Carpenter *currently coordinates and teaches within the Master's of Education—Experiential Learning and Development degree, which includes a study sequence in wilderness adventure programs. She also coordinates the Outdoor Education subjects within the Bachelor of Education degree at Victoria University in Melbourne, Australia.*

Correspondence

Anita Pryor
The Outdoor Experience Program
Jesuit Social Services
P.O. Box 1141,
Collingwood, Victoria 3066 Australia
Phone: 61-3-9415-8700
anita.pryor@jss.org.au

Cathryn Carpenter
Victoria University
School of Education
P.O. Box 14428
Melbourne, Victoria 8001 Australia
Phone: 61-3-9919-7518
cathryn.carpenter@vu.edu.au

Adventure Therapy as Complementary and Alternative Medicine (CAM)

Denise Mitten

■ ■ ■

Adventure therapy often is used as a complementary healthcare modality for people seeking growth and development in their lives. The notion that adventure therapy is a complementary and alternative medicine (CAM) and can be situated in the mind-body, the biologically based, and/or the energy therapies domains as defined by the National Center for Complementary and Alternative Medicine (NCCAM) will be explored. This paper defines and describes (CAM), and examines both the support for CAM and some constraints to the acceptance by some healthcare professionals of CAM. A connection is made between the public's growing use and acceptance of CAM and the public's use of adventure therapy. It also suggests ways to create visibility for our work in the greater area of healthcare.

■ ■ ■

The purpose of this paper is to create an understanding of adventure therapy as a complementary or alternative modality within complementary and alternative medicine (CAM). This paper will provide an overview of CAM and evidence for both professional and public support for CAM. Differences between CAM pedagogy and conventional medicine will be discussed in order to show how adventure therapy aligns with CAM pedagogy. Using the National Institute of Health's (NIH) description of CAM categories, adventure therapy will be situated within their system. It is hoped that the information provided in this paper will stimulate critical thinking that will help better inform our own practices of adventure therapy and help to create an understanding of how we can lay our work before a larger critical audience. Viewing our work through a CAM lens can increase our research opportunities and help our work grow and mature.

Some practitioners/authors call adventure therapy (also called adventure-based therapy) a "field," meaning a group of people who practice adventure therapy as a profession (Newes, 2000). Others define it as a therapy modality and still others as a therapeutic modality (Berman & Davis-Berman, 2000; Gillis & Thomsen, 1996) that might be used by professionals in a variety of fields. Gass (1993) describes three major types of adventure therapy (adventure-based therapy, wilderness therapy, and residential camping) based on where the program takes place, the length of time of the program and the specific type of programming used. In addition to being a therapeutic modality, adventure therapy can have a specific therapy component that includes psychotherapy or counseling. Gillis and Thomsen (1996) define "adventure (psycho)therapy as an active, experiential approach to group (and family) psychotherapy or counseling" (p.83).

For the purpose of this paper, adventure therapy will be defined as a therapeutic modality that includes the purposeful use of the natural environment and outdoor or other activities as a way to increase a person's state of health or well-being. Therefore, adventure therapy practitioners provide healthcare. Adventure therapy involves a treatment plan or program objectives on the part of the practitioner that involves a preplanned course of action specific to the population or person being served. This treatment plan includes updates and quantifiable measurements of the healing progress including health or behavior changes made (D. Berman, personal communication, March 30, 2004).

Adventure therapy is a therapeutic modality that may have its roots in medieval times. During these times there was an understanding of the benefits of physical exercise outdoors and being in nature, and medieval hospitals often were situated near monasteries. The monasteries had courtyards patients could use for walking and sitting outdoors as well as gardens where the medicinal and culinary herbs were grown (Irvine & Warber, 2002). Adventure therapy has identifiable roots in the United States as far back as the pre-1800s, when hospital patients were housed in tents (Davis-Berman & Berman, 1994). Tent housing provided beneficial exposure to fresh air, sunshine and exercise. At present, many people in the United States see Outward Bound as the organization that began using pedagogy and techniques and practices that currently inform many professionals' practice of adventure therapy.

While no government agency provides regulations specifically governing the practice of adventure therapy, the Therapeutic Adventure Professional Group (TAPG) of the Association for Experiential Education (AEE) has written a set of ethical standards for practice, for use by providers and practitioners (Gass, 1993). Crisp (2003) in Australia offers individual accreditation in wilderness adventure therapy (WAT) and some universities in the United States and Canada also offer specific training for people who want to provide adventure therapy. Such training is designed to help providers understand that integral parts of adventure therapy programming include the program design and the principles behind the design, an understanding of staff competency, access to clinical diagnosis, and an understanding and competency in programming procedures and processes (Crisp, 2003). Practitioners of adventure therapy also should understand the philosophy and theoretical foundations of adventure therapy and program design and should be trained in specific sets of interpersonal and clinical skills as well as outdoor or technical skills.

Participation in adventure programs (a broader category of programs that includes adventure therapy programs) is increasing. Up to 70,000 people a year may participate in the over 700 wilderness experience programs in the United States (Friese, Hendee, & Kinziger, 1998). Bly (2001) and Sugerman (2000) have found that participation rates are increasing, especially for women and older adults. Attarian (2001) confirmed that overall participation in adventure programs has increased in the last 15 years due to a number of factors, including socio-economic factors, more leisure time, media exposure, greater awareness of health and wellness, and wanting more time in nature.

Similar to more traditional forms of psychotherapy, people typically participate in adventure therapy programs for health reasons, including physical, emotional, and psychological concerns. Many participants are adolescents sent by the court or parents in the hope that they might achieve the emotional growth necessary for behavioral changes. Some of the most publicized programs use adventure therapy as a government funded alternative to juvenile incarceration (Newes, 2000). Trips and programs may be specialized for particular populations and/or issues (e.g., women with eating disorders, people with addiction problems, individuals recovering from brain injuries, or people in a life transition). Some adventure therapy programs have family groups as clients and are designed to facilitate better family functioning (Bandoroff & Scherer, 1994).

In the same way that there are different types and uses of massages in massage therapy (e.g., Swedish, deep tissue, trager, or shiatsu), there appear to be many different and valid ways adventure therapy is used and practiced. For example, adventure therapy can take place during a week-long backpacking trip or two hours each afternoon in a residential treatment facility. The practitioner could lead the process by "frontloading" the activities with information and/or metaphors, or the practitioner could allow the client to construct his/her own meaning from the activities.

Intent is an important concept when talking about adventure therapy just as it is in massage. A person could give a friend a massage and that could have therapeutic benefits. Similarly, people can rockclimb, participate in adventure activities, or go into the natural environment and reap thera-peutic benefits. Adventure therapy is separated from these personal uses of activities and the natural environment by the delivery of programs from trained, qualified practitioners with the intent of creating a space for the therapeutic benefits or therapy to take place. The intention is manifested in the treatment plan developed by the practitioner and specific for the individual(s) served.

CAM Defined

CAM practices, as defined by the National Institute of Health (NIH), "are those healthcare and medical practices that are not currently an integral part of conventional medicine" (http://nccam.nih.gov/health/whatiscam/).

From this definition one can understand that a list of CAM practices will be constantly changing depending on who compiles the list and when. Currently, there are over one thousand therapies considered to be CAM. A short sample list of these includes acupuncture, aromatherapy, Ayurveda, biofeedback, chiropractic, electromagnectic therapy, energy healing, herbal medicine, homeopathy, hypnosis/guided imagery, massage therapy, medi-tation, nutritional supplements, prayer/prayer healing, psychological coun-seling, relaxation therapy, spiritual healing, therapeutic touch, tai chi, tra-ditional oriental medicine/Chinese medicine, and yoga. The use and acceptance of CAM varies with populations. For instance some medical experts and practitioners consider biofeedback to be part of conventional medicine and not a CAM, while others consider biofeedback a CAM. Professionals in Germany have produced many studies and texts about herbal medicine, and therefore herbal medicine is more understood and mainstream there than in the United States. In the United States research and use of herbal medicine is lacking, in part because of patent laws which do not allow companies to patent herbal medicines.

The NIH National Center for Complementary and Alternative Medicine (NCCAM) is the federal agency in the United States that has defined and categorized CAM. The agency is dedicated to exploring CAM practices in the context of rigorous science, training CAM researchers, and disseminating authoritative information to the public and professionals (http://nccam.nih.gov/an/general/). NCCAM had a budget over $121 mil-lion in 2005 (http://nccam.nci.nih.gov/about/appropriations/). This large budget is indicative of public and professional support. While the NCCAM is a U.S. organization, professionals in many other countries have even broader understandings and use of CAM and have different organizations that define and/or regulate CAM.

Complementary medicine is different than alternative medicine. *Complementary* medicine is used *together with* conventional medicine. An example of a complementary therapy is using an essential oil (e.g., lavender, to help lessen a patient's discomfort following surgery. *Alternative* medicine is used *in place of* conventional medicine. For example, a person who has cancer may forego surgery, radiation, or chemotherapy that has been recommended by a conventional doctor and use Chinese medicine for treatment instead.

People also use the term integrative medicine. Integrative medicine, as defined by NCCAM, combines mainstream medical therapies and CAM therapies for which there is some high-quality scientific evidence of safety and effectiveness. Some people prefer the term integrative healthcare instead of integrative medicine. Their rationale is that the word medicine already implies a certain western perspective. Additionally, some people refer to CAM as CAT (complementary and alternative therapies) saying that the word therapies more accurately describe this group of modalities rather than medicine.

Support For CAM

In most countries including the United States there is both general public support and support from healthcare professionals for CAM. In fact, some estimates say that close to half of the United States' public uses CAM therapies (Astin, 1998). Eisenberg, in an article published in the *New England Journal of Medicine*, said that "In 1990, Americans made an estimated 425 million visits to providers of unconventional therapy. This number exceeds the number of visits to all U.S. primary care physicians (388 million)," (Eisenberg, Davis, & Ettner, 1998). Updating his information in 1998 in an article entitled *Trends in Alternative Medicine Use in the United States from 1990 to 1997*, Eisenberg et al. wrote that there was a 47.3% increase in total visits to alternative medicine practitioners during that period (guesstimated to be 629 million visits in 1997) and that an estimated $12.2 billion in costs for alternative medicine now exceeded the 1997 out-of-pocket expenditures for all U.S. hospitalizations. Additionally, many people undergoing serious medical procedures are choosing to supplement their care with CAM. For example, 88% of lung transplant patients use CAM therapies (Matthees, Kreitzer, Savik, Hertz, Gross, 2001).

Parents utilize CAM for their children, including massage, vitamins, herbs, meditation, chiropractic, homeopathy, prayer and spiritual healing, biofeedback, acupuncture, hypnosis, and nutritional supplements. Loman (2003) wrote that almost half of parents reported using CAM at some time, and one third reported the use of at least one modality in the past year. In general, parents older than 39 years were significantly more likely to report use of CAM with their children. An exception was that younger mothers were more likely to use infant massage.

Healthcare Professionals' Attitudes Toward CAM

A number of studies have assessed healthcare professionals' attitudes and practice patterns related to CAM. As early as 1983, Reilly (1983) surveyed 100 general practitioner trainees in Scotland to explore attitudes to alternative medicine among them. He found a positive attitude from 86 respondents. Global interest and awareness in CAM was evidenced by a literature review of 1980 to the present. Study results published in refereed journals indicate that practitioners surveyed in Austria, Australia, Canada, Denmark, Germany, Israel, Japan, Netherlands, New Zealand, Norway, Sweden, U.K. and United States have "somewhat positive" to "positive" attitudes towards CAM. Positive attitudes toward CAM, however, do not necessarily translate into using, providing, or referring clients to CAM practitioners. The importance of this distinction will be addressed later.

Some recent studies of physicians, nurses, and medical students' attitudes are briefly described below. In a regional survey of U.S. physicians conducted by Berman et al. (1995), over 70% of respondents indicated that they were interested in more training in areas including hypnotherapy, massage therapy, acupressure, herbal medicine, and prayer. A report of a subsequent national (U.S.) survey by Berman, Singh, Hartnoll, Singh and Reilly (1998) concluded that attitudes and training were the best predictors of the use of CAM in professional practice. In a survey of primary care and medical subspecialties practitioners, Crock, Jarjoura, Polen and Rutecki (1999) found that, overall, physicians demonstrated an open attitude toward CAM, but had low referrals for CAM therapies. Crock et al. (1999) suggested that increased referrals might come with increased physician access to CAM information. Studies surveying nurses generally show that nurses have even more positive attitudes towards CAM than physicians (McPartland and Pruit, 1999; Damkier, Elverdam, Glasdam, Jensen, and Rose, 1998). Nurses emphasized that information regarding unconventional therapies must be readily available for patients and health care providers (Fitch, Gray, & Greenberg, 1999).

Building on these previous studies in a paper entitled *Attitudes of Medical, Nursing, and Pharmacy Faculty and Students Toward Complementary and Alternative Medicine (CAM): A Comparative Analysis* (Kreitzer, Mitten, Shandeling, & Harris, 2002), we reported on the attitudes of faculty and staff toward CAM in medicine, nursing and pharmacy within the Academic Health Center at the University of Minnesota. We found that in general faculty and students within medicine, nursing, and pharmacy are highly receptive to the integration of CAM within education and clinical care. Specifically, over 90% of faculty and students believe that clinical care should integrate the best of conventional and CAM practices and that health professional should be prepared to advise patients about commonly used CAM methods. In contrast to the general public, we also found that both personal use of CAM and training in CAM modalities are limited by these heath professionals and that the lack of evidence is perceived by these health professionals to be the most significant barrier to integration of CAM into conventional medicine. As will be discussed later, these attitudes and their nuances are important to us as adventure therapy professionals who advocate for our healthcare modality of choice.

Understanding NCCAM Domain Designations for CAM

In order to see how adventure therapy might be considered a CAM, it is useful to understand the categories or domains into which NCCAM classifies CAM therapies. The information in this section can be found on the NCCAM website. Each category will described briefly and then in a later section, the ways in which adventure therapy fits into one or more categories will be explored. NCCAM categories of CAM are:

- Alternative Medical Systems
- Biologically Based Therapies
- Manipulative and Body-Based Methods
- Energy Therapies
- Mind-Body Interventions

Alternative medical systems.

Alternative medical systems are built upon complete systems of theory and practice that differ from the conventional western medicine system. Some of these systems were developed in western cultures, such as homeopathic medicine and naturopathic medicine, and others were developed in non-western cultures, including Native American medicine, traditional Chinese medicine, Tibetan, and Ayurveda. These alternative systems often evolved apart from and earlier than (some more than 5000 years ago) the conventional medical approach used in western culture.

Biologically-based therapies.

Biologically based therapies use substances found in nature, such as herbs, foods, and vitamins to cure or heal the body. These therapies include using dietary supplements, herbal products, and some other so-called "natural" substances (e.g., using organic tomato juice to treat prostate cancer or calendula to heal a wound).

Manipulative and body-based methods.

Manipulative and body-based methods are based on manipulation and/or movement of one or more parts of the body. Examples of therapies include chiropractic or osteopathic manipulation, and massage.

Energy therapies.

Energy therapies involve the use of energy fields. There are two types: biofield therapies and bioelectromagnetic-based therapies. Biofield therapies are intended to affect energy fields that purportedly surround and penetrate the human body. These energy fields are affected by one's own body movement, such as in Qi-gong. Other forms of energy therapy such as Reiki, therapeutic touch, and reflexology manipulate the body's energy fields by the practitioner applying pressure on the body and/or manipulating the client's body, or by placing the hands in, or through, their client's energy fields.

Bioelectromagnetic-based therapies involve the unconventional use of electromagnetic fields including pulsed fields, magnetic fields, or alternating current or direct current fields. Through the use of adhesive, velcro, shoe implants or as part of a mattress, magnets are applied to ailing body parts.

Mind-body interventions.

Mind-body medicine uses a variety of techniques designed to enhance the mind's capacity to affect bodily function and symptoms. Examples of CAM in this domain include movement therapies, art therapy, hypnosis, meditation, time in nature, biofeedback, mental healing, pet/companion therapy, prayer or spiritual healing, sound/music therapy, support group, Tai chi, visualization, and yoga. Patient support groups and Cognitive-Behavioral Therapy used to be considered CAM in the mind-body domain and now are considered part of conventional medicine.

Some CAM may fit into more than one category or at least not fit neatly into one category. For example Qi-gong is thought to affect the energy field surrounding the body. It also can be categorized into mind-body interventions as it is said to enhance the mind's capacity to affect bodily function and symptoms. Other mind-body interventions, including Tai chi, meditation, yoga and others may also affect one's energy field.

Mechanistic Thinking and Other Constraints to the Acceptance of CAM

One of the reasons that many people, including professionals trained in western medicine, have trouble integrating CAM practices into their work is that they are trained to treat symptoms using drugs and procedures that have proven mechanisms of performance. They know that "a" makes "b" happen and that "c" makes "d" happen. Usually the mechanism by which something works is proven using a double blind controlled research study that isolates one mechanistic variable. In contrast, many CAM therapies do not have a proven mechanism of action. Interestingly, many CAM modalities have been shown to be effective, even using double blind research when possible; however, their lack of a proven mechanism of action is a constraint for their use by many western physicians (Kreitzer et al., 2002).

Using conventional medicine, physicians tend to treat people one symptom at a time rather than holistically or as a whole being. Astin,

Shapiro, Eisenberg, and Forys (2003) conclude that western medicine has failed to move beyond the biomedical model. Basically, most conventional physicians do not seem to understand a biopsychosocial model or other models used by healthcare practitioners in other cultures: models that use systems of medicine or healthcare treatments that rely on an understanding that psychosocial factors influence physiologic functions and vice versa. Astin et al. (2003) say there is copious evidence that psychosocial factors can directly influence both physiologic function and health outcomes, and therefore using mind-body therapies can be very useful in treating a number of physical ailments. Even so, most conventional physicians rarely recommend these therapies.

Many healthcare professionals, especially those from non-western cultures, do not believe that one can cure or heal the person by eliminating their symptoms. These healthcare workers believe that one has to treat the whole person. This often includes lifestyle choices as well as using biologically based, energy, and mind-body therapies. Many healthcare professionals from non-western cultures do not believe that it is necessary to understand a mechanism of action before using the modality. In thinking mechanistically, some conventional healthcare providers have taken parts of alternative medical systems, such as herbs from Native American, Ayurveda, or Chinese medicine or body movement techniques (yoga) from Ayurveda and now use these as individual therapies. While many people benefit from using these therapies, some practitioners in Native American, Tibetan, or Chinese medicine believe that patients receive more benefits by living the whole medical or healthcare system, rather than by selective use of specific components.

Healing or Curing

Another underlying value of conventional medicine is that professionals "cure" their patients. This means that the condition or symptom(s) that the patient came to see the doctor about has been eradicated. Historically, that has also meant that the doctor "saving the patient's life" was the highest goal.

Many alternative medical systems have focused on healing and more recently, western European cultures have begun to understand more about healing. For example, there are a number of diseases for which there is no "cure." People who cannot be cured can still experience healing. Healing happens to the whole person while curing happens at the level of the body or the physical plane. Many CAM therapies contribute to healing. In part, the concept of healing is based on the fact that everyone will die even if it is from old age, and people prefer to die feeling a sense of well-being, completion, and connection. These outcomes tend to result from healing. In recent years hospice care and palliative care have become more prevalent and people working in these areas focus on healing rather than curing.

They know that their patients will die and have learned that their patients live a fuller life up to death when they experience healing. This healing often includes spiritual healing as well. Adventure therapy's fit with this concept of healing will be discussed later in this paper.

Rachel Naomi Remen, M.D., author of *Kitchen Table Wisdom* and a pioneer in understanding the mind body connection in health, says that there may not be a cure for all of us but there is a healing for all of us, "a healing that is rooted in mystery" (Remen, 1999). She says that healing is about hope and trust in life. She believes that the need for mastery and control in conventional or western medicine, which mirrors western cultural values, can limit the understanding of healing. Cultures that value mystery may be more open to holistic healthcare models and more open to understanding the value of healing (Remen, 1999). When one trusts life or can be in awe of the wonder and beauty of life and of the natural world, there tends to be a sense of well-being which includes hope and calmness. She notes that this is something that cannot be measured; it can only be experienced. Helping a person heal can include understanding and witnessing their stories and realizing that each of our stories is as unique as our finger prints. Remen (1999) wants people to know that life often is not limited by facts and that life is made up of stories, not facts. Stories are different than facts and, according to Remen (1999), facts can limit hope.

Remen (1999) also suggests looking at our wounds and the wounds of others and getting to know their stories. These stories often show vulnerability and courage, as well as the will to live. She says that our experiences in American culture tell us to put wounds behind us—unexamined—and to deny vulnerability. This attitude dates at least back to the North American frontier culture that valued competence, self-sufficiency, and independence. In her opinion these attitudes helped people learn not to deal with wounds, and therefore limit people from knowing and understanding our will to live. By examining our wounds with curiosity, seeing scars as symbols of survival, and seeing ourselves as survivors and not as victims, we can learn to trust life and increase our ability to have hope and courage. This process of sharing contributes to the healing process.

The following section will use the above definitions and discussion to define adventure therapy as a CAM and to situate it in NCCAM's therapeutic domains.

Situating Adventure Therapy in CAM

Adventure therapy has a number of similarities to other CAM modalities. Adventure therapy is a health care practice that is not currently an integral part of conventional medicine, thus fitting NCCAM's general definition of CAM. It was previously noted how the concept of healing is used in adventure therapy. Mechanistic thinking may not work to prove the effectiveness of adventure therapy, nor may there be a discernable direct relationship in which if a practitioner does "A" then "B" will always happen. Consciously, or perhaps unconsciously, adventure therapy practitioners use a biopsychosocial model. Our practices are multidimensional and people are often worked with in a holistic manner. For example, many practitioners understand that psychological healing affects the physical body and physical activity affects psychological and emotional health. Adventure therapy practitioners know that each person is unique, including their process for healing.

Additionally, there may be connections between the global move to CAM and the increase in the use of adventure therapy. It can be argued that people are turning to adventure therapy for reasons similar to those given for why people use other CAM modalities. For example, parents not satisfied with results from other forms of treatment send their children to adventure therapy programs in hopes that their children will achieve better mental health including changing behaviors, controlling addictions, and increasing self-awareness and self-respect. As mentioned earlier, many parents are turning to CAM as a way to supplement or replace conventional healthcare. Given this, in the United States there are a plethora of adventure therapy programs serving troubled youth. Such youth are often diagnosed with mental health problems.

As a complementary therapy, adventure therapy is often one component in a person's health management program, used in conjunction with other physical or mental health modalities. For example, a number of therapists in a metropolitan area have recommended participation in an adventure program for women as a component of their therapeutic work. In contrast to the aforementioned youth who are "sent" to adventure therapy programs, many other people self-select to go on adventure therapy trips for their own personal growth. They use these experiences to achieve better overall health and complement their other healthcare. The client may want to gain benefits listed in the preceding paragraph, achieve relaxation, or have other health goals. For some people some conditions have not been treated well by conventional western medicine and they try an adventure therapy experience.

Adventure therapy fits well into the concept of healing. Many adventure therapy practitioners agree with Remen that helping people through listening to their stories, stories that expose their wounds and the strength they have shown in coping with their wounds, leads to healing. Often adventure therapy practitioners help participants see themselves not as victims, but as survivors, seeing the courage in being vulnerable. Many adventure programs take place outside and participants are exposed to the beauty and awe of being part of the natural world, witnessing its mystery and feeling its wonder. Remen (1999) credits her experience with the natural world for her understanding of some of the ways that people use their strength to cope with their wounds. She tells us that we may need to know less and wonder more, and that real power lies not in mastery. Instead, it lies in an awareness of the possible and a willingness to be open to it and meet with it. Many adventure therapy programs use the outdoor environment to help people gain an awareness of the possible. In line with the goals of other CAM therapies, the healing accomplished through the use of adventure therapy has benefits for people's psychological-emotional, physical, social, and spiritual well-being.

Adventure therapy focuses on healing rather than curing. Curing may occur through adventure therapy experiences; however, this comes about through the healing experiences that clients have. Practitioners know that the growth and skills learned and gained through adventure therapy are part of an ongoing process of growth and healing. For example, some adventure therapy programs work with people with cancer. Tips of the Toes in Canada take youth with cancer on extended wilderness trips into a remote arctic region. Their staff, accompanied by a physician, expect that these experiences will contribute to the overall health and well-being or healing of the client, rather than cure the cancer. Power to Be in Canada and Wilderness Inquiry in the U.S. are two organizations that provide adventure therapy trips for people with physical and mental disabilities. These programs have goals that include increasing participants' self-awareness, self-respect, and general overall feelings of well-being. These organizations provide experiences that complement the medical or healthcare treatments already in place, adding greatly to the overall healing of the participants. In these examples, adventure therapy can clearly be seen as complementary medicine.

Adventure therapy probably does not have one mechanism of action. Instead, it may well be a system or a process that contributes to the curing or healing that the client attains. In the case of mental health issues, many therapists and psychologists see symptoms as a signal of dysfunction and treat the whole person (at least in the mental and emotional realms) rather than only the symptom. In Native American, Chinese, and Tibetan medicine systems, when a person has an ailment, the whole person is treated. This often includes a combination of diet, physicality, emotional work, and other biologically based substances. Similarly, through adventure therapy programs the whole person is treated. This includes health benefits from being in nature, from being physically active, and from learning about and experiencing relationship growth. In fact, the overall system of adventure therapy may be necessary for success and it may be that adventure therapy works through the integration of its components. Each specific component of adventure therapy, including the leader/client relationship, the therapeutic techniques used, and the natural environment can provide benefits to clients. When these three elements are used together in a skillful manner the benefits can be synergistic. As for many CAM therapies, how these components are used by the practitioner is as much of an art as a science.

As has been shown above, adventure therapy as a healthcare modality has many similarities to other CAM, including common CAM pedagogy. Using the NCCAM domain designations, one could view adventure therapy as a complementary modality in the mind-body interventions, the biologically based therapies, and the energy therapies domains. As will be discussed, adventure therapy has similarities to modalities in each of these NCCAM areas. Like many other CAM, adventure therapy does not fit only one category.

Adventure Therapy as a Mind-body Intervention

Mind-body interventions positively impact the well-being of people and strengthen their abilities to heal themselves in the physical, mental and spiritual areas. Components of adventure therapy that work as a mind-body intervention include physical movement, reflection, exposure to the wonder of nature, and support and interaction with other group members and practitioners.

Movement therapies are part of mind-body interventions, and in many adventure therapy programs movement is used. This may occur through initiatives or experiential activities, ropes courses, and/or outdoor pursuits such as backpacking, canoeing, or rock climbing. Movement is encouraged through exploring and adventuring in the natural environment. These are often new ways for some clients to use their bodies, helping to strengthen and heal in the physical, mental, and spiritual areas.

Often adventure therapy programs expose people to the awe and wonder of nature. Many programs are based entirely in outdoor and wilderness settings. Being in an outdoor setting often is meditative and stimulates healthy mind-body interactions. In fact, meditation is a mind-body intervention. A goal of mind-body interventions is to reduce stress. As there is copious research to support the efficacy of being in nature to reduce stress (Bardwell, 1992; Mitten, 1994; Irvine & Weber, 2002; Ulrich, 2002; Yankou, 2002), the connection is clear.

Interpersonal relationships can be an element of mind-body intervention. This occurs in support groups as well as the therapeutic relationship between a practitioner and client. Healing and growth occur in adventure therapy programs for some clients because of the support and interaction with the other group members. Additionally, many practitioners in adventure therapy have written about the importance of the leader/client relationship (Berman & Berman-Davis, 1998, Mitten, 1994; Newes, 2000). In psychotherapy the importance of the therapeutic relationship as a change mechanism is well acknowledged. In fact, psychotherapy research has shown the therapeutic relationship to be the strongest predictor of outcome (Orlinsky, Grawe, & Parks, 1994, cited in Newes, 2000). This healing through the therapeutic relationship between the leader/client also may be considered a mind-body intervention.

Reflection, used extensively in adventure therapy, fits well as a mind-body intervention. Reflection can lead to mental healing. Clients often reflect on their new relationships and their new way of being in relationships. Strengthened through reflection, these shared experiences and new relationship skills are integrated into clients' lives. These new experiences or new stories the clients have lived often have a healing effect on people and give people hope that they can have different relationships and be different in relationships.

Adventure Therapy as a Biologically Based Therapy

In biologically based therapies, substances found in nature are used for healing. Given that nature is at the core of most adventure therapy programs, adventure therapy clearly is situated within this NCCAM area as well. Healing occurs through the beneficial impacts of nature itself, including breathing fresh air, getting vitamins D, E and an increase in serotonin from the sunshine, and the increase in physical activity. Stress reduction, achieved through time in nature, is also a biologically based benefit of adventure therapy. Adventure therapy often takes place outdoors, sometimes for extended periods. Health benefits are gained during adventure therapy experiences and adventure therapy can lead to a healthier physical lifestyle. Many people return home from programs and incorporate more activity, more time in nature and a healthier diet into their lifestyle.

Adventure Therapy as an Energy Therapy

Energy healing and biofield therapies in particular also may be a part of adventure therapy. Energy fields that purportedly surround and penetrate the human body may be positively stimulated by nature. Therefore, people may be healed on an energetic level by being in nature. Clients may experience healing on the energetic level after they successfully complete activities in adventure therapy programs, especially if the activities are engaging and include exploring and adventuring. In addition, the healing that occurs through the therapeutic relationship between the leader/client, as described in the mind-body intervention, also may be an energetic-level intervention. Admittedly, measuring healing or changes in energy fields is difficult. Therefore, it is challenging to explain how or why being in nature or having positive relationships changes energy fields. There has been preliminary movement in this direction. There have been certain photography techniques that are said to photograph energy fields. However, at present the measure that is used most commonly is our basic human ability to sense a change in that person. On an adventure therapy expedition, this is most often described as "something is different and more wonderful about Jenny."

In addition to being a CAM as described above, adventure therapy also can be an integrated practice that uses or incorporates several complementary CAM modalities. For example, adventure therapy practitioners may incorporate visualization, meditation, diet, massage, pet/companion therapy, nature sounds (in person), mindfulness, and prayer or spiritual healing into their adventure therapy programs. The benefit for adventure therapy practitioners of incorporating other CAM into our practices and of networking with practitioners of other CAM will be discussed later.

How We See Ourselves as Adventure Therapy Practitioners

How we see ourselves as practitioners greatly influences our practices. It influences with whom we network, the direction of our research and the depth to which we can critically analyze and think about our practice. Therefore it influences how the rest of the world views us as well. The work in this paper is meant to encourage us to "try on" viewing ourselves as health practitioners who work in CAM, as well as to argue that adventure therapy is a CAM. By defining adventure therapy as a CAM, it will influence our applications of our work as well as how other professionals perceive its use. By defining adventure therapy as a CAM and more closely tying it into other healthcare fields, we expand our work and apply adventure therapy to an even wider variety of clients. Several examples follow showing how we can use adventure therapy to have a positive impact on the emotional and social well-being of many people in either a preventive manner or when people are in crisis.

Leisure has long been known to be important in developing cohesion in families. This includes between spouses and between parents and children. Camping and recreation in the outdoors has been shown to contribute more to family cohesion than other types of leisure (Freeman & Zabriskie, 2002). Using adventure therapy to build family cohesion can be preventive and thus be a logical part of health care.

As another example, eight million Americans have eating disorders. West-Smith's (1997) work indicates that that participation on outdoor trips influences women's body images. Therefore adventure therapy trips designed to work with women with eating disorders would be a positive complement to their other care. In addition it is less expensive and easier to maintain health rather than reclaim health. Therefore adventure therapy trips also can be used as a preventive measure for women and body image.

Adventure therapy could have an impact on the emotional and social well-being of couples in health-related crisis. Glantz (2001) reports that if one person in a married couple is diagnosed with Multiple Sclerosis (MS), then the divorce rate is 96%. If one person in a married couple is a cancer patient, then the expected divorce rate is 72%. There is gender difference. If the woman in the couple has the disease, she is more likely to be left by her husband, according to Glantz (2001). In fact, a woman is 12 times more likely to be left by her husband if she has a brain tumor, than if he has one. If a woman has MS, she is seven times more likely to be left by her husband than if the husband were to have MS. Medical providers understand that in cases of severe illnesses, the patient's marriage or relationships need attention along with the disease itself. People who are experiencing stress from many things, including severe illnesses, may benefit therapeutically from the elements of adventure therapy.

What To Do

This paper will conclude with some suggestions about how we, as people who practice adventure therapy in its many forms, could use the proposition that adventure therapy is a CAM to move our practices forward. These suggestions include:

- Network with and provide education for other healthcare practitioners
- Conduct and publish more research about the efficacy of adventure therapy
- Apply for research grants from health-related organizations such as NIH
- Learn about CAM, including other specific CAM modalities
- Integrate into our practices those CAMs that may have utility in complementing adventure therapy
- Work with third-party providers to cover the cost of adventure therapy healthcare
- Integrate a CAM perspective and CAM language into our work and practices

We need to do more networking with and providing education for other healthcare professionals, including making individual contacts, publishing informational articles in journals accessible to other health professionals, and inviting professionals to experience what we do. Presenting workshops and research papers at health-related conferences also can help educate other healthcare practitioners. Earlier it was reported that attitudes and training were the best predictors of use in professional practice, and that increased referrals might come with increased physician access to CAM information. Perhaps inviting healthcare providers to observe adventure therapy or participate in adventure therapy would help shift attitudes about referrals. There are opportunities for adventure therapy professionals to network with and educate healthcare practitioners in many fields.

We need to conduct more research about the efficacy of adventure therapy and publish this research. Lack of evidence is perceived by conventional healthcare workers to be the most significant barrier to integration of CAM into western medicine (Kreitzer et al., 2002). Because of the way that many CAMs work, there is now a better understanding that traditional research focusing on mechanistic controls is not always appropriate. We can look to other CAM fields to see how they explain and rationalize their work when it may not fit neatly into a mechanistic model. We can think creatively about research designs as well as our funding and consider applying for a grant from the NIH National Center for Complementary and Alternative Medicine. Publishing the results of more well-designed research studies in journals read by health professionals would help educate professionals. The following list is a sample of journals that have published articles about CAM: *Alternative Therapies Health Medicine, Arch Pediatrics Adolescent Medicine, Australian Family Physician, British Homeopath Journal, British Journal of General Practice, British Medical Journal, Canadian Family Physician, Cancer Prevention and Control, International Journal of Quality Health Care, Journal of Alternative and Complementary Medicine, Journal of Clinical Oncology, Journal of Nursing Education, Journal of the American Board of Family Practitioners, Journal of the Royal Society of Medicine, Journal of Women Aging, Medical Journal of Australia, New Zealand Medicine Journal,* and *Social Science Medicine.*

We need to explore other fields and other CAM therapies, including the existing evidence-based research, to see how our work fits into a larger healing picture. There are databases dedicated to CAM which can be used to find such research. For example, the Cochrane database publishes meta papers evaluating the research state of many CAM practices. AMED (Allied & Complementary medicine) is another database reporting articles about CAM. Sample questions to explore might be "Would the addition of meditation and yoga in programs help increase healing and give participants more skills to take home with them?" or "How might I incorporate journaling or art therapy more into my program?" As we learn about and integrate other CAM into our practices, we will become part of a larger healthcare community, creating opportunities for more networking and referrals.

We need to work to make a valid case for third party payment. In response to consumer demand, health systems have begun to offer CAM services (Astin, 1998) and some health plans are beginning to offer CAM benefits (Snyder & Lindquist, 2002). Again, we can network and provide information to insurance carriers. We can work in collaboration with healthcare providers who receive third party payment for their work. Networking with other healthcare practitioners in both conventional medicine and CAM, along with more research and information about adventure therapy in a variety of healthcare journals, can help provide the necessary validity and consumer support needed for possible third party payment.

Overall, we need to consider integrating a CAM perspective and CAM language into our work and practices. This includes taking the time to think critically about our practices, as well as participating in the workshop sessions and informal conversations that happen at conferences and symposiums. While the need for well-designed research is imperative, there is also a need to be able to explain the concept and systemic way adventure therapy works using other than mechanistic language. We need to think holistically about our work and understand that several dimensions, including the natural environment, the leader/client relationship and the program techniques may all contribute to the healing process. We can think about the kind of healing that occurs through adventure therapy experiences and how to describe and quantify those benefits. Important questions may include "Are there program components to which I am wedded (through history or early training), but really do not add healing value or may even detract from healing?", "What does it mean to contribute to someone's healing and how can that be accomplished through adventure therapy?", and "What are ways that we can integrate CAM language into our practices?"

Both individually and as a group, adventure therapy practitioners would benefit from reflection leading to decisions about how we situate adventure therapy in the healthcare arena. With focused attention we may be able to better inform our own practices, help inform other's practices, have access to a larger critical audience that can help our work grow and mature, and have access to more research funding. We must recognize that the more we examine our practices, the more likely our practices will increase in quality. In turn, we can better help our clients to achieve wellness, experience healing, and learn new relationship and life skills.

In summary, understanding adventure therapy as CAM may influence how we construct and understand our practices. Adventure therapy can be a powerful tool and an experience that has the potential to contribute to a person's healing in many ways. As professionals, we can do more to create visibility for our work in the greater area of healthcare. Simultaneously, we can begin looking inward to critically examine our work and better understand the systematic way in which adventure therapy contributes to healing for our clients.

References

Astin, J. A. (1998). Why patients use alternative medicine: results of a national study. *Journal of the American Medical Association, 279*(19), 1548-53.

Astin, J. A., Shapiro, S. L., Eisenberg, D. M., Forys, K. L. (2003). Mind-Body Medicine: State of the Science, Implications for Practice. *Journal of the American Board of Family Practice, 16*(2),131-147.

Attarian, A. (2001). Trends in outdoor adventure education. *Journal of Experiential Education, 24*(3),141-149.

Bandoroff, S., & Scherer, D. G. (1994). Wilderness family therapy: An innovative treatment approach for problem youth. *Journal of Child and Family Studies, 3*(2), 175-191.

Bardwell, L. V. (1992). A bigger piece of the puzzle: The restorative experience and outdoor education. In Henderson (Ed.), *Coalition for education in the outdoors: Research symposium proceeding.* Bradford Woods, IN: Coalition for education in the outdoors.

Berman, B. M., Singh, B. K., Lao, L., Singh, B. B., Ferentz, K. S., Hartnoll, S. M. (1995). Physicians' attitudes toward complementary or alternative medicine: a regional survey. *Journal of the American Board of Family Practice, 8*(5), 361-6.

Berman, B. M., Singh, B. B., Hartnoll, S. M., Singh, B.K., Reilly, D. (1998). Primary care physicians and complementary-alternative medicine: training, attitudes, and practice patterns, *Journal of the American Board of Family Practice, 11*(4), 272-81.

Berman, D. S., & Davis-Berman, J. (1998). *Tikkun olam: A model for healing the world.* Keynote address at the Heartland conference of The Association of Experiential Education. Camp Miracle, MI.

Berman, D. S. & Davis-Berman, J. (2000). Therapeutic uses of outdoor education. ERIC Document Reproduction Service No. EDO-RC-00-5.

Bly, L. (2001, February 23). You go, girls: Women-only groups are happily migrating towards adventure travel. *USA Today.*

Crisp, S. (2003). Retrieved February 1, 2004 from http://www.voea.vic.edu.au/pd/WAT _Intro_CourseMelb_2004.pdf.

Crock, R. D., Jarjoura, D., Polen, A., Rutecki, G. W. (1999). Confronting the communication gap between conventional and alternative medicine: a survey of physicians' attitudes. *Altern Ther Health Med, 5*(2), 61-6.

Damkier, A., Elverdam, B., Glasdam, S., Jensen, A. B., Rose, C. (1998). Nurses' attitudes to the use of alternative medicine in cancer patients. *Scand J Caring Sci, 12*(2), 119-26.

Davis-Berman, J. & Berman, D. S. (1994). *Wilderness therapy: Foundations, theory and research.* Dubuque, IA: Kendall/Hunt Publishing Co.

Eisenberg, D. M., Davis, R. B., Ettner, S. L., et al. (1998). Trends in alternative medicine use in the United States, 1990–1997: results of a follow-up national survey. *JAMA, 280,* 1569–75.

Fitch M. I., Gray R. E., Greenberg, M., Labrecque, M., Douglas, M. S. (1999). Nurses' perspectives on unconventional therapies. *Cancer Nursing, 22*(3), 238-45.

Freeman & Zabriskie (2002). The role of outdoor recreation in family enrichment; *JAEOL, 2*(2), 131-146.

Friese, G., Hendee, J., & Kinziger, M. (1998). The wilderness experience program industry in the United States: Characteristics and dynamics. *The Journal of Experiential Education, 21*(1), 40-45.

Gass, M. (1993). Ethical principles for the therapeutic adventure professional group. In Gass, M. A. (Ed.), *Adventure therapy: Therapeutic applications of adventure programming* (pp. 451-461). Dubuque, IA: Kendall/Hunt Publishing Co.

Gillis, H. L. & Thomsen, D. (1996). A research update (1992–1995) of adventure therapy: Challenge activities and ropes courses, wilderness expeditions, & residential camping programs, In L. H. McAvoy, L. A. Stringer, M. D. Bialeschki, A. B. Young (Eds.), *Coalition for education in the outdoors: Research symposium proceeding.* pp. 15-20. Bradford Woods, IN: Coalition for education in the outdoors.

Glantz, M. (2001). Till sickness do we part. In M. S. James (Ed.), ABC News Internet Ventures: Study: Husbands more likely to divorce ill spouses.

Kreitzer, M. J., Mitten, D. S., Shandeling, J., & Harris, I. (2002). Attitudes towards CAM among medical, nursing, and pharmacy faculty and students: A comparative analysis. *Alternative Therapies, 8*(6), 44-47.

Loman (2003). The use of complementary and alternative healthcare practices among children. *Journal of Pediatric Health Care, 17*(2), 58-63.

Matthees, B. P. A., Kreitzer, M. J., Savik, K., Hertz, M., Gross, C. (2001). Use of complementary therapies, adherence, and quality of life in lung transplant recipients. *Heart & Lung;* July/August: 258-268.

McPartland, J. M., & Pruit, P. L. (1999). Opinions of MDs, RNs, allied health practitioners toward osteopathic medicine and alternative therapies: results from a Vermont survey. *Journal of the American Osteopath Association, 99*(2), 101-8.

Mitten, D. (1994). Ethical considerations in adventure therapy: A feminist critique. In E. Cole, E. Erdman, & E. Rothblum (Eds.), *Women and Therapy.* (pp. 55-84). New York: Harrington Park Press.

NCCAM, National Institutes of Health. (February 5, 2004). NCCAM funding: Appropriations history. Retrieved February 10, 2004, from http://nccam.nci.nih.gov/about/appropriations/

NCCAM, National Institutes of Health. (May 26, 2004). What is complementary and alternative medicine (CAM)? Retrieved May 26, 2004, from http://nccam.nih.gov/health/whatiscam/

Newes, S. L. (2000). Adventure-based therapy: Theory, characteristics, ethics, and research; Unpublished manuscript, Pennsylvania State University.

Reilly, D. T. (1983). Young doctors' views on alternative medicine. *British medical journal (Clinical research ed.), 287*(6388), 337-9.

Remen, R. N. (1999). *Kitchen Table Wisdom.* New York: Riverhead Books/Penguin Putnam, Inc.

Snyder, M. & Lindquist, R. (2002). *Complementary/alternative therapies in nursing.* New York: Springer Publishing Co.

Sugerman, D. (2000). Adventure experiences for older adults: Examining current practices. *Journal of Experiential Education, 23*(1), 12-16.

Ulrich, R. S. (2002, March). Restorative gardens; Presentation for the Kermit A. Olson Memorial Lecture, University of Minnesota, St. Paul.

West-Smith, L. (1997). Body image perceptions of active outdoorswomen: Toward a new definition of physical attractiveness. (Doctoral dissertation, Union Institute and University, 1997). *Dissertation Abstracts International.* (University Microfilms No. 9736721).

Yankou, D. (2002). MorningStar: A place of restoration. *MorningStar Adventures, 18*(2), 3.

Author's Biography

*For the past 30 years, **Denise Mitten** has worked in adventure education. While working at the Center for Spirituality and Healing, Dr. Mitten did extensive research on complementary and alternative medicine in the areas of attitudes and efficacy. She is a writer and consultant in group dynamics, ethics, and gender topics and brings a comparative perspective regarding the value and uses of various leadership and motivation styles with many different groups. Currently, Dr. Mitten teaches at Ferris State University in Big Rapids, Michigan. .*

Correspondence

Denise Mitten, Ph.D.
Ferris State University
Leisure Studies and Wellness
SRC 102
401 South Street
Big Rapids, MI 49307
(231) 591-5317
mittend@ferris.edu.